# LENSES

# LENSES

## Applying Lifespan Development
## Theories in Counseling

### Kurt L. Kraus

Shippensburg University of Pennsylvania

**Lahaska Press**
Houghton Mifflin Company
Boston  •  New York

Publisher, Lahaska Press: Barry Fetterolf
Senior Editor, Lahaska Press: Mary Falcon
Senior Marketing Manager, Lahaska Press: Barbara LeBuhn
Associate Project Editor: Deborah Thomashow
Cover Design Manager: Anne S. Katzeff
Senior Composition Buyer: Chuck Dutton
New Title Project Manager: Susan Peltier
Editorial Assistant: Evangeline Bermas

Cover image: © Photodisc/Getty Images

For instructors who want more information about Lahaska Press books
and teaching aids, contact the Houghton Mifflin Faculty Services Center at
Tel: 800-733-1717, x4034
Fax: 800-733-1810
Or visit us on the Web at www.lahaskapress.com.

Photos on pages 2, 9, 10, 54, 84, 120, 166, 167, 200, 201, 230, 231, 263, 296, 297, 330, 364, 365, 390, and 425 courtesy of the authors.

Lahaska Press, established as an imprint of Houghton Mifflin Company in 1999, is dedicated to publishing textbooks and instructional media for counseling and the helping professions. Its editorial offices are located in the small town of Lahaska, Pennsylvania. *Lahaska* is a Native American Lenape word meaning "source of much writing."

Printed in the U.S.A.

Library of Congress Control Number: 2007938675

Instructor's examination copy
ISBN-10: 0-618-73200-4
ISBN-13: 978-0-618-73200-5

For orders, use student text ISBNs
ISBN-10: 0-618-37030-7
ISBN-13: 978-0-618-37030-6

123456789-EB-11 10 09 08 07

# Contents

## PART THREE
# Identity Development Lenses

# Preface

Welcome to a simple text with an exceptional intent: *Lenses* seeks to assist readers with the complex goal of better understanding both the clients we work with and ourselves as counselors. It falls squarely upon us to take responsibility for our self-awareness—a crucial mechanism of the counseling relationship. Readers will find that each chapter presents a particular perspective, a theory, or position that explains an aspect of human development worthy of our attention and understanding.

Three major goals directed the creation of this textbook:

1. To contribute a practical, clear, current text on often underrepresented human development perspectives and theories for the graduate education of counseling professionals.
2. To select from the wealth of human development models, theories, and perspectives that have practical applications for professional counselors by calling our attention to select aspects of our clients' lives.
3. To build upon, rather than merely repeat, the fundamentals of each of the robust theories and perspectives contained within.

My hope is that this text will imbue readers with real and rich case material through which complex issues of human development come to life. Here theory will be made meaningful through case examples. *Lenses* is written by scholar/practitioners, professional counselors, and college student personnel, each of whom utilize a particular theoretical or perceptual underpinning in their professional work with real people. I believe that they have much to teach us. Moving theory into action is not an easy feat. The chapters of this text will help you, the reader, in accomplishing that task.

The format for each chapter begins by addressing the question of relevance—"Why is this chapter important for the reader/student/learner?"—which is then followed by a relatively brief overview of that chapter's particular theory or perspective. Authors were invited to prepare chapters for this text because each has more than strictly academic expertise. Each is (or recently was) a counseling or college student personnel practitioner who has firsthand experience with a particular lens. This overview section presents (1) what aspect of human development the theory or perspective is attempting to explain; (2) how and when along the lifespan this theory-in-application is likely to be most evident; and (3) what the underlying assumptions of this theory or perspective on human development are. For those of you who are reading this text in a formal course, specific learner objectives will be articulated by your professor. The introduction each author has included is intended to capture your attention and foreshadow what benefits this theory or perspective has for the counseling professional.

In each chapter you will happen upon one or two brief biographies of a person or people whose contribution to this theory or perspective is particularly noteworthy. Authors have attempted to capture those elements of these people that best explain the emergence of their perspective or theory. It seems imperative that readers develop a sense of who contributed or continues to contribute to each lens. Perspectives and theories are not stagnant, rather they are dynamic and must embrace the forces of change that occur with time. (You will also find an equally short, annotated bibliography separate from the author's reference list, where interested readers can find connections to greater depth and resources for each lens.)

Each chapter goes on to present the theory or perspective firmly embedded in our professional context. In this section, authors comment on issues of particular relevance to students and practitioners. Complex issues are addressed, including (1) multicultural importance, gender, race, and culture; (2) practice considerations; (3) and the perceived value and trustworthiness of the theory or perspective and its potential shortcomings.

One or more case examples, the crux of each chapter, follow, allowing readers to truly appreciate the utility of each perspective in actual practice. The case illustrates through dynamic, anecdotal prose how our perspective from each of these lenses contributes to vital aspects of professional counseling (e.g., case conceptualization, assessment and evaluation, education, and intervention/treatment). Specifically, this section addresses: How does this theory inform my actual practice with this particular client. Thus, the case moves practice into "real life." As readers will learn, clients are encountered in a variety of professional settings, and each author is specific about the setting in which the case was encountered. Authors also present their case or cases embedded in a unique developmental context in order for the reader to experience the complexities of growth and development in the real world, not in some tidy office refuge where the client's world is minimized or escaped. Each case illuminates some otherwise shadowed aspect of the author's client or clients, and illustrates how one theory or perspective provides a valuable lens through which she or he viewed the client. I have asked each author to be vibrant in their descriptions to ensure that the language is active and engaging.

Each chapter summary reiterates the crucial elements of the theoretical or perceptual framework. It revisits how important each theory proved to be for practicing professional counselors, and hopefully leaves you, the reader, with a sense of the value and relevance of lenses in action.

As readers, I believe you will be interested to know that I have asked that each author to write in the first person where appropriate, to write in a scholarly yet understandable and engaging prose, and to rely on the terms professional counseling, counselor, and client (student) rather than psychotherapy, therapist, patient, or consumer. I share this "behind the scene" information with you so that you understand the perspective I have imposed on the chapter authors. Although the text is clearly written for counseling professionals, it is likely that others in the mental health and human service disciplines will enjoy the utility and readability of *Lenses*. I certainly hope the counseling perspective, which is the overarching, guiding perspective throughout this text, assists readers in graduate counseling programs to further define their professional orientation as that of a professional counselor.

As often as possible, chapter authors have emphasized the paramount use (i.e., pragmatism, utility, application, value, and necessity) of their particular lens in their conceptualization and subsequent work with clients. Clients, my selected term for this text, is broadly encompassing; children, school students, clients in private practice setting, university students, and adults at various places along their life journey are represented here. I have asked authors to write with teaching applications in mind. *Lenses* does not purport to teach the basics of human development theory, nor does it offer the definitive word on any one theory or perspective, for many excellent texts are readily available for those readers who seek additional opportunities to learn more about any of the perspectives and theories introduced in this text. *Lenses* simply offers readers sight into a variety of human identity development theories and insight into how such theories inform counselors' professional practice. I truly hope you enjoy the text.

My most sincere thanks to: the twenty chapter authors whose scholarship and personalities this book showcases; the progenitors, theorists, and scholars whose theories and models and often whose life's work was selected for inclusion in this book; nearly 100 graduate students from Shippensburg University and across the country who were generous to send ample direction, critique and feedback on chapter drafts; many faculty members who piloted chapters in their lifespan, human growth and development, and socio-cultural counseling courses, and who sent wonderful feedback; numerous professionals from the fields of counseling, psychology, and sociology who reviewed this manuscript for Lahaska Press—your efforts were incredibly valued and are obviously reflected in this text; my colleagues and students at Shippensburg University of Pennsylvania. I am indeed a very fortunate man to surround myself with your company. Most importantly, thank you, Sally, Jocelyn, Emily and Ian—my inspirations.

—klk

# CHAPTER ONE

# Introduction: Establishing a Meaningful Context

## Kurt L. Kraus

The profession of counseling is securely rooted in the broad human development landscape. Amongst allied mental health professions, counseling is in many ways a maverick in its choice to place particular importance and value in clinical practice upon what is "right" with individuals who become our clients rather than on what is "wrong." Although such dichotomous language is frequently limiting, it captures an essential essence of professional counseling's identity. Our nonconformity clashes at times when we are asked by third-party payers to present or clarify a diagnosis or when we compete among other mental health providers for ever shrinking health care dollars, which often seem reserved for "the sick."

Counselors' consideration of clients' strengths proves to continually inform and potentially transform a client's growth and development. Attention to one's weaknesses, while undoubtedly informing, is *not* likely a professional counselors' first fascination or inclination for action. Consider how limiting and confining looking only at either side— strengths or challenges—would prove to be if you yourself were seeking the services of a mental health professional. Symptoms (diagnostic identifiers), events (changes, traumas, awakenings), behaviors (more readily noticed by concerned others), and "states and traits" (reflecting course and duration and potentially a host of other judgments the profession may make regarding a person) that emerge as the focus of a client's presenting concern or concerns are best viewed as nestled importantly within the individual, within his or her immediate and ever

## A NOTE FROM THE AUTHOR

My hope is that this text will imbue readers with rich, real case material where complex issues of human development come to life. Here, theory will be made meaningful through case examples. *Lenses* is written by scholar/practitioners, professional counselors, and college student personnel, each of whom utilizes the theoretical or perceptual underpinnings in their work with real people. I believe that they have much to teach us; moving theory into action is not an easy feat. The chapters of this text will help you, the reader, in accomplishing that task.

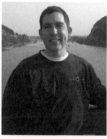

**Kurt L. Kraus**

Kurt L. Kraus is an associate professor of counseling at Shippensburg University of Pennsylvania. His path there included teaching English and special education at the middle and secondary levels in central Maine. He went on to become a school counselor and continued his education at the University of Maine, where he earned his doctorate in 1996. Dr. Kraus's current clinical, teaching, and research interests include counseling children and adolescents, group work, and identity development. He has a profound interest in traditional Chinese medicine—particularly the mind-body integrating exercises of qigong and taijiquan as health promoting and preserving practices. Much of this text was compiled and edited while he was a visiting faculty member at Beijing Language and Culture University in Beijing, the People's Republic of China. Dr. Kraus resides with his family in Carlisle, Pennsylvania.

expanding environment, and within a larger, more global context. Each realm exerts its own unique force, and the result is inevitably complex.

Counselors practicing in a wide variety of settings—from schools to outpatient hospitals, from college campuses to private practice—are continually cognizant of the complex context from which each client emerges. The variables that contribute to one's context seem innumerable. Throughout the rich history of mental health practices across disciplines (such as clinical social work, psychiatry, faith-based systems of care, and psychology), professionals have grown more and more careful to be thorough in their consideration of what "context" actually means.

In the eras past, when in a distinctly Western worldview a "patient's" mental health had to fit snuggly within the scope of general medicine, the biological realm of a client was viewed as wholly sufficient. The mental health of a patient, however, confounded early medical practice. (I will refrain from the temptation to editorialize this perspective.) More than a few disease processes or injuries escaped detection; moreover, social and psychological explanations were held in suspicion because insufficient rigor defined their early contributions to the mental health field. Therefore, many sources of valuable understanding about a person's mental health and well-being fell out of the purview of general medicine and were not considered. By and large, what was not seen was not considered. The use of a vision metaphor to capture this historical point of view is purposeful here, as the book's title reveals.

If we consider our history as suffering from myopia, we can celebrate that those myopic views of what constitutes mental health (including mental illness) have expanded. The profession of counseling and many of the allied mental health professions now actively consider an exceptionally wide sphere of influence on the development of a human being. Counselor educators and other commentators are guilty of speaking the obvious when we offer as an insight that human beings are complex and therefore require our equally complex efforts to understand them. But, it is in an attempt, I believe, to remind ourselves of the dangers inherent in retreating to the relative safety of that old myopic vision. If, after all, we could condense the human experience into nifty or convenient, clean, transparent packages, our work would be immeasurably less challenging. Life, however, is not reducible, and everyone in the helping professions is embracing the complexities.

Phenomenologists emphasize that the "lived experiences" of people are best accessed by others through a careful, respectful "entering" of the other's world. We (whoever "we" are) must thoughtfully (i.e., consciously) suspend our preconceptions, becoming aware of our judgments and biases in order to become open to a glimpse into another's world, one in which we do not really reside, one in which we are at best visitors. A traditional and often slightly myopic "bio-psycho-social" approach to "seeing" people fully proves insufficient. The vast complexities under the too-wide heading of biology far exceed what one might hope to bring to an individual understanding of what results from one particular person's biology. In a similar vein, psychology is an enormous vessel containing innumerable aspects of the self, which renders it nearly impossible to consider each and every ramification of a client's "psychology" as a counselor attempts to grasp a full understanding of a client with whom they work.

Residing alongside or perhaps deeply imbedded within biology, psychology, and sociology are discrete arenas worth particular attention. The enormity of "race" traditionally receives attention across all three areas—bio-psycho-social—but deserves specific, separate attention. Here race is offered as a unique worthy-to-stand alone construct as do sexual orientation identity development, cognitive development, and some others. *Lenses* does not cover all theories worthy of our attention; on the contrary, it is severely limited. Limited though it may be, it is limitless in the sense that its intent is to increase the readers' obligation to consider theoretical perspectives, perceptions, and insights beyond the easy reach of those few exclusionary positions we often settle for as sufficient.

The book is composed of three major sections: global lenses, theory-specific lenses, and identity development lenses. The purpose of this design is purely pedagogical, meaning that I have made decisions that I believe will, in a logical (Western) structure-bound, content-dependent way, increase readers' understanding of a wealth of information. An array of lenses into human development is provided in the following chapters. Read it as you wish (or, for many of you, as it is assigned). My expectation is that you will probably be drawn to one or more perspectives or theories and disinclined to see the significance of others. For example, if you rarely, if ever, work with gay men, Marszalek and Pope's chapter may seem less informing to your daily practice. But I would hope that by reading it, by truly working to understand the insights offered into the process of gay male development, you open yourself to the rich possibilities that should you hear a presentation from a client in the coming year that sounds somehow similar to John's (the client in Marszalek and Pope's chapter), you would have a modest foundation from which to step into your client's world that you would not have had if you had never read the chapter. I encourage you to see the value of this and other chapters not immediately relevant in your mind. It is our "job" to be competent. Being open, welcoming, and skilled are prerequisites to forming effective counseling relationships with clients, but these alone are not adequate. You and I must be knowledgeable to be competent. As one reviewer of an early draft of this text wrote, "Kurt, I believe it is our job to impose a developmental lens on our work." I agree.

I've recently begun wearing glasses. As I neared 50 years old, my ophthalmologist pacified me without a speck of incredulity, telling me that glasses were inevitable. I'll spare readers any disclosure of what these new bifocal spectacles mean to me; suffice it for me to write that I am not pacified. Glasses are inconvenient, challenging to get used to, and a powerful, ever-present, personal reminder that I'm not quite who I once was. These lenses are merely the eye care professional's tool used to offer me some relief from my own visual limitation. They are "corrective lenses," and I am learning slowly to appreciate their utility.

Maybe had I worn "noncorrective" lenses earlier in my life, I would have had a less tumultuous adoption of the "inevitable" corrective lenses. But clear and nondistorting lenses we call *windows*. We encounter windows daily and are relatively certain that they do not influence that which is seen beyond. In the late 1970s, Violet Oaklander titled her now classic text *Windows to our Children* (1978). "Windows" referred, then and now, to the numerous ways people are able to view (here to mean: access and assess the complex Gestalt of the child client) a child in counseling. Windows, in her analogy, afford a means of seeing clearly from the outside in. With *"Lenses,"* the analogy I have selected for this text, talented authors offer thirteen relevant lenses, through which counseling professionals are able to focus specifically on a particular aspect of their client, the goal being to carefully consider the effect that focal area may bring to the work the counselor and client do together. It became my goal through this text to offer a handful of valuable lenses to practitioners. An astute reader will quickly find perhaps equally valuable lenses missing! Undoubtedly true. Nevertheless, this baker's dozen is worthy of our attention—in fact, it requires our attention. Perhaps other lenses will be added to future editions of this text, but for now allow me to expand on the analogy I have selected.

Lenses come in a multitude of shapes, configurations, and combinations, and they are used for an equally wide variety of purposes. Telescope and microscope lenses are ostensibly the same, but arranged differently to achieve vastly different objectives. One would not conceive of viewing distant planetary objects with a magnifying glass; a stamp or coin collector would not select a telescope to aid in identifying a noteworthy purchase. Likewise, if one needs a particular lens to aid in a particular activity but doesn't have it available, there is no substitute.

The notion of utilizing lenses in the counseling profession is similar. If a counselor attempts to enter the world of a client without knowledge of an appropriate theory or perspective, one that would increase the counselor's understanding of the client's lived experiences, the counselor is limited. Misapplication of a lens will also prove limiting, if not outright inappropriate or potentially harmful. The antiquated notion that one size fits all—one theory is sufficient in conceptualizing a client— is thankfully a notion of the past. To imagine that an African American's lived experience is sufficiently viewed through a lens of a White

American or European is foolhardy, but sadly not uncommon. Neither should one believe that a woman's development is adequately explained through applying a developmental theory built to explain a man's development—regardless of the countless other variables that may emerge from this example. If as a counselor I have a good number of lenses available to me, I have the opportunity to consider each as the need arises. Like the ophthalmologist or optometrist, I can flip a variety of corrective lenses down in front of my eyes. I can consider whether and how each affects my perceptions and beliefs, how each clarifies or distorts my "being with" each and every client I encounter.

Finally, to take this analogy just a bit farther, the reader will find that several chapters here are short, several medium, and others pretty long. Like lenses themselves, authors present their selected theories and perspectives in vastly different ways. Each, although adhering to my requests for format and content, speaks (writes) with his or her own unique voice or voices. Each offers the reader a lens for your consideration. Some, not surprisingly, emphasize one aspect of the theory that guides them and short-changes others. To be honest, it might be tempting to say, "Oh, this little chapter is obviously simpler or less complex or less important than another of greater length or with a more scholarly lexicon." Please do not be so easily persuaded. Each chapter is rich and informing. Each author shares a case, shares the real lived experience of a client or clients with whom she or he worked. There is great respect in these disclosures; and each is deserving of a debt of gratitude not easily paid to our clients other than thanking them for the opportunity they provided us to travel with them in their growth.

So, there is less parallel construction between chapters than I had originally imagined, and that has proven to be just fine. After all, I was quite surprised when my ophthalmologist informed me that I needed different corrective lens strengths for each eye, both near and far. I know now why I am adjusting slowly to my new glasses; it is taking considerable time figuring out how to use them. After all, I had grown rather accustomed to seeing things simply through my naked eyes, although perhaps not quite clearly. I'm determined to value the correction. I am ever so hopeful that the readers of this text will benefit greatly by having new lenses at their disposal. May you always see your clients through the lens or lenses that acutely adjust your vision so that you may see them, experience them, value them, and bring to them the deepest, most growth-promoting accuracy that you are able.

# CHAPTER TWO

# A Social Constructionist View of Development

## John Winslade & Anne Geroski

During the writing of this chapter, I (John) saw a play performed about the life of Miguel, a twelve-year-old Latino boy from an unnamed Central American country. The play, *¡Bocón!* by Lisa Loomer (1998), was about a transition from adolescence into adulthood. The features of life that defined the developmental pathway for Miguel were the cadences and grammar of the Spanish language, stories of mythical figures such as *La Lorona* (the weeping woman), the harshness of poverty, manual labor picking coffee in the fields, political rebellion and civil war around his village, his parents' incarceration, his own eventual journey to the United States to seek a life for himself in Los Angeles, and his cultural positioning in the United States as an unwanted immigrant. It was a moving story of the transitions that accompany the crossing of borders (both political and psychological), and it invited an appreciation of the forces that shape many lives that are so often left out of the textbooks that describe the developmental challenges of adolescents.

In this chapter, we seek to respond to some legitimate questions about human development that are raised by Miguel's story. Does Miguel's life really go through the same stages of development as a child brought up in a middle-class, urban context? How does development in poverty, in an urban ghetto, on a reservation, or in a third world country differ from what is usually mapped out in human development theories? How do the contextual features of Miguel's life impact on his development along with the biological blueprint for his growth? What impact does culture have on development, and how can it be included in our theories of development? We take these questions seriously and seek to include them in a developmental account of Miguel and his life.

A social constructionist view of development attempts to address these questions. It is an evolving viewpoint rather than a clear model and is built upon the postmodern shifts in social theory in recent decades. This view argues that the study of human development should not only focus on what is universal in human development, it should also include a strong emphasis on the cultural forces that shape human development differently in different contexts. For example, wars, migration, traumatic experiences, major disruptions to family life such as death and divorce, unemployment, parental incarceration, and many other events can have powerful shaping effects on the developmental paths of a person's life. Or cultural patterns of family life may emphasize or diminish the experience of "sibling rivalry." Culture is indeed universal, but it is not uniform. Therefore, an account of human development should account for the differences that each cultural context imposes on the development of the individual person. A model of development should not be a completely unified model but should leave room for local influences to define developmental pathways.

A social constructionist approach also takes seriously the effect of power relations in the production of local influences. It encourages us to be curious about such local influences rather than to impose extrapolations of models drawn from elsewhere. People know more than professionals about what is happening to them. Therefore, it is respectful to listen seriously to the meanings they make, including to folk theories of human development.

What is the value of this approach for counselors? It is in the nature of counseling work to take account of the contextual and cultural features of our clients' lives and to use those understandings as a map for clinical direction. A social constructionist perspective offers a map that recognizes complexity rather than conformity and invites curiosity rather than expertise. We invite you to join us in this journey across these intriguing ideas. Development happens in the midst of sociocultural practices, the practices of living. We believe that the ideas here are very practical, even though based in demanding philosophical arguments. We have, therefore, sought to show this practical value in the story of Cori and his developmental struggles in the context of life on a reservation.

## ABOUT THE CHAPTER AUTHORS

### Anne Geroski

I was drawn to narrative and social constructionist ideas in my quest for a theoretical orientation and counseling approach that seemed appropriate working across cultures and in schools. When I first began the study of social constructionism, it felt a little like reading a new language. I had to work hard and patiently to really grasp these new ideas. I was not always patient enough, but I was lucky to find some even-more-patient teachers like John Winslade and Kathie Crockett at the University of Waikato in New Zealand to scaffold my learning. I continue to study this body of work. I continue to witness the richness and depth that it offers my teaching and the practice of counseling. It is truly a gift to find something that has a radical impact on one's life and work; I feel privileged to have accessed the work that is described in this chapter. These ideas give me tools to work with integrity across cultures and in a variety of practice settings. I hope that you will be as inspired by these ideas as I have been.

Anne Geroski

Anne Geroski, Ed.D., is an associate professor at the University of Vermont. Her professional work has included working as a school and mental health counselor in a variety of settings in the United States and overseas. She lives with her partner, three children, two cats, and four fish . . . and they all (the humans, at least) like to travel and play sports!

### John Winslade

I am always interested in ideas that stretch my thinking into new areas. And I guess I have to own to a certain impatience with the status quo, which I have to keep under control at times. I am also concerned that critical perspectives from the margins should be taken seriously. A commitment to social justice has not always been the concern of psychological theory, but I think it should be. So this chapter on social constructionist ideas in human development is not just a piece of intellectual dabbling; it is an expression of a commitment on my part. At the same time, it was not easy to write. It involved thinking through material from a variety of sources that have not often been brought together in one coherent document and articulating them from a different angle than I had done in the past. Anne Geroski invited me to join in this project, and I have 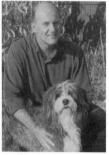 also enjoyed working with her compassionate commitment, which is evident in the story of her work that is contained here.

John Winslade is a professor at California State University San Bernardino, where he coordinates the Educational Counseling Program. Before 2003 he was a senior lecturer at the University of Waikato in New Zealand. His background is in counseling in school and family contexts in New Zealand, and he

**John Winslade**                    has particular interests in conflict resolution work and grief counseling. He has co-authored four books on narrative therapy and narrative mediation and has two more in process at the time of writing.

## Overview and Context

This chapter is about human development from a social constructionist perspective. It is not so much a theory of human development, complete with a series of formal theoretical propositions, as it is a perspective on calling a person's development "human." The word *human* in human development immediately suggests a universal psychological pattern of development across a vast range of different contexts. It pulls our thinking away from social and cultural influences on a person's development and toward the general, more biological, features of development. In this chapter, we would like to broaden the focus to include more cultural influences on development, adding them to our biological inclinations.

The social constructionist perspective proposes that childhood and adulthood are not just naturally occurring life stages but are constructed in interpersonal, cultural, historical, and political contexts (Burman, 1994). In order to work effectively with people in counseling, it is necessary to include this wider focus. This requires starting from an acceptance that there just is not an accepted universal body of knowledge of human development that necessarily applies to all people in all places (Drewery & Bird, 2004). Current knowledge is not as compelling as that.

A social constructionist account is therefore an attempt to make sense not just of natural processes of human development but also of the various ideas that have become naturalized in our knowledge of human development. That is, the ways that we talk about human development influence that very development. The words and the ideas themselves, therefore, need to be studied. We are seldom studying pure "nature-in-the-raw." We should be cautious, therefore, of the assumption that human development is primarily driven by a biological time clock and that the developments that take place in children are to a large degree inevitable. However, we do not advocate throwing out all existing ideas of human development. We can still observe changes or developments in people's lives. Such change is clearly not random, and the study of human development should help us identify patterns to development and understand the processes that shape it. It should also bring to light the assumptions that undergird our ideas about these processes.[1]

## Social Constructionism and Post Modernism

The name we are adopting for this approach, *social constructionist*, is by no means an agreed-upon term. There are many who would prefer to call what we are talking about *constructivist*, or *poststructuralist*, or *postmodern*, or *narrative*, or even *critical psychology*. We are not particularly invested in the correct name. According to Vivien Burr (1995), social constructionism: (1) takes a critical stance toward conventional knowledge or taken-for-granted assumptions about the world, (2) treats knowledge (our understandings about the world) as historically and culturally specific, and (3) is based on the assumption that common ways of understanding are constructed through social interaction rather than resulting from objective observation or natural selection. Language, then, rather than, say, pure experience, is considered to be a precondition for the development of knowledge. Scientific ideas about human development can only be expressed in language, and the language world (which is a cultural world) may be said to shape the ideas that develop

---

[1] It is difficult to attribute the authorship of social constructionist theory and narrative practice to a few individuals. These ideas are in continuous development in a wide intellectual discourse. When ideas are understood as constructed though discourse, it becomes difficult to identify the roots of every idea. In fact, we contend that no idea is ever really completely unique because understanding is constructed in a social interaction. Identifying key theorists is, therefore, somewhat antithetical to social constructionist thinking; to name specific contributors risks leaving many others unmet, unrecognized, unknown. Having said this, throughout the chapter we offer brief introductions of several key individuals who have shaped our personal understandings.

among scientists just as it does in lay thinking. Also salient is the post-structuralist idea that there is no determined nature or essence to people (nor to meanings or objects in the world). Instead, personal and social essences are thought of as constructed through discourse.

Questioning the assumptions that have dominated the field of human development is typical of postmodern thought, in which social constructionism is firmly rooted. The term *modernism* refers to the period of the last few hundred years in which the scientific agenda that began with the Enlightenment has come to dominate our understandings of truth. During this time, we have largely assumed that the truths established through scientific methods in the universities take precedence over other methods of claiming that something is true. Postmodernism, then, invites us to deconstruct (Derrida, 1976), or tease apart, the assumptions of the modernist period and to bring many of them down to earth by viewing them as products of local and historical conditions rather than as grand universal truths.

## Nonlinearity of Development

One such assumption in much of the literature on human development is that development will always be positive. It will always be moving toward greater maturity and ability. Postmodern critics challenge us to recognize the idea of inevitable progress as one of the grand narratives of modernism (Lyotard, 1984), that is, as a cultural and historical perspective rather than as an essential truth about life. Common ideas about human development often amount to some version of personal progress, echoing on the individual level our modernist beliefs about the inevitability of social progress (Seidman, 1994). But this is a questionable assumption that deserves greater scrutiny.

Perhaps people often do develop in positive directions, but perhaps also they sometimes go backwards in their developmental paths (perhaps in response to an illness, for example) or develop down a pathway that proves not so helpful for their lives (such as involvement with drugs). The pathway of development may not always be in a straight line from birth to death. In fact, many cultures do not share this linear view of development (Drewery & Bird, 2004; Morss, 1991).

## Multiciplicity of Identities

A linear account of human development is based on an assumption that individuals have a stable singular identity that is constantly integrating new experiences and information into a single whole person. We all know, however, the feeling of being a different person when we move from one context where we know the rules of the game to another where we do not know these rules. For example, we may be an accountant or professor in the office, a patient when we visit the doctor, a consumer when we go shopping, a tourist when we travel, while at home we are a mother, father, spouse, daughter, or son. Or more subtly, within each of these social roles, we are at one moment an active participant in a conversation, at another moment a complainant about some injustice, at another moment the helpless bystander being washed over by social forces that we do not quite comprehend. With each of these identities, we enter into different ways of speaking and different relational positions from which we connect with others.

Social constructionists do not lament the fragmentation of the whole person that results. Instead, they celebrate this situation as evidence of the multiplicity of identities, and therefore of multiple developmental paths. This idea of personhood as made up of multiple developmental narratives (Gergen, 1991) that are always responsive to the contours of the social landscape is central to a social constructionist account of human development. A one-size-fits-all approach, by contrast, might lead to a distortion of some people's experiences of development, or even of some aspects of everyone's development. Instead, we would call for developmental theories that are more flexible and that recognize in theory as well in practice that there are often multiple divergent pathways of development.

It is also worth considering the possibility that the sense of self that is developing in people not be regarded as "stable" at all and that the study of human development need not be about a search for such stability (Drewery & Bird, 2004). Hence, social constructionists are likely to be constantly commenting on the various theories of human development that specify a more or less invariant set of stages that people go through by saying, "Wait a minute, you're leaving out many people's experience, and it's a lot more complicated than that." Such critique is not intended to be negative so much as to be inclusive of more people and more aspects of developmental experience.

## Discourses and Development

Social constructionist writers are, nevertheless, still cognizant of the patterns that appear in people's developmental pathways. But they account for these patterns in different ways. They tend to look for explanations of these patterns not just in the influence of nature but also in the influence of discourses that circulate in our social worlds. The term *discourse* here refers to the socially organized ways of interpreting meanings in a given context (e.g., a given society) that define categories of under-standing and specify the domains in which things are generally accepted as truths (Burman, 1994). This use of the term *discourse* was developed by Michel Foucault. For example, in various cultural traditions, there are different emphases in the discourses of "family" that specify the pat-terns of personal relations that family members are expected to learn and practice. That is, we understand "family" and act as family members according to the discourse through which "family" is understood in our cultural context. We all develop within the parameters of various dis-courses. Discourses are shared as we use them to engage in social exchanges of all kinds, to help us make meaning of our experiences, and to establish normative ideas that provide us with direction and instruc-tion. Because discourses are shared, it would not be surprising that we would find lots of similarities from one person to another, provided that they share at least some aspects of a cultural context.

A social constructionist perspective rejects the assumption that psy-chological knowledge is ever neutral (Drewery & Bird, 2004; Foucault, 1969, 1972, 1978, 1980) and that critical inquiry into the foundation of this knowledge is warranted. Foucault argued that psychological knowledges were both products of the dominant cultural discourses out of which they originated and also that these knowledges served a pro-ductive, not just a descriptive, function. They do not just represent in a neutral way the condition of things in the real world. Instead they work to shape and constitute the world in particular ways. Erica Bur-man (1994) suggests three ways in which we might question standard research knowledge about human development:

1. By uncovering the circumstances in which research was conducted. Research is always conducted in a social and political context that exerts an influence on the research findings.
2. By inquiring into the social and political circumstances that made a piece of research seem relevant. Research usually gets funded according to historical and political agendas of the day, and the find-ings will to some extent reflect those agendas.
3. By tracing the role of the research in a particular social context and its impact on that context. Research that is taken up has a social impact because it fits with the social agendas already at work in that context.

The work of Jean Piaget has been hugely influential on the whole field of developmental psychology. His studies of the cognitive structure of human thinking seemed to offer what John Morss (1991) referred to as "something like a mental X-ray" (p. 17). On the basis of this cognitive structure, Piaget proposed that the development of children's thinking could be traced through a series of stages negotiated through processes of accommodation and assimilation. These ideas were elaborated into areas such as moral development (Kohlberg, 1984) and are still to be found in many textbooks on children's learning and development.

Since the 1970s, some researchers have set out to show that Piaget's ideas do not always stand up in practice (for example, see Bryant, 1974; Donaldson, 1978). But the social constructionist concern is not so much about what Piaget got wrong as about what he left out and about the unwitting assumptions from his own worldview that have become entwined in human development theory. A criticism of this work is that the social contexts in which children were doing the thinking were mostly left out of Piaget's universal account of the structure of children's thinking. As John Morss (1991) argues, it was not that Piaget was ethnocentric in a crude sense. It was more that his work embodied a commitment to certain discursive values that are not universal and yet are assumed in his work to be so. These values are most evident if we look at the rational kind of person that was the endpoint of his process of development. This adult appears to live a comfortable, middle-class, European life that does not always compare with how many people live. A social constructionist account of development focuses much more on what people take in from their surroundings in the development of their thinking. In learning to think, they must respond to the demands of these surroundings in both thinking style and in the content of their thoughts.

For example, when teachers have in their minds a Piaget-derived concept about a child's "cognitive readiness" to progress to a new developmental stage, they might subtly guide children, through granting social recognition, into the expression and development of the signs of readiness that will be accorded value in the wider culture to which they belong. Valerie Walkerdine (1988) has demonstrated this with regard to the development of children's mathematical concepts. She argues that the processes by which children are produced as knowers of mathematical concepts is part of a larger educational project of the "mastery of reason" (Walkerdine, 1988) through which children develop the abilities that are recognized in the modern world as necessary for economic and social participation. Being a particular kind of stable, rational person, with the right degree of emotional expression (but not too much), is highly rewarded in our universities, professions, corporations, markets, politics, and courts. Schools and families are the primary institutions charged with

producing in children the abilities, personal qualities, styles of performance, and habits of thinking that will be rewarded in later life. Counselors also participate in this production of young people's identities as
reasoning individuals when they invite young people to reflect upon their
experiences and emotions and to bring them under rational control. Thus
when particular forms of rationality and of reasoning abilities are assumed
as desirable outcome qualities of human development, models of development will focus on and highlight qualities that appear to illustrate
progress toward these.

# A Social Constructionist Theory of Development

## The Production of Development

From a social constructionist perspective, development is not read as primarily natural in a biologically determined sense (Walkerdine, 1988).
Social constructionists read development from the start as *produced* within
social practices (i.e., produced in connection to social discourses). Therefore, to study development, we need to take an interest in what is happening within such social practices. We need to analyze the power
relations associated with a given practice in order to appreciate who is
influencing whom, or "who is in a position, allowed, and permitted to say
what to whom and with what effects" (Walkerdine, 1988, p. 12). From a
social constructionist perspective, such influences are negotiated in the to
and fro of discourse as well as in the unfolding of inbuilt biological blue-
prints. Even before we are born, even before we do something that gets
recognized as a developmental task, we are "always-already-social" (Walkerdine, 1984, p. 16), that is, there is no task we can do that is not already,
before we do it, part of a social relation and therefore needs to be understood in terms of the influences of power relations on its production.

But there is another issue that arises at this point. Should we be
focusing so much on individual human development at all (Bird, 1999)?
Social constructionists have suggested alternatives, such as focusing
more on the development of social interactions or on the development
of group or collective identities (Bird, 1999; Burman, 1994). Certainly
there are many cultural traditions around the world that do not place
the same intense degree of emphasis on the individual as does the dominant liberal-humanist Western worldview. More collectivist cultural
traditions might share greater affinity for a developmental psychology
that was less myopic about the development of the individual to the
exclusion of collective, tribal, or family development.

## ABOUT ERICA BURMAN AND VALERIE WALKERDINE
### Constructionism in Human Development

Erica Burman and Valerie Walkerdine have applied many of Foucault's ideas to the domain of human development. Burman has written extensively in feminist psychology, with a special interest in critiquing the psychology of human development. In 1994, she published her groundbreaking text, *Deconstructing Developmental Psychology.* She describes herself as a critical psychologist and lists a series of possible identity descriptions that may be ascribed to her own path of personal development "as child, daughter, sister, aunt, child-free, childless, daughter of a single parent, feminist, child-centred, woman centred . . ." (Burman, 1994, pp. 7–8). She is a senior lecturer at Manchester Metropolitan University (MMU), in England, and the co-founder of the Discourse Unit, which is an "interdisciplinary space that focuses its critical activity mainly on the discipline of psychology, but which also includes researchers working on the intersection of politics and subjectivity" (retrieved from the Discourse Unit website on October 26, 2004). Burman is also the co-convener of the Women's Studies Research Centre at MMU and is an accredited group psychoanalyst. Her current research interests include the study of constructions of "race" and gender in psychotherapy, and in the facilitation of a more democratic, participatory vision of mental health services.

Valerie Walkerdine was the Foundation Professor of Critical Psychology and director of the Centre for Critical Psychology, University of Western Sydney in Australia, and has recently moved to Cardiff University in the United Kingdom. She is the editor of the *International Journal of Critical Psychology.* Her research features a strong interest in gender and class perspectives in human development, and her approach to these subjects is influenced by her reading of Michel Foucault and also the poststructuralist psychoanalyst, Jacques Lacan.

## Historical, Cultural, and Social Contexts in Development

There has been a trend in developmental psychology to move away from the study of "the child" in isolation, as something like a lone little scientist, busily solving the cognitive problems. The move away from an

abstraction of "the child" has led to the study of "the context." But the
definition of the context has tended to halt at "the family" and could
pay more attention to the historical, political, economic, and cultural
influences on any child's development (Burman, 1994). Erica Burman
argues that an intense interest since about the 1950s in attachment theory
and the implications for normal development of a satisfactory bonding
with the mother have been associated with a strong public interest in
good and bad mothering, which in turn has served the social purpose
of producing (or reproducing) restrictive social roles for women. The
construction of normal developmental milestones can also be said to
structure mothers' observations of what their children are doing and to
create worry about being found guilty of "faulty mothering" (Burman,
1994, p. 58) if the children do not match the norm. Meanwhile, other
relationships are not accorded the same degree of attention. As Valerie
Walkerdine (1988) notes, it is mothers who, in dominant discourse, are
"held responsible for the emergence of the natural" (p. 213) in children's
development.

The abstracted nuclear family (mother, father, and two to three children), which tends to be assumed in most child development studies,
also does not match the experience of family that many children know.
Child development study families tend to be white and middle class,
for a start. And the many children who are brought up by sole parents,
grandparents, or aunts and uncles, in divorced or blended families, or
in poverty deserve greater recognition in the developmental narrative.
Perhaps psychological studies could treat race, culture, gender, class, or
other demographic features less as confounding variables to be screened
out of their results and more as highly influential contextual features of
the development of most of the world's children. Rather than controlling for cultural influences, developmental studies should more often
treat them as central to what is being studied. This might lead to a
wider range of children having their experience constituted as "normal."

The emphasis on culture and discourse leads to the key position from
which social constructionists view personal development. It includes
more fully the work that culture does to set out paths for development
(Drewery & Bird, 2004). As mentioned earlier, rather than understanding development as evolving naturally, we would start by thinking
of it as a process of *production*, that is, our lives are not just patterned
naturally and then we encounter a series of cultural factors that apply
the brakes to the natural path of development. The constructionist position is that our lives are produced by the mix of competing discourses,
dominant knowledges, power relations, social practices, and narrative

trajectories among which we live. These discourses constitute much of what we consider to be natural. They govern our development into specific pathways and provide us with rites of passage to negotiate. We experience developmental challenges along the way as we perform the acts of living in relation to the norms that are established by these discourses.

The notion of adolescent rebellion is an example of a normative idea that sits in current historical contexts. Normative ideas usually start out as descriptions and later become prescriptive. In European or Western traditions of thought, adolescence is assumed to be a "natural" stage of growing up. As a result of the prevalence of talk (both lay and academic) about adolescent assertion of identity and their "need" to separate from their parents and become independent adults, young people are assumed to go through a stage of development called *adolescence,* which is natural and normal. The natural quality of this developmental stage is grounded in the biological events of puberty. Sometimes it is even constructed as a crisis (i.e., an "identity crisis"). Social constructionists would not necessarily argue that this idea is wrong or that it is not real. For many young people and their parents, it is sometimes painfully real. However, assuming that "identity crisis" is something that every adolescent—across all cultures—will go through has the danger of dismissing the fine nuances of specific contexts and specific cultures within which the "adolescent" ideas, behaviors, and characteristics we are witnessing are produced and nurtured.

To study adolescence from a social constructionist perspective, then, we would have to take into account the cultural context in which young people are produced to go through a series of rituals and social practices that we recognize as typical of adolescents. We would have to look at how their lives are governed by the adult world so that they progress through a series of cultural rituals and tests in order to be initiated into adult participation in the world. We are referring to such things as learning to pass school tests, gain driving licenses, participate in popular culture and sporting activities, open bank accounts, form relationships with their own and the opposite sex, establish readiness to leave home, and enter the paid workforce.

The precise shape of this development is always changing in accordance with historical changes. When we were young, adolescent development did not require the acquiring of personal cell phone numbers, chat room identities, relationships with distant e-mail buddies, or website addresses in the way in which our children are required to develop now. Nor did we need to avoid being labeled as ADHD or learning disabled. (There were, of course, other identity descriptions that we had to avoid.) In this sense, we grew up in a world that produced and governed the development of young people in ways that were different from the context in which young people live now. The point here is that there are particular historical aspects of the cultural world in which adolescent human development takes place, and to study it we should take account of how young people negotiate a path specified for them in ways that keep on changing.

## The Politics of Development

The resulting study of personal development from a constructionist perspective is a study of difference as much as it is of homogeneity. It is a study of the work done by specific discourses and stories to produce people's lives in particular directions. Who governs the process of development considered in these terms? It is clear that there is no central control room, no child development politburo, no governing board that decides on what will be produced in children. Rather, we all participate in the ongoing production and reproduction of the meanings that come to dominate our understanding. We do this on a daily basis as we engage in social practices and talk about what we are doing. Our talk is always built on the foundation of a network of assumptions.

These assumptions, however, achieve privileged status in our understandings through being granted legitimacy and sanction in places that matter in a particular social world, such as in academic journals and textbooks, in laws, in courtrooms, in school policies, in social welfare systems, and so on. Foucault (1991) therefore developed the concept of *governmentality* to describe the process by which people's lives are produced (see also Rose 1990, 1998). The word is a combination of the concepts of government and rationality. It describes the ways of thinking, or the discursive assumptions, that get built into the social technologies that influence the patterns of identity development. He also urged the paying of attention to the power relations involved in the ways in which lives were governed. By power, he meant the ways in which people were being produced in patterns that accord some people privileged access to opportunity in life and excluded others from the same opportunities.

If current abstractions of normal human development are skewed toward a representation as "natural" of the experience of the White, middle class, two-parent family, they privilege those who can see themselves in this image. They also risk pathologizing those who do not.

## ABOUT MICHAEL FOUCAULT

Michel Foucault, born in Poitiers, France, in 1926, was a philosopher by academic training. After a series of other academic appointments, he was elected to the College de France, in 1970, where he held the position of professor of History of Systems of Thought. Foucault was a major contributor to postmodern social theory, which serves as the backcloth for social constructionist thought and narrative practice. His early work focused on understanding the conditions under which knowledge is produced. A second focus was on the genealogy of power, with careful articulation of discursive and nondiscursive practices in power relations. Foucault's work in the mid 1970s was on amplifying the voice of marginalized groups, and his prestige at the time helped establish a public forum for discussion of issues of social justice. Later, Foucault began to shift from an investigation of power and knowledge to the topic of subjectivity and subjective practices, and the ways in which individuals cultivated what he called the "care of the self." Foucault died in 1984.

This may create a sense of entitlement among those who are so privileged and a sense of deficit in those who are not. Personal development is better seen, we believe, as an interaction between biological influences and the cultural possibilities that are urged upon a person by the economic, political, and cultural worlds. Often, the study of human development has begun with biological influences and treated cultural influences as of secondary importance. A social constructionist perspective turns the tables. Along with Jerome Bruner (1990), we would view the cultural world as both opening up and closing down specific possibilities for development and the biological influences serving as a constraint on what is possible to be culturally produced.

A more recent emphasis on the lifespan notwithstanding, human development has focused mostly on the development of children. Implicit in this focus is always a set of assumptions about what the child is developing toward, that is, the study of child development always assumes an abstracted adult self that is regarded as the target of normal development. While it is never completely clear just what kind of adult is the potential ideal, we can sometimes deduce it from the particular developmental pathways that we select for emphasis. Carol Gilligan (1982) is famous for deducing that the developmental pathway envisaged in Kohlberg's (1984) theory of moral development was skewed toward the production of male identity and left most women stranded without being able to reach the higher stages of moral development. Social constructionists are interested in just what kind of imagined finished product guides the study of development. It is in this sense that Erica Burman (1994) states that "definitions of childhood are relational, they exist in relation to definitions of adults" (p. 59). She goes on to point out that the dominant image of "the adult" that shapes understandings of children's development is located in a North American or European version of middle-class life.

## Diversity Issues in Development

How does a social constructionist perspective embrace diversity? Before answering this question we need to comment on the word *diversity* itself. What exactly is diversity? What images come to mind when the word *diversity* is used? What kind of person leaps to the front of your imagination? Often, the word is used to lump together various groups of people who do not have access to social privilege on account of social divisions created by those who have easier access to privilege. These are the social divisions based on gender, race, disability, social class, sexual orientation, national origin, religious belief, and such.

Unless we are careful about how we frame this issue, the perspective we can easily slip into is a view of some people as diverse (as in different from) those who are not diverse, that is, "us" and "them." The "us" that is assumed is usually the dominant group with regard to gender, race, class, and the like. In thinking about diversity, therefore, the challenge is not to start always from the position of the dominant group, especially if we already belong to that group.

## The Location of Culture in Development

Focusing only on the "human" in "human development" raises the real danger of falling into the trap of mapping out pathways for human development for people in each of the many diverse cultural contexts around the United States or around the world only from the perspective of dominant culture. Social constructionists seek to avoid this danger by also taking into account people's own cultural perspectives on their development. They seek to open up space for voices from diverse cultural positions to make their own developmental claims for people in their own communities (Drewery & Bird, 2004). To do this requires a great deal of caution with making universal claims about human nature.

The challenge is to accommodate diversity without trying to unify all cultures (Drewery & Bird, 2004). Only emphasizing the commonalities between cultures is problematic because it tends to render people's diversity invisible. Rendering diversity invisible then clears the path for those from privileged cultural positions to slide past issues of diversity under the pretext that, "We are all human underneath." A related challenge is to think about diversity without considering diversity within cultures. There are often subtle ways in which cultural discourses operate to produce different developmental pathways within a shared cultural context. We also need to account for these exceptions. For example, there are those who are affected by particular cultural traditions but go to some effort to reject or modify them, or seek to take up leadership roles in bringing about social change within a cultural community. The history of feminism contains many examples of women who were not content to have their lives produced within the dominant specifications for being a woman. They consciously set about challenging and modifying these specifications for themselves and their daughters. As a result, the pathways for female development in many (although not all) contexts has changed considerably.

Rather than creating an impression of a homogenous human core that is coated around the outside with cultural flavoring, social constructionism suggests that culture plays a more central role. Sometimes, cultural issues are treated as *content* detail in a person's development while the more important *structure* is treated as homogenous and biological. The impression created is that culture is tacked on rather than crucial to what makes us human. Social constructionists would argue that human development is diverse by nature. Bruner (1990) proposes that the central concept of human psychology, the process of how individuals come to know and understand their experience in the world, is shaped by intentional states that are formed through participation in "the symbolic systems" of culture (p. 33). In this way, culture can never just be an "'overlay' on biologically determined human nature" (Bruner, 1990, p. 20).

## Folk Psychology in Development

Bruner (1990) introduced the concept of *folk psychology* to explain how understandings about the social world are communicated and reproduced. Folk psychology refers to a set of normative descriptions about how

---

## ABOUT JEROME BRUNER
### Narrative Theory

Jerome Bruner developed a compelling articulation of how individuals produce meanings and how knowledge is constructed through social interactions and discourse. Born in 1915, Bruner was a professor of psychology at Harvard and Oxford universities, and is currently a research professor of psychology and senior research fellow in law at New York University. Bruner was first known for his articulation of cognitive psychology in the 1950s and 1960s when behaviorist theories dominated psychology. Bruner focused on how individuals categorize information to generate understandings. Suggesting that children play an active role in the construction of knowledge made Bruner a key figure in educational reform in the United States and in Britain.

Later, Bruner became increasingly influenced by Lev Vygotsky. He became critical of the "cognitive revolution" and began to identify with cultural psychologists and with the development of a narrative perspective in psychology. These ideas have been significant in the practice of narrative therapy.

---

"human beings 'tick' " (p. 35) that is culturally specific rather than generalizable to a universal human nature. They are drawn from people's own thoughts about their own lives, rather than from expert knowledges. They provide an idea about what people are like, how one should act, how one's actions and ideas will be interpreted, what possibilities exist for being in the world, and how one can commit to those ways of being. Basically, folk psychology is a "system by which people organize their experience in, knowledge about, and transactions with the social world" (p. 35). Folk psychology also describes normative ideas about what will happen when someone violates accepted discourses. Rather than screening such folk psychology out of our studies, or treating it in an oppositional way as lower level knowledge that must be overcome and replaced by higher level abstractions based on more scientific methods, Bruner is advocating that we take this knowledge seriously and study it, precisely in order to better understand human development.

Apfelbaum (2002) reminds us that the historical accounts of a community provide the "foundational legitimacy for making sense of personal experience and, therefore, for constructing one's identity" (p. 80). On this view, the "self" does not grow from an inner essence or biological predisposition that is overlaid by culture; it is constructed from experiences that are given meaning through language. The task of developmental psychology, from this perspective, becomes one of tracing the impact of specific cultural influences on people's development.

## Culture and Power

Deconstructing cultural developmental influences involves much more than celebrating diversity. The study of cultural development needs to include a focus on power relations. Cultures are not discrete entities but exist always in relation to each other and are constantly exerting influence on each other. But dominant Western cultures are usually in positions of much greater influence on the lives of people from indigenous or minority cultures than the reverse.

It is arguably more accurate to speak as if we are all sites where multiple cultural narratives intersect rather than essentially linked to one culture by "nature." The anthropologist Renato Rosaldo (1993) suggests that we should pay more attention to "border identities" in order to understand how different cultural narratives interact in the construction of identity. Focusing on "border identities" refers to a focus on relations between shifting cultural positions rather than core identities within them. It seeks to be more inclusive of those who cross back and forth over the dividing lines of race, ethnicity, and culture without requiring them to make forced identity choices. It avoids essentializing people on the basis of singular group membership and recognizes instead that we all are diverse creatures within ourselves as well as between us. We are all hybrid products of the influences of a multitude of discourses, and we are all positioned within complex intersections of power relations. But this does not mean that we all have consistent access to privilege. Nor does it mean that we are totally excluded from the exercising power either. A social constructionist position is interested in how people often achieve particular personal developments in the face of the operations of power in their lives. (See Table 2.1 for a summary of the assumptions made by the major human development theories.) The study of human development can take on the task of studying such complexity rather than abstracting a simpler view of human nature, or of culture itself.

TABLE 2.1  Social Constructionism and Human Development

### Common assumptions of major theories of human development

| Universal | Many people's experiences don't fit—everyone does not develop in the same ways. |
|---|---|
| Naturalistic | Assumes what exists is what must be. |
| Unified | Developing identities are not so uniform or so stable. |
| Focus on individual development | Suggests development without a context. |
| Biological-based | Omits the very important influences of culture on development. |
| Eurocentric model | The assumed mature adult is Western man. |

### A social constructionist approach is based on

| Epistemological critique | Conventional theories are too positivist. |
|---|---|
| Historical critique | Dubious foundations in social Darwinism and colonizing practices. |
| Feminist critique | Favors a male model of development. |
| Cultural critique | Leaves out experiences of non-Western cultures. |
| Critique of function | Used to create social norms and then to govern people in relation to these. |

### A social constructionist approach emphasizes

| Discourse | Discourse sets the parameters for development. |
|---|---|
| Power relations | Dominant discourse privileges some developmental pathways. |
| Production | People's lives are shaped by cultural forces rather than evolving naturally. |
| Knowledge and power | Scientific knowledge is never neutral or free from discourse. |
| Cultural psychology | Culture is not a coating around what is human but at its core. |
| Narrative | Stories link norms with personal experience. |
| Nonessentialism | There are no essences of people, developmental stages, or cultures. |

### Narrative counseling practice based on social constructionism emphasizes

| Deconstruction | Unpacking the work done by discourse and power in culture. |
|---|---|
| Externalizing | Objectifying problems rather than people. |
| Curiosity | Asking questions to open up fresh meanings rather than relying on established truths. |
| Multiplicity | Exploring multiple possible developmental pathways. |
| Folk psychology | Emphasizing local, indigenous, or common sense knowledge ahead of expert "universal" truths. |
| Alternative stories | Building counseling partnerships to re-author stories of personal development. |
| Thickening stories | Weaving stories into alternative developmental pathways. |

# Critiques of Social Constructionism

It has become commonplace in human development and counseling textbooks for one particular criticism of social constructionism to keep on appearing. It is the critique that social constructionism is too relativistic. For example, Anita Woolfolk's (2004) text on educational psychology argues that social constructionism, "when pushed to the extreme" (p. 325) renders all beliefs and all knowledges meaningless because they all become equal since they are all socially constructed. Similar ideas are expressed in relation to counseling practice by Sam Gladding (2004).

We propose that the criticism is a weak one because it misrepresents social constructionist viewpoints, and we worry that it comes from an unquestioning acceptance of traditional human development ideas that are unsettled by social constructionist thinking. As Michael White noted (personal communication, August, 2004), he has never met a single person interested in a postmodern viewpoint who would agree that everything is relative and that one idea or belief is therefore as good as another. It appears that the notion of complete relativism is an interpretation by critics more than a position argued by the advocates of social constructionism. Social constructionists are too interested in the ethics of knowledge and power to be so naïve. The critique only holds water if we start from the assumption that knowledge should be free from all ethical contestation. And it is the concern with ethical questions, which cannot be solved by appeal to empirical data, that drove writers like Foucault and nourishes narrative practitioners. And so while this critique about relativism is logically flawed, it seems hard to dispel, and it occupies a lot of energy. Perhaps it is better resolved in practice than in theory.

Ken Gergen (1999) acknowledges the persistence of this critique of social constructionism. He lists a series of strident accusations that have been leveled at this perspective ranging from "nihilist" to "anti-scientific" to "morally bankrupt" (p. 221). For a thoroughgoing treatment of various questions about social constructionism, we refer readers to Gergen (1994). His response to these critiques argues:

> Social constructionism doesn't try to rule on what is or is not fundamentally real. Whatever is, simply is. However, the moment we begin to articulate what there is—what is truly or objectively the case—we enter into a world of discourse. . . . (Gergen, 1999, p. 222)

## ABOUT KEN GERGEN

Ken Gergen is a leading exponent of the social constructionist movement in psychology. He is a professor of psychology at Swarthmore College, Pennsylvania, and has been a major influence in social psychology since the late1960s. Despite a wide-ranging interest in the implications of social constructionist ideas, Gergen is modest about his own position as a writer. He acknowledges the limitations in his personal experience and therefore on what he is able to write about.

> My words will inevitably carry the traces of nationality, gender, age, and sexual preference. . . . My experiences in life are also limiting. I have lived a life of some privilege: I have had a steady job, never fought on a field of battle, and never lived in poverty. Yes, I have had my share of suffering but I cannot write out of the depth of fear and pain that has affected many families during my lifetime.   (Gergen, 1999, p. vii)

While principally taking up the role of general theorist on social constructionism, Gergen has also investigated applications of these ideas in therapy, in organizational development, and most recently in positive ageing.

More important are the critiques that identify gaps in the development of social constructionist work. Advocates of social constructionism have not yet developed studies in the field of human development in great detail. To date, they have been mostly concerned with making the necessary philosophical distinctions on which more detailed studies can presumably be built. Vivien Burr (1995) notes that there is much work for social constructionists to do to detail a revised psychology of personhood. Such a psychology needs to go beyond the philosophically robust but overly generalized accounts that we currently have.

Another problem that social constructionists wrestle with has to do with the basis for claiming that people can be agents in making changes in their own lives. Foucault's efforts to erase the humanistic subject from our assumptions may have led to some widespread confusion. Even Foucault, in his later work, sought to correct this emphasis. The question is about the basis on which individuals can hold intentions and decide on actions if discourse and culture are so powerful in structuring people's inner experience. Vivien Burr acknowledges this as a problem that various social constructionist writers provide answers for but on which there is no strong consensus.

It seems therefore that social constructionist thinking is still emergent. There is not even consensus on the name. Our belief is, however, that it represents such freshness of thinking that it is well worth exploring further. Current examples of this seem to hold out much promise. In the meantime the jury is still out and needs to remain so.

## Implications for Counseling

So what does all this mean for counseling practice? The approach to counseling that has most fully embraced this social constructionist perspective is called *Narrative Therapy.* It was developed initially during the 1980s and 1990s in Australia and New Zealand by Michael White and David Epston, and has been taken up by many practitioners in North America and other parts of the world. We shall outline some of the main aspects of a narrative approach that can be linked to a social constructionist view of development.

Michael White's (1989) aphorism, "The person is not the problem; the problem is the problem," is a good place to start. It speaks to an effort to step out of the patterns of thinking through which people are frequently categorized by normalizing discourse in positions of deficit or pathology. Those who differ from the established developmental norms in terms of their cultural positioning are particularly likely to have such processes of evaluation applied to them. By contrast, the narrative perspective, drawing on Bruner's folk psychology, directs our interest toward a person's own intentions for their lives in the face of the various cultural and discursive influences at work. This means viewing a person's development as a personal and cultural narrative more than as a predetermined, biological process of evolution. Again, a narrative is a cultural product that is shaped by its author but also by the narrative conventions of its context of production. So, a narrative counselor would be interested in helping people deconstruct, or unpack, the discursive or cultural influences on their developmental paths. Some of these influences may be producing limited opportunity. In this case, the role of power relations in the production of the path may also be deconstructed.

The linguistic move that narrative practice in counseling is most well known for is that of "externalizing." This is a practice of speaking of the problems that people encounter in life as external objects or forces that exert a shaping influence on the narrative they are striving to construct. It creates a linguistic space in which people can consider the cultural forces at work in their development and exercise their own expertise with regard to the narratives that will work for them, rather than relying on psychological experts to specify developmental pathways.

The knowledge of the client as an expert in the process of addressing a problem is not, however, always immediately available for narrative counselors to work with. It often lies neglected in the unstoried aspects of experience that have not been granted authority or legitimacy in the dominant cultural discourse. Hence, it becomes necessary to scaffold a conversation in which such knowledges can be reconstructed. To do so, conversations need to be linked together as viable narratives based on "unique outcomes" (White & Epston, 1990). A unique outcome is then tied with other plot events through attributions of meaning and woven into a story that has salience in the cultural world of the client. This is achieved mainly through the counselor taking up a stance of curiosity and asking questions designed to generate particular local knowledge, rather than through taking up a didactic stance based on expert scientific knowledge of universal human development theories.

As clients consider the previously unstoried aspects of their lives, they produce their lives in slightly different ways. We spoke earlier about development as produced in social practices. The counseling conversation produces development through bringing these other events into sharper focus and making them a part of a broader scope of understanding. From this understanding, a client can draw a richer or more desirable identity conclusion. This practice is built on Jerome Bruner's (1990) notion that as people make meaning of their experience, they organize story elements into a sequence that can serve as the basis for identity conclusions.

On the basis that human development is always produced in social practices, narrative counselors recognize that particular personal developments can never be separated from larger systems of meaning embedded in language, culture, politics, and history. So when we ask clients to consider the meaning of specific events, we also need to examine the discourses that influence the stories that are told to and by our clients. This inquiry calls for a nonneutral and active counselor stance. From a position of interest and curiosity, the counselor works to access the expertise of the clients in resisting dominant discourse and expressing more fully their own intentions for their lives.

## ABOUT MICHAEL WHITE AND DAVID EPSTON
### Narrative Therapy

Michael White, co-pioneer of narrative therapy, has lived all his life in Adelaide, Australia. White was initially drawn to Gregory Bateson's ideas about information processing and family systems. But he also had a strong commitment to social justice and was influenced by feminist critiques of psychology. This commitment led him to the critiques of institutional care and expert discourses that were developed by Michel Foucault and Erving Goffman. Reading such writers encouraged his exploration of the epistemological basis of family therapy. White also drew from anthropologists Barbara Myerhoff and Edward Bruner and the narrative psychology of Jerome Bruner. With David Epston and Cheryl White, Michael White began to argue for the value of deconstructing dominant discourse in therapeutic practice.

Michael White travels widely around the world and teaches in many countries. In recent years, his work has focused on applying narrative principles to community work as well as therapy. He continues to work as a therapist at the Dulwich Centre in Adelaide, Australia. The Dulwich Centre also maintains a publishing house that has produced many books and several journals on narrative practice. White likes to cycle and swim regularly and enjoys flying small planes.

David Epston, a Canadian-born family therapist who practices in Auckland, New Zealand, worked extensively with Michael White in the original co-authorship of narrative therapy. He is the co-director of the Family Centre in Auckland. His engagement with the narrative metaphor began through the study of anthropology and a keen interest in literature and storytelling. He is known for his creative engagement with clients. Epston has authored many publications on therapeutic letter writing in the documentation of alternative stories. He has also pioneered the development of "leagues" or groups of individuals who have worked against similar problems (e.g., the Anti-Anorexia League of New Zealand). Like Michael White, David Epston is an enthusiastic cyclist.

Re-authored stories take hold when there are people to notice and appreciate them. So, the work of recruiting and engaging an audience interests the narrative therapist. There are many ways of engaging an audience of others in the construction of new stories. These may include inviting significant others into counseling sessions to bear witness to new developments and providing written documentation of success, such as writing letters, issuing alerts, and giving awards and statements of proclamation.

All of these practices often afford people who consult counselors the chance to develop identity around stands of refusal of what the dominant cultural context expects. Narrative practice is often about inviting people to refuse to locate their development in relation to standard accounts of human nature. Let us end this section with a quotation from Michael White (2002) that underlines this position:

> Many questions can be raised about how it could ever be possible to sustain any account of identity, including of human nature, that would not be a social, cultural and historical product, and that would be outside of language and beyond the systems of understanding and discursive practices that shape people's existence. (p. 47)

## Practice Settings

Narrative approaches to counseling first emerged in family therapy circles in New Zealand and Australia in the work of Michael White and David Epston in the late 1980s and early 1990s. Narrative therapy has continued to develop in family therapy domains worldwide. A growing cadre of clinicians has begun to use these ideas creatively to work with individuals, adults, and children in relation to a variety of problems. That this approach is of use in the management of even severe psychiatric problems is attested to by work in psychiatric settings, such as that of Glenn Simblett (1997), and James Griffith and Melissa Griffith (1994).

There is also a growing literature of narrative group work (see Silvester, 1997) as well as interesting work in the area of conflict resolution and mediation (Winslade & Monk, 2001). The field of grief therapy is also being offered transformative thinking in a social constructionist and narrative mode (Hedtke & Winslade, 2004; Klass, Silverman, & Nickman, 1996; M. White, 1989).

Of particular noteworthiness for a set of practices that focus explicitly on power relations and social justice are the developments of narrative community work. This has developed in a number of domains, such as in AIDS prevention in Africa; in immigrant Latino communities in the United States (Bracho, 2002; C. White, 1998a); in relation to deaths in custody in South Australia (McLean, 1995); in trauma responses in Palestine (M. White, 2004); in health promotion among Maori in New Zealand (McKenzie, 1997); among the homeless (C. White, 1999); among consumers of mental health services (Jackson, 2002; C. White, 2003; M. White, 2003; Power to Our Journeys Group, 1997); among people living with HIV (C. White, 2000); and in many other areas.

In school counseling, narrative ideas are not yet as widely recognized in the United States as in New Zealand and Australia. However, narrative conversations can be particularly suited to brief engagements with students in schools, especially those who have been storied in ways that silence their desire to make changes. In this domain a social constructionist perspective on human development can help the counselor avoid getting caught by totalizing assumptions about a young person's developmental path. There is a small but growing literature on school counseling from a narrative perspective (see Beaudoin & Taylor, 2004; Besley, 2002; Cheshire & Lewis, 2004; McMenamin, 2004; C. White, 1995, 1998b; Winslade & Monk, 2007).

## Cori's Story: Recovering Local Knowledge

We shall now introduce a story of narrative practice that embodies the social constructionist principles explained so far. The intention of this story is to illustrate how these ideas are not just of intellectual interest but have very pragmatic implications for counseling work. This story comes from Anne's work with a mental health agency on an Indian reservation in the United States. The commentary on the case is written by John and Anne, reflecting on Anne's work.

> My (Anne's) first introduction to Cori was when he was already "in trouble" at school. In fact, Cori had developed quite a reputation as "a problem" by the time his mother had followed up on the school's referral to the public mental health clinic in town. Cori came to me with the label "Depression, Rule-out ODD." His mother, Salina, came with a reputation, too. Her quiet refusal to fill the prescription for sertraline (Zoloft®) from the clinic psychiatrist earned her this reputation as a "noncompliant" parent. These were the somewhat formidable circumstances surrounding my first encounter with Cori.

My work with Cori began with the mapping of the stories that were part of his narrative of identity. Cori was born the first son of his mother, initiating his membership in the Beaver Clan. He was also the first-born great grandson of the esteemed tribal healer, Arden Waikedo. Cori's child-clan was Turtle, originating from the clan membership of his father. While the long history and stories of the Turtle clan were somewhat lost to him because his father no longer lived on the Indian reservation, Cori did enjoy close relations with his maternal grandparents and other members of the maternally linked Beaver Clan, which was a large and active clan in his community.

Because notions of clan membership are not a part of dominant discourse about human development, one might be tempted to ignore, or perhaps pathologize, the role of clan membership in Cori's identity construction. At best, dominant discourse about human development might lead Anne to consider his clan membership as a coating around the outside of the development of his individual nature. When we think of human development, however, as a process of production through the interplay of competing discourses, power relations, social practices, and narrative trajectories, it becomes critical to understand more about Cori's clan membership.

What is the significance for Cori of being born into the Beaver Clan, and what are the responsibilities for him that are inherent in this affiliation? What role, too, does the child-clan membership potentially play in Cori's life, and how does paternal alienation affect Cori's connection to Turtle clan? How does clan affiliation encourage and produce personal qualities and behaviors? How does Cori's lineage as a descendant of Arden Waikedo get storied into his family's, clan's, and tribe's stories of who he should be? What are the hopes and dreams that his ancestors and family have for Cori, given this lineage and clan affiliation? These are some of the questions that Anne carried into her work with Cori. They stand in contrast to uniform ideas about individual development formed in scientific communities that bear little relation to the context of Cori's existence.

It is also important for Anne to understand the influence of Western cultural traditions on Cori's development. Indian culture is and has been interpreted for dominant culture in non-Indian authored stories. Decontextualized Indian images and a history of unequal power relationships characterizes many crosscultural interactions. Anne must therefore be mindful of how these stories will influence her work across cultures.

Appreciating the concern that Indian secrets and stories are in danger of being traded and sold like commodities, Anne makes no assumptions and works hard maintain her nonexpert position. With this come new questions: What questions are okay to ask? To whom should they be asked? What understandings would be helpful for non-Indian helpers who work with Cori? How might the words Anne uses and any taken-for-granted knowledge systems that she brings into her work, risk the reproduction of cultural dominance? How can Anne respectfully honor ways of being that she does not fully understand? How is Anne perceived by Cori and his family and clan and tribe, given the legacy of power and dominance that is also an unwitting partner in their relationship?

Anne's very presence in Cori's life is based on a referral from school to the mental health center. Both institutions are administered by individuals who are outside of Cori's culture. Should Anne work with models of therapy that categorize individuals into boxes of normal and pathological and that locate pathology as something internal to individuals, when these normative and contextual ideas are far removed from Cori's experiences and the beliefs of his people? Anne worried that locating depression and ODD inside Cori, for example, would be contrary to cultural ways of thinking about health and disease. She was also concerned that these ideas might invite Cori to see himself as damaged, implicating his mother as well. For the actual counseling work with Cori, how should Anne acknowledge and account for the legacy of power and privilege that has long existed between the White people and the Indian people of Cori's tribe for centuries? What might be the repercussions for Cori and his family if they chose to work with ideas that privilege Western notions about medicine and mental health over tribal ways of healing? What might be the repercussions of not doing so? Can these two systems co-exist?

> Cori's mother, Salina, was living in a new mobile home on the land behind the house of her parents. Cori was in the seventh grade in the local mission school and his younger sister was in the fifth grade there, too. Salina had attended this same school when she was a child, and she felt that the "strict" behavior polices in this school would be good for her children. When Salina had attended this mission school as a child, she had been prohibited from speaking her native language and from discussing her spiritual stories and celebrations. Despite this, Salina said that her family had believed that this particular school was the best in the community. Now she wasn't so sure.

Salina had finished college. Only 15 percent of her people living on the reservation had a college degree, an honor that was
revered more from outside the village than from within. She had
a well-paying job as an administrator of the community Head
Start program and was now able to support herself and her two
children without government assistance. But Salina's job required
frequent travel off the reservation for meetings and conferences,
which is not uncommon for professionals working in rural areas.
When Salina was away, Cori and his sister simply moved into
grandmother's house next door. Also living with Salina and her
children was her new boyfriend, Emmet, who also worked in the
community, and his two children.

Salina told me that when she was away on a recent business
trip, Cori had been suspended from school for fighting and his
return to school had been delayed because she had been away and
because of Cori's refusal to return to school. Salina felt that Cori
had been singled out in school.

Anne wondered about Salina's comment that the mission school was
the best school for her children despite the fact that the school had
required her to put aside her cultural traditions and language when she
had been a student there. What did it mean that her family wanted to
send their children to the "best" schools, even when those schools did
not validate their own cultural truths? What did this ask of Salina and
of her parents who were so deeply connected to the spiritual life of their
community? And what of Salina's academic and employment "success,"
measured in Western ways. Were these accomplishments also perceived
as a "success" in tribal eyes? What costs in terms of her native culture
were involved in achieving this academic success? What values, hopes
and expectations did Salina's parents have for their children and their
grandchildren? Which of these notions did Salina want to carry forward in her parenting of Cori? What stood in the way of her doing so?

I asked Salina to talk a little about the beliefs that she wanted to
bring into raising her son and daughter. Salina told me that she
was raised by her mother in the home of Grandfather Arden
Waikedo, the tribal healer. She was raised on the traditional stories of her people about the mountains, the rivers, the winds, and
the Creation Story. They were part of the everyday understandings in her home, told both in the native language of her people
as well as in English. These stories always gave her comfort and

a sense of place and meaning. Salina told me that her brothers had continued to be very active in religious tribal life and had mentored many Beaver Clan children into their different fraternities.

Gergen's (1991) idea of personhood as made up of multiple developmental narratives seems most relevant here as we begin to understand Salina's development as a professional woman juxtaposed to her development as granddaughter of one of the most distinguished tribal healers in modern time. We wonder about the discourses within each culture that shape those identities and how she reconciles the contradictions between those discourses.

> "You have gone to college and you have a job at Head Start," I noticed, "and you are a single parent of two children. How is all of this for you?"
> Salina teared up and confessed that she thought that she was "a bad parent." "If I was home more," she said, "Cori would probably not act up. The school told me that Cori only misbehaves when I am away and that it's probably because I am not around enough."

Kaethe Weingarten (1995) says, "Mothers still suffer from a maternal discourse that holds them responsible for the fate of their children and simultaneously renders them powerful enough to harm them but powerless to protect them" (p. 11). This discourse is woven into many models of developmental theory (see Erica Burman, 1994, for an account of this). For example, attachment theorists emphasize "secure" mother-child attachment bonds as the model for subsequent healthy child development. From this perspective, mothers are implicated whenever their children experience difficulties, as if mothers are solely responsible for the development of their children. As social constructionists point out, however, we are never subject to a singular discourse. Salina is positioned by multiple discourses about childhood and parenting. We wonder if some of her tribal ideas about parenting have been silenced within her self-critique. A narrative approach to counseling inclines us to inquire into her local knowledge rather than to impose a dominant knowledge. It invites us to be curious about Salina's knowledges about parenting that have helped her and Cori be so successful in the past, particularly during difficult times.

> "And your family . . . your mother and sisters and brother . . . what do they think?" I asked. "What do they think about how you are parenting Cori?"

"My mother," Salina said, "is happy to have Cori stay with her whenever I am away. Cori has always been with her."

Anne wondered if this meant that in Salina's tribal culture, caring for children did not fall solely on the shoulders of the mother. Salina was raised in the house of her parents, which was also the house of her grandparents. The Western notion of the nuclear family might position Anne to think of Salina as the sole parent of her children. However, in Salina's culture, parenting appeared to be a family and community responsibility. Anne wondered if this accounted for why Salina was so enraged that the school would not allow Cori's grandmother to be the one to re-enter him in school in her absence. Was this also why Salina grappled with a bad parent identity conclusion? Yet, careful listening makes it apparent that Salina's bad parenting story does not fully capture her parenting experiences.

"What ideas do you have that you think are important for raising children?" I asked.

This question positioned Salina as more active in the construction of herself as a parent, rather than leaving this task in the hands of medical or educational authorities.

Although not wanting to give the bad parent story too much undeserved attention, Anne wondered if Salina's decision to stop taking Cori to see his father was a plot event that was storied into her "bad parent" identity conclusion. Anne asked Salina about this decision.

"It was a hard decision," Salina said. "I used to drive Cori to see his father every weekend, and it was a very long drive. His father never offered to meet me half way, nor did he ever agree to pick him up or take him home. It was just me, driving back and forth each weekend, for 3½ hours. But I did it because I thought it was right. It is important for a son to know his father." "But then, about a year ago, Cori began to say that he didn't want to see his dad anymore. I encouraged him to go anyway. He would come back from the weekends frustrated, saying that his dad didn't pay attention to him, and always went out. Cori's sister also complained about going and she often tried to make arrangements to be with her grandmother on the weekend, rather than go to see her dad. I asked some friends at work what they thought I should do and I even bought a book about divorce. They all seemed to think that I should continue to take Cori to see his dad. Everyone knows that kids need their dad. So, I insisted."

"Then I noticed that Cori was pretty sad when he came back from his dad's and he told me that his dad was drinking again. We used to fight when I'd insist that he go. Finally, I realized that I was doing all the work, and no one—not Cori, not his dad, not me—no one seemed interested in it anymore. It was so hard to see him come home so sad, and he never seemed to want to talk to me. It was as if he was mad at me for making him see his dad. So, I said that I'd take him only if he wanted. I stopped taking him a few months ago because he convinced me that he really didn't want to go."

Self-help books and television talk shows provide lots of advice about how not to damage children in the context of divorce. Conventional psychology offers many ideas about parenting and notions about navigating divorce abound. The ideas presented in Salina's thinking appear aligned with some of the dominant Western discourses about divorce and custody agreements that remind us that fathers are important in the development of children. They also suggest that children who grow up without an active presence of their fathers are somehow damaged. We do not disagree that the connection between children and their parents after divorce is a good idea. However, this idea did not seem to be working for Cori and Salina.

Salina's story about encouraging Cori to be with his father stood in stark contrast to the bad parent identity conclusion she had first offered me. Anne wondered how one could be so mindful of the experience of her child, so literate of popular ideas about divorce and boys and what they need, be able to make a reasoned decision about their child, and still hold on to totalizing descriptions of herself as a bad parent? How did this action of reason stand in juxtaposition to an identity conclusion of failure? Anne wanted to bring more voices to this new development:

"So, your decision for Cori to *not* visit his dad was a decision that took you a while to work out. You didn't just jump into it. You tried to have him go, but it just wasn't working . . . you asked some friends, you got a book, and you gave it a lot of thought, but in the end, you felt that it was not a good idea to force Cori to go," I noticed.

"Yes," she agreed.

"So," I said, "It sounds like it was kind of a thought-out decision?"

"Well, I guess it was. I guess it was kind of reasoned," she said, seemingly surprised at our conversation.

"What does that say about your ability to make parenting decisions? How does "reasoned" fit with your idea that you are a 'bad parent'?" I asked.

These questions invited Salina to contour the story of reason into her landscape of identity and to entertain the possibility of identity conclusions that were contrary to the "bad parent" notions she had carried into our conversations. Anne also wanted to invite Salina to reexamine divorce ideas in light of her cultural knowledges and traditions, and her family experience.

> After a while I asked Salina to talk about how tribal knowledges consider divorce and separation. I wondered how divorce and child custody were traditionally handled in her tribe. She sat puzzled for a minute, and then said, "There is no word in our language for divorce . . . nor for custody of a child. It isn't a part of our native language."
>
> "How do you account for that?" I asked.
>
> "In our ways," she told me, "children don't just belong to their parents, they are part of both parental families and also of their clan and child clan. Children have two whole clans of parents to watch over them. And when our boys get older," Salina continued with some excitement, "it is an uncle or compadre who initiates them into the fraternity. Then that fraternity is also family for them."
>
> Salina paused, and then added, "Our people never needed custody agreements. Children were raised by the people."
>
> "What do you take from this in your own parenting?" I asked.
>
> "I don't take any of this in my own parenting," she said quickly. "I used to be more like this, though. That was what it was like when Cori and his sister were little, and how it was when I was born, too. But somewhere it all got lost to me. I don't think in these ways anymore. It seems like these days it's all divorce and custody and I just can't seem to get it right for Cori. These days, it just seems that from all of the books I read and what everyone tells me—I'm doing it all wrong."

How had these tribal and family ideas been lost to Salina? Could it be that "the books and everyone" got in the way of her parenting? We think that the "bad parent" identity conclusions that were located inside her might better be placed back in the discourses (outside of her) where they belong. Externalizing questions do this.

> "I wonder if sometimes 'books and everyone' get you thinking that you're a bad parent?"
>
> "Well," she said, "when they say that boys can't grow up without their Dads then I know that I have done something wrong."
>
> "Yes, and yet I wonder what happened to the ways of your people—that the community takes responsibility for parenting children? Do 'books and everyone' get in the way of remembering these other ideas?"
>
> "Lots of things get in the way," she said. Salina explained that when her children were young, she had worked hard to pass on the stories of her people to them. But, it was hard to do because she always felt self-conscious about her ability to speak in her native language, especially around her father and grandfather. Later she struggled to find a way to coax Cori and his sister away from the temptations of television and video games to be interested in the stories of their people. These struggles worsened during the time of fighting and separation from Cori's father, and as the children grew older, they seemed uninterested in the stories of their people. She said that she didn't know what to do.
>
> I reminded her that she had told me that those stories had always given her comfort in troubling times. She agreed.

The multitude of ideas about how Salina should live her life as an Indian woman, a parent, a professional is evidenced in the rich and diverse stories that she has shared. We suspect that being immersed in two distinct cultures where one is dominated by the other, challenges Salina's efforts to afford them both equal currency. Yet, within these stories lies the narrative of a young woman who dares to take a stand. The story of taking a stand also features in the narratives of her great grandfather who carried wisdom and healing, her grandfather who left the village to work because he had to, and her parents who sent their kids to the mission school because they wanted the best education for them. We wonder if taking a stand also offers Salina a position from which she can make reasoned parenting decisions and if taking a stand also can position her to wrestle loose from some of the strong "bad parent" identity conclusions that sometimes made it difficult for her to parent her children.

These questions invite consideration of how parenting notions are situated in context and culture. Asking Salina to call upon her Indian wisdom bank privileges her native knowledge over dominant discourses. Engagement in these meaning-making and parent-identity conversations shifts her from the constrained and totalizing notions of "bad parent" to the construction of stories that produce the kind of parent identity that Salina wanted to carry forward in her relationships with her children.

Cori refused to return to school after the suspension—a position that aroused much concern for Salina as well as among school personnel—but he did agree to talk with Anne in his home with his grandmother. His mother, Salina, was out of town, so Anne had only been able to speak to her briefly by phone before this home visit.

> I had met him one time before at the school, but I wasn't sure if he remembered who I was. When I arrived at the home, I thanked Cori for inviting me, and Cori's grandmother and aunt joined us in the living room.
>
> "So, Cori," I began, "here you are at home when your teachers and everyone else would like you at school. What has happened?"
>
> "I'm not going back there," he said. "They don't like me there."
>
> "Help me understand what you mean," I invited.
>
> When Cori did not respond to my question, I asked him permission to ask his grandmother how she understood what was happening. I was hoping that his grandmother's care and concern would be communicated in her response.
>
> Grandmother responded in her native language and Cori's Aunt translated, "She don't know why Cori won't go back to school. She thinks it's because he thinks the teachers don't like him any more."
>
> "You know Cori pretty well," I noted, looking at grandmother. "Do you think that the teachers don't like him?" I asked.
>
> The question generated a short conversation between grandmother and Auntie that I did not understand. In the end, the response came—apparently shortened and again translated through the Aunt—that it was time for Cori to return to school.

Anne tentatively understood Cori's refusal to return to school as a stand against a positioning of "bad kid . . . Depression, Rule-out ODD" that circulated in his school and at the mental health clinic. Was his refusal to respond to Anne's questions also a stand against a pathologized mental health assessment that she represented? Anne did not fully understand the meaning of grandmother's comment that Cori should just return to school, and she wondered what meanings might have been lost in its simplified translation. Was it a refusal to take a position against the school that had storied him as bad? How might power and history have shaped the story? Anne wanted to find a way to bring out grandmother's caring and confidence toward Cory, and she hoped to reveal alternative stories about Cory that grandmother also held on to.

> "What does your interest in having Cori return to school say about your confidence in his ability to be successful there?" I asked.
>
> "He is a smart boy and if he can just behave, he will be fine," she responded, again, translated through the aunt.
>
> Noting that Cori appeared to be listening to what his grandmother had to say, I asked Cori again for permission to ask his grandmother another question. Permission was granted with a nod.
>
> "I hear that these few weeks have been a difficult time for Cori. How are you understanding what is going on with Cori?" I asked grandmother.
>
> Grandmother responded, talking for a while in her native language again. This time I asked Cori if he would mind translating what she said.
>
> "She says," he almost whispered, "the people at the clinic think that I am sad because I don't see my dad and so she guesses that's what's wrong with me."

Anne was intrigued by grandmother's story about Cori's difficulties. It reminded her of the diagnostic story that came from the clinic with the still unfilled prescription for Zoloft® and the diagnosis of "bad kid . . . Depression, Rule-out ODD." Anne suspected that grandmother held on to other stories about her grandson, but was at a loss for how to bring them forward. Realizing that Cory was very much listening to what his grandmother was saying and also able to translate for her, Anne decided to focus on Cori again.

> "Hmm . . . Is that how *you* see it?" I whispered to Cori, encouraging (perhaps, hoping for?) the possibility of a different opinion.
>
> "No," Cori responded. Firm and quiet.
>
> "You see it differently," I affirmed. "I'd be interested in hearing your ideas about this."
>
> Cori was not interested in talking to me any more that day, however. But he did agree to talk with me again in a few days.

If we reject the "bad kid" metaphor, there might still be a story of the production of powerlessness, but it is not about a powerlessness inside of Cori. Instead, social constructionists might understand Cori's behavior as a social practice that is meaningful in a set of power relations. Anne began to wonder if Cory was responding to a story that was inconsistent with how he would like to see himself. She wanted to rejoice in his stand against an institution that was not working for him, but she also realized that his story of who he wanted to be was very fragile. This is not to say that Cori's violent behavior at school should be excused, nor that he shouldn't be held accountable for it. It only suggests that such behavior exists in a context that is still unknown to us. Cori needs to be accountable to himself and to his community. The work of his counselor is to help him continue at school in ways that are more consistent with the kind of student he and his family would like him to become.

> When we did talk a few days later, Cori was back at school, at his mother's and grandmother's insistence. We talked about some of the troubles at school. Cori said, "The teachers say it's me that's bad, but they don't see that it's the other kids. They just bug me—the kids do. They don't stop and the teachers just see me when I do something wrong. Sometimes they just get me up against the wall and there is nothing I can do. I just get so mad."
>
> "So, things happen that get you up against the wall?"
>
> "Yeah, the kids bother me. The teachers bother me. I wish that they would just leave me alone."
>
> "Bother you?"
>
> "They tease me."
>
> I asked Cori to tell me about the last time that teasing happened and when he was finished, I asked, "So, what did teasing get you to do?"
>
> "I hit him. That was why they suspended me."
>
> "So, teasing got you up against the wall, and you hit him. Then you got in trouble?"
>
> "Yeah."
>
> "Is that a position that you like to be in at school, up against the wall and then in trouble?"
>
> "No."
>
> "What would you rather have happen in school?"
>
> Cori told me that he'd rather be playing ball at recess. He also said that he preferred to be "not known" at school than to be known as a "bully." He said that he didn't much mind being a bully, really, but that it upset his mother and grandmother that he was so bad, so he wanted to change that and just be "not known" at school.

I was curious what "not known" might look like? What "not known" might do? And how "not known" might be perceived by the other kids. Soon it became obvious to us that "not known" really was "one of the kids" rather than not known by anyone.

# Summary

The challenge of counseling from this perspective, then, is to help young people (and also their parents and caregivers) situate themselves in stories of development that are sustaining and enhancing. Rather than lining up these stories with conventional accounts of human development, Anne worked to build on the stories that came from Salina's and from Cori's world. This is not to say that normative ideas about development are wrong. But a narrative emphasis focuses more on the social and cultural processes that produce personal development. Anne was working with the complexity of Cori and Salina's lives because their personal narratives of identity were being embodied in the midst of a complex interplay of discourses and cultural narratives.

We believe that counselors need to use both theoretical and practical ideas that are flexible enough to serve the purpose of handling the complexities of social existence. The practices of narrative therapy are one such attempt to achieve this goal. They invite practitioners, first of all, to take a reflexive position in relation to their own power. They also invite a stance of curiosity with regard to the knowledges at work in the production of experience. They invite the externalization of internalized identity conclusions based on norms established by dominant cultural discourse. And they open up new or previously unnoticed and understoried possibilities that are based on client preferences for their own identity stories. The developmental paths that emerge do not necessarily fit into the textbook but stand a good chance of fitting with the actualities of people's lives.

# Annotated Bibliography

## Social Theory

The postmodern literature on which a social constructionist approach is based is a rich and diverse canon that is often challenging to read. We shall restrict ourselves here to suggesting some starting places for those who are not familiar with this literature. Rather than leaping into a reading of some of the major philosophers who have contributed to postmodernism, we would recommend starting with some secondary sources such as:

Lyotard, J. F. (1984) *The post-modern condition: A report on knowledge.* Cambridge, U.K.: Cambridge University Press.

Seidman, P. (1994) *The postmodern turn: New perspectives on social theory.* Cambridge, U.K.: Cambridge University Press.

Michel Foucault's work is not easy to access. One way to do so is to read some commentaries on his work such as:

McHoul, A. W., & Grace, W. (1997). *A Foucault primer: Discourse power and the subject.* New York: New York University Press.

To begin reading Foucault's writing itself, it is worth reading one of the collections of interviews with Foucault. They are more conversational and give a more informal introduction to the way he thinks. A text that includes a range of these interviews is:

Foucault, M. (1989). *Foucault live (Interviews 1966–84)* (S. Lotringer, Ed.) (J. Johnston, Trans.). New York: Semiotext.

Counselors might find the following Foucault books most relevant to the work outlined in this chapter:

Foucault, M. (1978). *Discipline and punish.* New York: Vintage Books.

Foucault, M. (1980). *Power/knowledge: Selected interviews and other writings.* New York: Pantheon Books.

## Social Constructionism

The best introduction to social constructionism in psychology is:

Burr, V. (1995/2003). *An introduction to social constructionism.* London: Routledge.

An introduction to Ken Gergen's work on social constructionism can be found in these two books:

Gergen, K. (1994). *Realities and relationships: Soundings in social constructionism.* Cambridge, MA: Harvard University Press.

Gergen, K. (1999). *An invitation to social construction.* London: Sage.

## Narrative Theory

Jerome Bruner's narrative perspective in psychology is outlined in:

Bruner, J. (1990). *Acts of meaning.* Cambridge, MA: Harvard University Press.

Bruner, J. (1986). *Actual minds, possible worlds.* Cambridge, MA: Harvard University Press.

## Social Constructionism and Human Development

The social constructionist study of human development is still fairly young but has been marked out by Erica Burman in a text that is critical of traditional viewpoints:

Burman, E. (1994). *Deconstructing developmental psychology.* London: Routledge.

Valerie Walkerdine studied children's development of mathematical concepts.
Walkerdine, V. (1988). *The mastery of reason: Cognitive development and the production of rationality.* London and New York: Routledge.

An introductory textbook on human development that incorporates a social constructionist perspective is Wendy Drewery and Lise Bird's book on human development in New Zealand.
Drewery, W., & Bird, L. (2004). *Human development in Aotearoa: A journey through life* (2nd ed.). Melbourne, Australia: McGraw-Hill.

## Narrative Therapy

The seminal and most widely known text on narrative therapy is Michael White and David Epston's book:
White, M., & Epston, D., (1990). *Narrative means to therapeutic ends.* New York: Norton.

Michael White's latest text on narrative conversations will undoubtedly become a landmark text in the narrative literature.
White, M. (2007, in press). *Maps of narrative practice.* New York: Norton.

A series of books have elaborated and explained narrative practice, such as:
Freedman, J., & Combs, G. (1996). *Narrative therapy: The social construction of preferred realities.* New York: Norton.
Monk, G., Winslade, J., Crocket, K., & Epston, D. (Eds.). (1997). *Narrative therapy in practice: The archaeology of hope.* San Francisco: Jossey-Bass.

Some texts have related narrative ideas to the practice of counseling in schools and working with children:
Besley, A. C. (2002). *Counseling youth: Foucault, power & the ethics of subjectivity.* Westport, CT: Praeger.
Freeman, J., Epston, D., & Lobovits, D. (1997). *Playful approaches to serious problems: Narrative therapy with children & their parents.* New York: Norton.
Winslade, J., & Monk, G. (2007). *Narrative counseling in schools: Powerful & brief.* Thousand Oaks, CA: Corwin Press.

Finally, readers interested in keeping up to date with developments in narrative practice should access the journal:
*The International Journal of Narrative Therapy & Community Work.*

# References

Apfelbaum, E. (2002). Uprooted communities, silenced cultures and the need for legacy. In V. Walkerdine (Ed.), *Challenging subjects: Critical psychology for a new millennium.* New York: Palgrave.

Beaudoin, M., & Taylor, M. (2004). Breaking the culture of bullying and disrespect, K-8: Best practices and successful strategies. Thousand Oaks, CA: Corwin Press.

Besley, T. (2002). *Counseling youth: Foucault, power & the ethics of subjectivity.* Westport, CT: Praeger.

Bird, L. (1999). Towards a more critical educational psychology. *Annual review of critical psychology, 1*, 21–33.

Bracho, A. (2002). Pedagogies of hope. *The International Journal of Narrative Therapy and Community Work,* (4), 56–58.

Bruner, J. (1960). *The process of education.* Cambridge, MA: Harvard University Press.

Bruner, J. (1986). *Actual minds, possible worlds.* Cambridge, MA: Harvard University Press.

Bruner, J. (1990). *Acts of meaning.* Cambridge, MA: Harvard University Press.

Bruner, J. (1996). *The culture of education.* Cambridge, MA: Harvard University Press.

Bryant, P. (1974). *Perception and understanding in young children: An experimental approach.* London: Methuen.

Burman, E. (1994). *Deconstructing developmental psychology.* London: Routledge.

Burr, V. (1995/2003). *An introduction to social constructionism.* London: Routledge.

Cheshire, A., & Lewis, D. (1994). Young people and adults in a team against harassment: Bringing forth student knowledge and skill. In D. Paré & G. Larner (Eds.), *Collaborative practice in psychology and therapy* (pp. 121–132). Binghamton, NY: Haworth Press.

Derrida, J. (1976). *Of grammatology* (G. C. Spivak, Trans.). Baltimore, MD: Johns Hopkins University Press.

Donaldson, M. (1978). *Children's minds.* Glasgow, U.K.: Fontana/Collins.

Drewery, W., & Bird, L. (2004). *Human development in Aotearoa: A journey through life* (2nd ed.). Melbourne, Australia: McGraw-Hill.

Epston, D. (1989). *Collected Papers.* Adelaide, Australia: Dulwich Centre Publications.

Epston, D. & White, M. (1992). *Experience, contradiction, narrative and imagination.* Adelaide, Australia: Dulwich Centre Publications.

Foucault, M. (1965) *Madness and civilization: A history of insanity in the age of reason* (R. Howard, Trans.). New York: Pantheon Books.

Foucault, M. (1969). *The archaeology of knowledge* (A. M. Sheridan Smith, Trans.). London: Tavistock.

Foucault, M. (1972). *The order of things: An archaeology of the human sciences.* New York: Pantheon.

Foucault, M. (1978). *Discipline and punish* (A. Sheridan, Trans.). New York: Vintage Books.

Foucault, M. (1980). *Power/knowledge: Selected interviews and other writings.* New York: Pantheon.

Foucault, M. (1989). *Foucault live (Interviews 1966–84)* (S. Lotringer, Ed.) (J. Johnston, Trans.). New York: Semiotext.

Foucault, M. (1991). Questions of method. In G. Burchell, C. Gordon, & P. Miller (Eds.), *The Foucault effect: Studies in governmentality* (pp. 73–86). London: Harvester Wheatsheaf.

Gergen, K. (1991). *The saturated self: Dilemmas of identity in contemporary life.* New York: Basic Books.

Gergen, K. (1994a). *Realities and relationships: Soundings in social constructionism.* Cambridge, MA: Harvard University Press.

Gergen, K. (1994b). *Toward transformation in social knowledge* (2nd ed.). London: Sage.

Gergen, K. (1999). *An invitation to social construction.* London: Sage.

Gergen, K., & Gergen, M. (2003). *Social construction, a reader.* London: Sage.

Gilligan, C. (1982). *In a different voice: Psychological theory and women's development.* Cambridge, MA: Harvard University Press.

Gladding, S. (2004). *Counseling: A comprehensive profession* (5th ed.). Upper Saddle River, NJ: Pearson Prentice Hall.

Green, A., & Keyes, S. G. (2001). Expanding the developmental school counseling paradigm: Meeting the needs of the 21st century student. *Professional School Counseling, 5,* 84–95.

Griffith, J., & Griffith, M. (1994). *The body speaks: Therapeutic dialogues for mind-body problems.* New York: Basic Books.

Hedtke, L., & Winslade, J. (2004). *Re-membering lives: Conversations with the dying and the bereaved.* Amityville, NY: Baywood.

Jackson, V. (2002). In our own voice: African-American stories of oppression, survival and recovery in mental health systems. *The International Journal of Narrative Therapy and Community Work,*(2), 11–31.

Kohlberg, L. (1984). *The psychology of moral development.* New York: Harper & Row.

Loomer, L. (1998) *¡Bocón!.* Woodstock, IL: Dramatic.

Lyotard, J.-F. (1984). *The postmodern condition: A report on knowledge*: University of Minnesota Press.

MacKenzie, B. (1997). Health promoting conversations. In G. Monk, J. Winslade, K. Crocket, & D. Epston (Eds.), *Narrative therapy in practice: The archaeology of hope* (pp. 275–295). San Francisco: Jossey-Bass.

McHoul, A. W., & Grace, W. (1997). *A Foucault primer: Discourse, power and the subject.* New York: New York University Press.

McLean, C. (1995). Reclaiming our stories, reclaiming our lives. *Dulwich Centre Newsletter,* (1), 1–40.

McMenamin, D. (2004). Talking about 'knowing with' (Like a team!). In D. Paré & G. Larner (Eds.), *Collaborative practice in psychology and therapy* (pp. 97–108). Binghamton, NY: Haworth Press.

McNamee, S., & Gergen, K. (1991). *Therapy as social construction.* London: Sage.

Monk, G., Winslade, J., Crocket, K., & Epston, D. (Eds.). (1997). *Narrative therapy in practice: The archaeology of hope.* San Francisco: Jossey-Bass.

Morss, J. (1991). After Piaget. In J. Morss & T. Linzey, *Growing up: The politics of human learning* (pp. 9–29). Auckland, New Zealand: Longman Paul.

Myers, J. E., Shoffner, M. F., & Briggs, M. K. (2002). Developmental counseling and therapy: An effective approach to understanding and counseling children. *Professional School Counseling, 5*(3), 194–202.

Power to Our Journeys Group (1997). Power to our journeys [Special issue]. *Dulwich Centre Newsletter,* (1), 25–33.

Rosaldo, R. (1993). *Culture and truth: The remaking of social analysis.* Boston: Beacon Press.

Rose, N. (1990). *Governing the soul: The shaping of the private self.* London: Routledge.

Rose, N. (1998). *Inventing ourselves: Psychology, power and personhood.* Cambridge, U.K.: University of Cambridge Press.

Seidman, P. (1994). *The postmodern turn: New perspectives on social theory.* Cambridge, U.K.: Cambridge University Press.

Silvester, G. (1997). Appreciating indigenous knowledge in groups. In G. Monk, J. Winslade, K. Crocket, & D. Epston (Eds.), *Narrative therapy in practice: The archaeology of hope* (pp. 233–251). San Francisco: Jossey-Bass.

Simblett, G. (1997). Leila and the tiger. In G. Monk, J. Winslade, K. Crocket, & D. Epston (Eds.), *Narrative therapy in practice: The archaeology of hope* (pp. 121–157). San Francisco: Jossey-Bass.

Todd, L. (2000). Letting the voice of the child challenge the narrative of professional practice. *Dulwich Centre Journal,* (1 & 2), 72–79.

Walkerdine, V. (1984). Developmental psychology and the child-centred pedagogy. In J. Henriques, W. Hollway, C. Urwin, C. Venn, & V. Walkerdine, *Changing the subject: Psychology, social regulation and the development of language.* London: Wiley.

Walkerdine, V. (1988). *The mastery of reason: Cognitive development and the production of rationality.* London and New York: Routledge.

Walkerdine, V. (2002). *Challenging subjects: Critical psychology for a new millennium.* New York: Palgrave.

Walkerdine, V., Lucey, H., & Melody, J. (2001). *Growing up girl: Psychosocial explorations of gender and class.* New York: New York University Press.

Weingarten, K. (1995). Radical listening: Challenging cultural beliefs for and about mothers. In K. Weingarten (Ed.), *Cultural Resistance: Challenging beliefs about men, women, and therapy.* Binghamton, NY: Harrington Park Press.

White, C. (Ed.). (1995). Schooling and education [Special issue]. *Dulwich Centre Newsletter,* (2 & 3).

White, C. (Ed.). (1998a). Creating respectful relationships in the name of the Latino family [Special issue]. *Dulwich Centre Newsletter,* (1).

White, C. (Ed.). (1998b). Taking the hassle out of school: And stories from younger people [Special issue]. *Dulwich Centre Newsletter,* (2 & 3).

White, C. (Ed.). (1999). Homelessness [Special issue]. *Dulwich Centre Newsletter,* (3).

White, C. (2000). Living positive lives [Special issue]. *Dulwich Centre Journal,* (4).

White, C. (Ed.). (2003). Mental Health [Special issue]. *The International Journal of Narrative Therapy and Community Work.*

White, M. (1989). *Selected papers*. Adelaide, Australia: Dulwich Centre Publications.

White, M. (2002). Addressing personal failure. *The International Journal of Narrative Therapy and Community Work,* (3), 33–76.

White, M. (2003). Narrative practice and community assignments. *The International Journal of Narrative Therapy and Community Work,* (2), 17–55.

White, M. (2004). Working with people who are suffering the consequences of multiple trauma. *The International Journal of Narrative Therapy and Community Work,* (1), 45–76.

White, M., & Epston, D. (1990). *Narrative means to therapeutic ends.* New York: Norton.

Winslade, J., & Monk, G. (2001). *Narrative mediation: A new approach to conflict resolution.* San Francisco: Jossey-Bass.

Winslade, J., & Monk, G. (2007). *Narrative counseling in schools: Powerful & brief.* Thousand Oaks, CA: Corwin Press.

Woolfolk, A. (2004). *Educational psychology* (9th ed.). Boston: Allyn & Bacon.

CHAPTER THREE

# Bronfenbrenner's Ecological Model

## Shirley A. Hess and Jill M. Schultz

Bronfenbrenner's model of human development starts with an initial mapping of the settings where most social interactions occur, those settings where we interact with people on a face-to-face basis. From this micro-level analysis, it is possible to explore how we are shaping the people around us and how we are concurrently being shaped. But if the mapping of human development ended at this point, the scope of influences on our development would be disastrously incomplete. Other questions would persist: How does the relationship between and among our experiences in different settings where we interact with other people impact our development? What is the impact on our development when significant events and interactions occur in settings that we do not occupy but someone in our circle of family and friends does? And possibly most important, in what ways does an increasing complex and interconnected cultural, economic, and political world reach into our lives in ways that impact our development? Bronfenbrenner answers these questions by producing a model that reveals how our development is inseparable from our environments throughout our lives. After explicating the multiple interconnected and interlocked rings of influence surrounding us as developing individuals, Bronfenbrenner helps decode the complex ways these rings of influence advance and restrain our development.

In trying to grasp the concepts of Bronfenbrenner's model, counselors and counselors-in-training may find it useful to consider the ways they have been shaped by the world around them. Although the following list is just a miniscule sampling of the types of questions Bronfenbrenner's model evokes, they are representative of questions an ecologically oriented theorist enjoys asking. The questions all start with this lead in, "In what ways is or has your development been shaped by," and end with one of the following:

. . . interactions with your parents and siblings?

. . . interactions with your peers and teachers?

. . . interactions between your parents and teachers?

. . . interactions between your parents and other adults in their workplace, their family, or their community?

. . . your racial, gender, sexual, and religious identities? For example, what cultural experiences and messages constructed your beliefs about people both like and unlike yourself?

. . . living in a country organized by capitalism? For example, in what ways are your beliefs about poverty, academic achievement, human worth, and individual merit shaped by the norms of an economic system?

. . . Supreme Court decisions? For example, have you thought about how you would have been influenced differently if you attended a school that was legally segregated on the basis of race, that is, before Brown v. Board of Education?

. . . not having been born in the year 1800?

Ecological approaches to development require us to deeply consider the impact of the social world on the development of the individual. In some ways, moving beyond personal experiences to uncover other possibly even more powerful influences on development is a radical approach because it goes against most of our western cultural training of seeing ourselves as autonomous individuals.

Once the fairly visible forces and the macro forces on development that often remain unexplored are known, another important question arises: What does it mean for the ethical practice of counseling if the scope of human development is partially the product of specific social, cultural, geographic, and historical contexts?

## Bronfenbrenner's Ecological System

While Bronfenbrenner's work opened new ways of conceptualizing child development, we find that the model resonates within the broader context of lifespan development as framed by Baltes (1987). Moving away

## ABOUT THE CHAPTER AUTHORS

Throughout your graduate studies and beyond, we encourage you to make it your practice to study outside of your discipline as a means to broaden and deepen your understanding of your chosen field. Efforts to seek a multitude of complementary and even conflicting interpretations of the human experience, a worthy goal accomplished by the editor of this text, are usually richly rewarding intellectual experiences. It seems to us that Professor Bronfenbrenner encourages each of us to look further behind, around, over, and under any explanation of human development that seems too inflexible, too isolated or specific, or simply not inclusive enough.

### Shirley A. Hess

Shirley A. Hess, Ph.D., LPC, NCC, is an associate professor of counseling at Shippensburg University of Pennsylvania. Her professional interests include dreamwork, the training and supervisory processes, loss and bereavement, and qualitative research. Shirley has practiced in college counseling centers, outpatient facilities, and in college student personnel settings. She enjoys the outdoors, especially hiking on the Appalachian Trail.

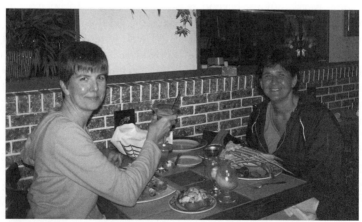

**Jill M. Schultz (left) and Shirley A. Hess**

## Jill M. Schultz

Jill M. Schultz, Ph.D., is an associate professor of social sciences at Frederick Community College in Maryland. She teaches and creates interdisciplinary courses in the social sciences. Jill's professional interests include the development of the sociological imagination, social justice issues, and qualitative research. She enjoys trying new restaurants and reading new authors.

from the limited explanatory power of singular theories and pulling together the dominant themes in contemporary developmental psychology, Baltes provides a framework that can be utilized by counselors working with clients from an ecological theoretical perspective.

One of most interesting aspects in the field is the acknowledgement that humans continue to develop after childhood and adolescence (*lifelong process*). The research on child development and schooling has suggested the malleability of childhood, which means by extension that adults, too, do not have fixed and determined life paths but are actively producing their own experiences (*plasticity*) while being influenced by the sociocultural conditions of their time (*historical embeddedness*). Our understanding of development is also enhanced by the recognition that development, like most things in life, is not a linear progressive process of accumulation but a phenomenon that may include zigzags, swirls, accelerations, quick stops, and reverses (*multidirectionality* and *gain/loss*). And, one of the most promising perspectives is the value placed on embracing multiple ways of knowing that is garnered when all academic disciplines are invited to participate in the dialogue about human experience (*interdisciplinary*). Baltes's themes serve as a background to understanding the specific ecological model created by Bronfenbrenner discussed in this chapter.

Bronfenbrenner's theory is an analytical tool for understanding individual development within complex social systems. A client conceptualized through the ecological perspective is an individual invisibly linked and deeply embedded in a specific cultural context. Every person develops within many deeply interconnected rings of influence, much like the way a stone dropped into water is connected to and surrounded by concentric rings. Bronfenbrenner (1977, 1979) names the five interconnected rings encircling the developing person the *microsystem, mesosystem, exosystem, macrosystem*, and *chronosystem* (see Figure 3.1).

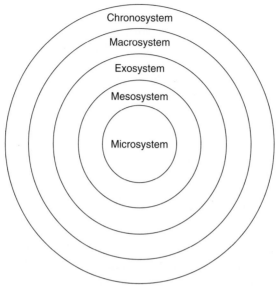

FIGURE 3.1    Rings of Influence
Source: Bronfenbrenner (1977, 1979)

# Spheres of Influence

## Microsystem

The *microsystem* is Bronfenbrenner's term for the multiple settings in which we interact with others on an everyday, face-to-face basis. In these settings our development is influenced by direct participation and inter-action with other people. Unlike models suggesting an unfolding of certain stages and normative sequencing, ecological approaches presume that human interaction—and the stage upon which it unfolds—play a primary role in growing or in waning our development throughout our lifespan. At this level of the system, the key idea is that all members of the system are actively influencing each other and shaping the world around them. This focus on the bidirectionality of influences in face-to-face encounters acknowledges the agency of every individual in any setting and is significant in the helping professions because counselors use interactions to co-create change with clients.

Most child developmentalists focus on the family as the first setting in which children relate to other humans. As the child grows, the microsystem expands to people in other settings such as childcare and caregivers, schools and teachers, playgrounds and peers. Then as the child becomes an adolescent, new settings and people emerge for inter-action and engagement. The adolescent interacts in work situations and with bosses, athletic teams and coaches, and club affiliations and adult leaders. By young adulthood, the primary settings for face-to-face inter-actions may shift again, this time to a residence hall and roommates, peers and professors, and new jobs and new bosses. Throughout the lifespan, primary settings for interpersonal interaction continue to change as the developing person adopts and adapts to the different set-tings and to the different people with whom the person lives, works, and plays.

Ecologically, the microsystem is significant because of the concept of bi-directionality. For example, the new infant in the family is not conceptualized as the only important, active, and developing member of that microsystem. Interactions with the infant will impact the devel-opment of parents, siblings, pets, and other household members. As the child ages, each significant setting in the microsystem produces a web of interconnected people whose interactions may give rise to devel-opmental concerns or triumphs for any of them.

When the presumption is incorrectly made that only "other" people are impacted by external influences or when individuals are viewed in only one of the settings of the microsystem, their character as well as attending influences may seem obvious to an observer, the way a client's "issues" may initially appear obvious to a counselor. For example, when we as professors stand in front of the classroom or work with students in our offices, our microsystem consists of each of us and our students. From the vantage point of a student, the influences creating us as mem-bers of the faculty probably seem easy to read. We obviously have been influenced by advanced training in our fields, and we value and are attentive to words, texts, and meaning. We are perceived, generally, as the authority in the classroom (despite our attempts to co-construct the classroom experience), and students often extrapolate that our parents taught us to value education early in life and that we are intelligent people (or we wouldn't be in the front of the room). Yet, this picture of our development is entirely partial and only touches on what can be gathered from our interactions on one stage, an academic setting.

Those same students might do a double-take and rethink what they know about their professors if they could see us in a different setting. What assumptions might be made if a student saw us in other isolated settings related to our lives? What could be "known" about us and the path of our lives if we were observed, not as professors in a classroom, but as actors in other settings (e.g., sister/daughter celebrating holidays

---

## ABOUT URIE BRONFENBRENNER

Urie Bronfenbrenner was a world-renowned scholar in the field of developmental psychology and human ecology, a discipline he created. He was born in the United States and spent most of his professional career as a professor of human development and psychology at Cornell University. His ideas and research affected social policies through the creation of the Head Start program in 1965 and his Ecological Systems Theory transformed the approach used to study human development through the lifespan. His interdisciplinary conceptualization of development had international influence on research, programs, and policies affecting children and families. Bronfenbrenner was the author, co-author, or editor of more than 300 articles and chapters and 14 books, most notably *Two Worlds of Childhood: U.S. and U.S.S.R., The State of Americans, The Ecology of Human Development*, and *Making Human Beings Human*.

---

with our families, diners eating at restaurants, shoppers buying wine or medicine, vacationers relaxing on the beach)? Similarly, we know that our perspective of human development must be based on more than what we "see" before us in any setting and that we acknowledge through our interactions with others that we, too, are influenced.

## Mesosystem

Most people routinely move through various settings that constitute their microsystem. Bronfenbrenner's mesosystem captures the idea that individuals develop by relating and interacting with others within multiple settings in their microsystem (e.g., familial, academic, recreational, and employment settings). Because people must learn to simultaneously manage experiences in more than one setting, a synergy is created across settings that affects the developing person. This is the *mesosystem,* which captures the developmental significance created by the connections across settings.

Consider the importance of the mesosystem in child development. Children typically experience the behavioral expectations of at least two sets of adults (e.g., parents and teachers) in two different settings (e.g., home and school). Parents and teachers must interact with each other so that their independent interactions with the child communicate identical expectations about routines at home that can impact school performance, such as homework, nutrition, and television viewing. Likewise, what occurs in the school setting (e.g., bullying, an argument with a school friend, feeling inadequate) influences a child's behaviors at home.

The mesosystem of an adult has an equally important impact on shaping the course of development. For example, within a day the roles assumed by an adult woman in different settings may change from student, to employee, to mother. As she interacts with the people populating these different settings in her microsystem, the interpersonal dynamics and expectations she experiences across these settings may be complementary or conflicting. As a student, she finds that her professors structure their course expectations around the schedules of eighteen-year-old students living in resident halls. She is expected to meet with other students several hours outside of class several times during the semester to complete group projects. She is also an employee, and in the work setting, her employer presses her to demonstrate loyalty and career potential by working extra hours and picking up additional projects. At home, as a mother, she has children who share her enthusiasm for school and have created a special daily routine of completing their studies together that reduces her exhaustion and builds her relationship with her children. So while an exploration of interactions in the microsystem reveals how discrete settings can impact development, the mesosystem broadens the developmental perspective to take into account how the interplay of experiences in multiple settings shapes individual development.

## Exosystem

The exosystem also involves a connection or linkage between two or more settings, but unlike the mesosystem, the developing individual does not participate directly in one of those settings. Initially it might seem both obvious and developmentally inconsequential that the people who populate our lives have experiences in settings that do not include us. After all, how can we be shaped by events that are at least one time removed from our own interactions?

Bear in mind that a child and a parent share the same setting of home in their microsystem but both the parent and child have experiences in other settings in their microsystem that affect life in the home. For the child, a parent's workplace may influence experiences in the home, such as when a parent's income rises or falls with promotions or demotions, or when a parent must travel away from home for work for extended periods. Similarly for the adult, a child's interactions in school may indirectly influence interactions in the home setting. A child's report card, a starring role in the school play, or encounters with peer groups are examples of influences on the setting of home that happen outside of the parent's sphere. These experiences, external to the child and parent's shared setting of home, impact their experiences at home and thereby shape the development of the people in the shared setting.

The impact of the exosystem on our development can be devastatingly powerful and examples abound across the lifespan. If the person who co-pays the rent loses a job, everyone in the household is impacted, even if they have nothing to do with the reasons for the loss (e.g., layoff or a fight with the boss). If lack of adequate intellectual stimulation at work makes one partner depressed, then a couple can find their personal relationship suffering. However, if the partner wins the lottery with colleagues from work, their lives and hence the direction of their potential development is impacted.

The context and processes of human lives are powerfully shaped in the exosystem through the decision-making authority of legislative bodies at the local, state, and national levels. Although the developing person is most likely not directly interacting with the officials determining legislative outcomes, legislation on economic and social issues (e.g., the federal minimum wage, civil rights, international treaties, and licensure requirements) work in powerful but possibly less visible ways to shape the experiences of the developing person. For example, passage of the Title IX of the Education Amendments of 1972 shows the impact of the exosystem. This legislation prohibits sex discrimination in federally assisted education programs and has created educational and related job opportunities for millions of young Americans. This legislation focused attention on the preparation of girls for college, opened up opportunities in athletics, and altered expectations about the achievement potential of girls and women. The setting for the decision was a government body and through the relationship of the legislature and the schools (e.g., administrator, teachers, coaches), students are impacted. It is significant to recognize that nearly all of the young women whose current lived experiences have been remade by Title IX were not remotely involved in the decision making that produced these effects.

## Macrosystem

The *macrosystem* is Bronfenbrenner's term for the overall cultural patterns in society. This component of the model reflects the understanding that any explanation of human development must situate knowledge about people in the pervasive cultural context. Like the exosystem, the macrosystem is external to the individual and extremely influential on development. The centerpiece of the theory for use in counseling is the idea that attending to the client's situation makes sense only if it is done in light of the social context in which it is occurring.

This system tends to be the most invisible when the focus in on any one individual. For example, in a society structured through a complex linking of capitalism, White privilege, and patriarchy, individuals can be expected to be overprivileged or disadvantaged on the basis of gender, race, class, and other divisions reflective of a society characterized by hierarchies. Thus any unequal power relation that exists in the macrosystem can be expected to be an integral part of the human experience at the micro-, meso-, and exosystems.

## Chronosystem

The *chronosystem* is less a system than an accounting for the variable of time on all the four other systems. The passage of time gives contour to processes of human development in spectacular ways that are worthy of marvel. For example, the historical markers of places such as Colonial Williamsburg in Virginia, the memorials at New York's Trade Center, or the Alfred Murrah Federal Building in Oklahoma City invite us to reflect on the ways, both known and yet unknown, in which we are, partially, products of our times.

Fully acknowledging the absurdity of identifying here every possible way time manifests in human development, we will simply look back in time to identify three ways historical events and historical patterns of change have influenced us as faculty and hence permitted the creation of this chapter. We would point to the invention of communication technology from the printing press through to today's e-mail attachments, which allow us to communicate with our editor while he enjoys a well-earned sabbatical overseas; the passage of the Morrill Land-Grant College Act of 1862 by the U.S. Congress, which allocated federal land to states for the creation of public colleges and universities, including our alma mater, the University of Maryland; and the invention of multiple medicines and vaccines, which have lengthened our lifespans. Obviously, we could just as easily have focused on the advances in the education of women, the rise of capitalism, the outcomes of wars, and so on.

Time produces shifts in our ideas about truth and reality; hence time impacts the experience of our development. The impact of the social world on our development occurs during a specific time of our lives and under a specific set of conditions. To be young or old during various periods will define a life shaped by opportunities and expectations commensurate with the norms of the day. Imagine, for a moment, the ways people two hundred years from now will conceive of the people on this planet as the products of our time here. What current concepts that we embrace will be overhauled or dismissed as old-fashioned? What parts of our lives will seem barbaric or particularly enlightened? And to return to the idea of human connectivity, what aspects of our condition do we attribute to those who lived generations before us and what human condition will future generations attribute to our doings?

## Utility of Theory

Traditional models of development typically focus on stages (e.g., biological, cognitive, or physiological states such as puberty or menopause) or individuals' environmental contexts. Bronfenbrenner and Crouter (1983) labeled these environmental contexts *social addresses* (e.g., social class, geographic location, ethnicity). Although widely used, these models are limited because they only consider one discrete aspect of the individual or the environment. Even models that explore the person–environment interaction are limited because they do not define the "processes through which properties of the person or the environment function to produce a particular developmental outcome" (Bronfenbrenner, 1988, p. 31). Bronfenbrenner (1988) asks us to move from these more simplistic models of development to consider the advantages of viewing development through more complex ecological models. For example, ecological models include not only the context in which development is taking place and the personal attributes of the persons present in that context, but also the process through which their development evolves (Bronfenbrenner, 1988). The process is fluid and is moderated by the interplay between the characteristics of the person and the structures of the environmental context yielding positive or negative influences and effects.

At times, influences can have both moderating and mediating effects (Bronfenbrenner, 1988). For example, a client comes to the counseling center (or community setting) feeling depressed because he is torn between being at school and moving back home to help care for his ill grandmother. His parents want to avoid a nursing home, so they have taken on additional employment to help pay for home care for his grandmother. He is worried, feels guilty, and is unable to sleep. To bring some relief, he begins using alcohol and valium that put into action (mediating effect) a series of negative effects on several arenas (e.g., academics, relationships with friends, job). The student's continued use then accelerates the downward spiral (moderating effect) leading to more problematic outcomes (e.g., poor grades, deteriorating relationships, fired from job).

Ecological models ask us to discover what is most salient to the client. In this sense, ecological models are inclusionary of cultural considerations (e.g., age, race, class, gender). These components are then viewed within the context of the multiple systems interacting with the client's life, rather than exploring one issue or one aspect of the client and excluding everything else. As with the client who is now abusing substances to bring on sleep and alleviate anxiety, if we focus only on the immediate and apparent situation of the student (e.g., his substance use, anxiety, what is happening with the student in his immediate environment: academics, social interactions, job) and ignore other important influences (e.g., parents' stressors, parents' expectations of their son's role, unavailable home health care for his grandmother), we miss the complexity of the student's condition. Here we see the mesosystem (the connection and interaction among the student's microsystem of academic, social, and occupational settings), the effect of the exosystem (parents' employment and financial situation), and the influence of the macrosystem (aging in a capitalist system). All are important to consider in working with this student.

The previous example highlights the theory's effectiveness with adult populations in university counseling centers and mental health facilities. However, ecological models have utility in a variety of settings and with populations across the lifespan. The theory is particularly useful in work with children by school counselors. The student's microsystem is readily visible to those who are supervising students as they go through their day moving from setting to setting and interacting with their environment (e.g., classroom, cafeteria, library, playground, extracurricular activities). Here the key is not to rely solely on the observed interactions and behaviors but also to notice the processes that produce the observed products. This more complex observation leads to the awareness of the student's mesosystem where settings such as school and home interact. A student who receives academic support and encouragement at home is more likely to be successful at school. On the contrary, a student who is mistreated at home may be withdrawn and anxious at school or get into fights with peers. Likewise, being aware of the student's exosystem can be useful in understanding the many factors and situations influencing students. For example, a father losing his job may cause tension at home that may indirectly affect the student's ability to concentrate on homework assignments. On a macro level, the availability of firearms, school shootings, and the threat of other forms of terrorism affect students' sense of security and safety and may cause increased anxiety and fear. Given the complexity of the interconnected rings of influence, we cannot make assumptions about the origin and nature of a student's anxiety without attending to these interconnected systems of influence.

Although grasping this concept of interconnected systems is critical to counselors' work with clients, so, too, is Bronfenbrenner's idea that all people bring complex histories and experiences with them to every situation. Counselors using this approach believe that their clients are not "blank slates" waiting to be written upon, but people with deep resources of experience and histories to uncover and connect. Ecology theory suggests that counselors who listen to their clients are able to uncover a vivid and nuanced interpretation of the forces shaping and reshaping their clients' development. Identifying the ecological factors associated with clients' situations helps clients see themselves as enabled and constrained by the influences within systems as well as the equally important dimension of seeing themselves as active shapers of other people's experiences within the ecological systems.

This theory helps map how clients unravel the relationship between social structure and their personal experiences. Clients do not share a common set of experiences nor do they respond to their experiences uniformly. Each client experiences a unique set of factors that shapes experience and each client responds in individual ways to the social world. Clients' ranges of responses to situations are not independent actions but bound by social relations and regulations. The theory posits multiple influences that affect the developing person and structure individual experiences. Counselors and clients are encouraged to detect how social structures and social engineering influence personal experiences.

## Challenges to the Theory

As with any theory, ecological systems theories face limitations and constraints. This theory challenges the counseling profession to embrace the complexity of a theory oriented toward seeing clients in the context of society. Seeking an understanding of how the order of the social world influences personal development is challenging because it requires sharp analytical ability to make visible invisible structures that shape lives. This process of reading the social world may seem too daunting, or even unnecessary, to some professionals who then resort to more familiar unitary and less comprehensive models. And a further difficulty is that clients as well as counselors must be educated to situate their experiences against the backdrop of a larger social world. Counselors can help clients make sense of their lived experiences through social and cultural interactions and against the backdrop of many other influential and interlocking systems within and well beyond their family. Often clients have not had experience connecting or stepping outside the personal attributes model, particularly in Western cultures where ideas about personal choice are inculcated in ways that obscure other social influences on personal experience. Although the original incarnation of Bronfenbrenner's model focused on children's development, the strength of using this model with adults may be that adult clients (unlike children) are more equipped to "read" their social world and hence engineer ways to shape their experience in various settings.

## Implications for Practice

Counselors-in-training are typically asked to self-explore and to consider the effect of the family unit on their personal development. However, application of the ecological model also demands the purposeful training of counselors to read their social environment and to deeply explore the societal sources they draw on for their explanations of human behavior and experience. Specifically, by focusing on the macrosystem, social structures that maintain inequality by treating individuals differentially in accord with the economic, political, and social needs of the dominant society are revealed. From that knowledge counselors can move forward in their thinking about the "other" and why the "reality" offered by their own situated experiences may be markedly different from the lived experiences of their clients. This process requires that counselors be open to the emergence of an alternate reading of the social world by their clients.

So just how do people acquire the ability to see the larger social forces that structure individual experience? The raw materials that can lead to the development of insight into the social world comprise the fabric of daily life, yet the degree to which people unravel these threads varies. As Lemert (1997) says, when people "begin to look critically in the right place" (p. 22), abstract social structuring comes into focus. This critical insight originates in a curiosity, a questioning stance, or an inability to overlook common justifications. This can happen only if an individual does not dismiss emotions, particularly emotions that are incongruent with prevailing expectations, as irrational sources of knowledge. For example, the woman who puzzles over the difference between her positive feelings associated with her attraction for another woman and the anger and outrage it evokes in other people and groups may find in her emotions the catalyst for further inquiry in the prevailing social order.

How then can counselors and clients acquire the ability to perceive and evaluate the constraining and fostering elements operating in the social world? The now classic term *sociological imagination* was coined by Mills (1959) to describe an individual's ability to differentiate "between 'the personal troubles of the milieu' and 'the public issues of social structures'" (p. 8). This "quality of mind," or honed insight, results from knowing how to look beyond personal conditions to the larger social structures that organize and regulate human experiences.

Counselors and clients must think through and beyond their individual experiences to discuss the impact of the greater social world on their lives. Counselors can assist clients in acquiring the ability to see that the conditions of their lives flow from the interrelated nature of the social world. In working with clients, the counselor is trying to develop clients' sociological imagination to help them see that the conditions of their lives are in some ways structured around them and that their experiences are not completely the products of their own free will and choice, that is, to some extent they, like all of us, are the product of larger social forces.

The role of the counselor is to see through the clients' eyes and help clients accurately conceptualize their understandings of their many worlds. Then the counselor can work with clients to understand the processes by which clients came to reject or embrace particular views about themselves and about their experiences. In doing so, counselors utilize client's contextualized experiences to facilitate the process of uncovering salient linkages among Bronfenbrenner's systems.

To make these interlinking processes more vivid, two cases studies are presented. In the first we provide the developmental context for the case, tell the client's story, describe the counselor's and client's work together, and discuss the case within the context of Bronfenbrenner's systems. In the second, we describe members of a grief group, focus on one client's story, and provide a series of questions to encourage the use of the ecological perspective for client conceptualization.

# Marie Hart

## Developmental Context

Marie is a forty-three-year-old, White lesbian and the oldest of five children (two sisters, ages thirty-nine and thirty-six; two brothers, ages thirty-four and thirty-one). Growing up in a traditional agrarian community as the oldest sibling, Marie assumed both childcare and farming responsibilities. A strict work ethic was enforced and fundamentalist religious doctrine was practiced. All the children were active in the church and highly involved in music and athletics. Family and religious rules were clear and the consequences of breaking the rules understood and expected. Although neither of Marie's parents graduated from high school, they supported their children in pursuing successful careers. Marie and her sisters entered the teaching profession, and her brothers chose careers in landscaping and carpentry.

Marie described her parents as modeling hard work, proud of their children, but emotionally distant, especially her mother. Additionally, her father was described as very involved with the children's athletic activities but also critical and physically and verbally abusive at times. She thought of her parents as giving, willing to do anything for their children. Similarly, Marie said that although she and her siblings did not often verbally or physically express their love and affection for one another, she believed they would not hesitate to "drop everything" and be there if anyone in the family needed them.

All of Marie's siblings are married, with children, and reside close to the home where they were raised. Marie lived near her family for a short time after graduating from college but then secured jobs between two and six hours from her home. After some failed relationships with men, Marie found her "true self" in college when she had her first relationship with a woman. Although it was difficult to negotiate this new identity because of the vocational, religious, and familial barriers at the time, Marie had two long-term (about six years each) lesbian relationships. Both relationships were maintained in secrecy under the guise of close friendships. At times she and her partner "dated" men to protect the external image of their relationship. Her first partner took a job on the west coast and the geographic distance became too great for them to negotiate. Her second relationship ended amicably when they realized they were growing in different directions.

Currently, Marie is in the midst of a career change, pursuing a master's in school counseling after a twenty-year career as an elementary school teacher. Marie entered the teaching profession because she felt it was her calling. As a child, she remembers "giving lessons" to her younger brothers and sisters (e.g., reading to them on the porch stairs, making arithmetic flash cards) and feeling very comfortable in the role of "teacher," instructing them on how to ride a bicycle, throw a ball, hoe the fields, or drive a car. For as long as Marie could remember, she wanted to be a teacher, and it felt like a natural move to enter the field of education. During her high school and college years, Marie was active in athletics. As an educator, she was very involved with the school district's athletic program and served as coach of the varsity softball team. This involvement as a teacher in both the classroom and on the athletic field gave her a more holistic view of students' lives.

Marie has reached a point in her career where she wants the training needed to offer more substantial assistance to the many students who come to her for emotional support and guidance. Although teaching and coaching have been fulfilling, she wants to have a more direct impact on students' development. Despite her nontraditional status, she has made a smooth transition to graduate school, doing well academically and making connections with a range of students in her program. Just as entering the field of education felt natural 20 years ago, this evolution toward the counseling profession seems to "tap the core of who I was meant to be."

## Finding Her Voice

Marie was in the first year of her school counseling master's program when she was first seen by me (Shirley) in the University Counseling Center. Marie initially entered counseling feeling fatigued, unable to sleep, distracted, sad, and incapable of "controlling" bouts of tears and despair. Although Marie was able to perform at work and in her classes, she reported having increasing difficulty "pushing through" the pain and emptiness, feelings that were beginning to take a toll on her, both physically and emotionally. The death of Marie's mother, after a long illness, had triggered a struggle with depression and suicidal ideation. Additionally, her partner of two years had recently ended their relationship, although they remained friends.

Initially our work focused on symptom management and the grief that was complicated by the depressive symptoms and suicidal ideation. After a few sessions, Marie and I decided a medical evaluation was in order and an antidepressant was prescribed to relieve some of the problems associated with the depression (e.g., lack of sleep, poor concentration, lethargy).

As the counseling relationship developed over the first few months, Marie focused on acknowledging and expressing her grief through journaling and exploring her dreams. In many of her dreams, she was a passive bystander, watching helplessly and emotionless as disasters happened around her. What we came to understand was the influential and stifling nature of Marie's cultural norms around the expression of emotion and grief. For example, she learned that certain types of emotions must be minimized (e.g., anger, rage, despair) because of the beliefs that death is part of God's plan and that the departed is at peace in a better place. By example she was shown that death is faced with stoicism and strength (e.g., not crying) and the bereaved rely on faith in God to get through the loss, almost denying the reality of the effect of the loss.

The following is a sample interchange between Marie and me (Shirley) as we explore various influences on Marie's ideas about grief.

*Shirley:* "What messages have you received about how you are supposed to grieve?"

*Marie:* "Well, you are supposed to be strong, and not to make things worse by crying. I remember when I was really little I went to my great-grandmother's viewing. No one was crying and people kind of looked not real. When I looked at my great-grandmother in the casket, my grandmother said, 'Doesn't she look good? She's at a better place, now.' I remember feeling confused because I knew she was dead but people were saying things that didn't fit with her being dead. I wondered what my grandmother meant when she said, 'she's at a better place now.'"

*S:* "People's actions and words didn't make sense to you. What your grandmother modeled for you was that you were supposed to keep a stiff upper lip and focus on things other than feelings? That didn't seem to fit with you, even as a child."

*M:* "Yeah, when I think back on that now, especially the part about being in a better place, of course I know my grandmother meant that my great-grandmother was now in heaven. So, being in heaven makes her death okay, which for some reason, being in heaven wipes out feeling sad, upset, or even angry. There is no room for those feelings."

*S:* "Very powerful messages."

As Marie began to grasp the nature of these cultural messages, her observations became more vivid and her comments more poignant and personal as she talked about her mother's death.

*Marie:* "I can see that everyone is very sad and even angry that our mother died but no one dare talk about those feelings, let alone express them. It reminds me of how angry I felt when my father told us he didn't want my mother to know she was dying. He said, 'There could be a miracle; no one really knows for sure how long she has, only God knows.' I really wanted to tell her that she was dying but I also didn't want to go against my father."

*Shirley:* "Like earlier in your life, the message didn't fit for you. You were told to pretend, to stuff your feelings and go along with your father, even though that is not what you wanted to do."

*M:* "It wasn't right that he kept that information from her; It was her life, not his. I would certainly want to know if I was dying. I understand that he was protecting himself in some ways, he was in denial. But, it just wasn't right to take that away from her."

*S:* "He asserted his position as the head of the family; he made the decision to deny her the truth and his position of authority silenced your voice. What was that like for you?"

*M:* "I had to back off. I felt helpless. I wanted to tell her. It would have been hard, but she had a right to know. It just wasn't okay to go against him."

*S:* "Like in your dream, all of this was going on around you and you felt helpless to do anything."

*M:* "Yeah, kind of trapped in a way. Every part of me knew what I should do and wanted to do, but I just backed off."

*S:* "What might have happened had you gone against his wishes?"

*M:* "I've been wondering about that, about what she would have done differently or would have wanted had she known her prognosis. Why didn't I just tell her; why did I listen to him? I knew it wasn't the right thing to do."

*S:* "Hmm, you tell me—how do you understand what kept you from telling her?"

Marie began to question the validity of many of the cultural messages she received about the expression of emotion as well as who holds power in relationships. And, in talking about her experience of feeling silenced, Marie began to notice that this theme of voicelessness permeated much of her life. Not only were there cultural rules about grieving and expressing emotions, there were strong religious messages about heterosexuality and the sinfulness of being a lesbian. Marie understood the necessity of silence as she spoke of hiding her sexuality as an elementary school teacher in the late 1970s and 1980s because of the fear and threat of losing her job. Marie acknowledged the silencing yet had difficulty viewing her development as negatively influenced by external social and cultural forces. Marie bought into the message that she was different, that she was the problem. Even when Marie began to question these messages, it was difficult for her to imagine how being out as a lesbian or voicing her opinions or concerns to people in authority would make her life better. The prospect of standing up to powerful institutions that perpetuate oppression seemed daunting.

To counterbalance her experience of oppression and silencing, I asked Marie if there were any areas in her life where she did have voice. When Marie thought about this question, her response was astounding in that experiences of being heard were in settings external to the institutions previously cited as silencing. Now as an adult woman, she was beginning to find her voice in the lesbian community where she had access to books, music, and like-minded friends. Her voice was also heard and reciprocated when she had a partner. Also, contrary to the times when access to alternative information was limited, as a master's student, Marie was learning that there were other systems where she could be accepted and affirmed (e.g., higher education). In hearing and sharing the voices of others, she began to see her problems in a different light. Marie began to say, "Oh, this isn't just about me. I'm not the main problem here." Her voice moved from the individual as the problem to a more systemic understanding of the constraints. In talking about missing a spiritual community, she said, "Well, I guess if my church doesn't accept me then I'll find a new church that embraces who I am and what I believe."

Through the initial grief work and the process of reclaiming herself, Marie's symptoms improved. However, the grief Marie experienced was more complicated than first appearances indicated. The anticipation of, and anniversary of, her mother's death devastated Marie. She was haunted by disturbing nightmares that carried over to her waking life. Increased startle responses, fear of being alone, not wanting to be in darkness, dread of impending doom, and flashes of memory became typical occurrences. As we began to explore the nightmares and dreams, and the feelings and realities associated with them, a heaviness began to smother us as the ugliness of Marie's past poured over us. To present a picture of Marie's pain, I include two passages from her journal.

I don't know who I am anymore—nervous, afraid, frozen, every breath a struggle. The nightmares are terrifying as pictures flash quickly in front of me, shadowy outlines off to the side. I feel scared, motionless, dead, but alive with pain. The nightmares come more frequently now: chases, rape, mutilation, tidal waves, bullets rifling through my body. When I awaken, I am disoriented, feeling sick in my stomach, and my head is pounding. I can't breathe, my whole body is tense and flooded with waves of feelings inside of me. The nausea is overwhelming. I feel a presence in the room that is frightening, an anticipation that something awful is going to happen. I try to remember where I am as I begin to focus on the familiar objects in the room that bring me back to an awakened state.

My soul is stripped raw as the anger flows out of me, salt-filled tears burning at the very core of who I am, or was, or am to be. Every part of me—disjointed, scattered and separated from the center. I feel like my insides are pulling inward away from my skin. I feel so empty, so alone. So many feelings inside of me, each screaming to come out. The internal tension is unbearable. At times, the feelings begin to seep out, escaping, and I feel out of control. Inside I hear, "Be quiet, be still, don't move, stay inside, protect." I can't sort it all out.

What emerged from our work during this time, and the memories that materialized for Marie, was the realization that Marie as a child was sexually abused by her uncle (father's brother), now deceased. An awful secret was released that rocked Marie's sense of emotional stability, distorted her idea of herself as a human being, and devastated her trust in the world as she had known it. Confusion and disbelief paralyzed Marie. As she put it, "The bottom has fallen out and I am caught in a downward spin, spiraling out of control into an endless sea of darkness. I can't make it stop."

Although this new realization temporarily set us back therapeutically, it also inspired our work to move to a deeper level of trust, insight, and understanding of the structural constraints of Marie's social world. Because Marie had previously done some of the hard work of questioning the cultural messages that bound her, she was able to view this new information through that familiar thematic lens of power and oppression. She understood more clearly the societal process that trained her to internalize her status as "victim" by identifying herself through the eyes of her oppressor (e.g., worthless, weak, helpless), where Marie was neither heard nor seen. Her earlier work in counseling took on new meaning and served as a catalyst as Marie once again took on the arduous task of finding her voice and redefining and reclaiming her "self." Here again, it was important to situate the problem within a societal context (system of oppression and victimization), not within the individual (Marie).

*Marie:* "I didn't tell anyone what he was doing to me. I should have told someone . . . but I doubt they would have believed me. I was just a child and he was a respected deacon in our church—no one would ever have believed me."

*Shirley:* "So only those with power are believed, have a right to a voice."

*M:* "That's not how it should be but that is how it was."

*S:* "What does your voice have to say about what happened to you?"

*M:* "I didn't want any of it but he made me do it. He knew no one would believe me; he even told me that no one would ever believe me. When I think of him I feel so angry, I could just scream. He made me a victim. I hate him for making me a victim."

*S:* "Yes, he victimized you, abused you; he hurt you and silenced you. At that time you could not have done anything different—you were a child . . . Yet here you are now, as an adult, speaking your truth."

*M:* (Lets out a scream)! "That felt good."

*S:* "It's freeing to be heard."

*M:* "Yes, to be finally heard."

*S:* "You know Marie, it seems like you learned at an early age to be helpless and silent at the hands of more powerful forces."

*M:* "Yeah, that is exactly how I felt when my dad didn't let us tell our mom she was dying—helpless and silenced. It seems like this has been a happening throughout my whole life, not being able to speak the truth, my truth."

Within the safety of a trusting counseling relationship, Marie worked on grieving the many losses this trauma resurrected (e.g., childhood, expectation of safety and protection, innocence) by acknowledging and expressing the myriad of emotions (e.g., anger, despair, profound sadness) through modalities such as journaling, art, music, and dreamwork. Bibliotherapy increased her knowledge of the phenomenon of victimization, contextualized her trauma, and eased her perception of aloneness. Likewise, group work and attending workshops and conferences for survivors of trauma normalized her thoughts, feelings, and reactions, and helped her relocate blame and contempt from self to abuser and to a society that tolerates, and even perpetuates, victimization of individuals with devalued status. Through these interactions with others, and the experience of finding her voice, Marie began to not only notice the changes within her but also the influence she was having on those around her.

## A Systems Conceptualization of Marie's Case

To understand Marie's current situation in an ecological context, we must work to unpack the complex interlocking systems shaping and influencing Marie and Marie's role in shaping her world.

**Microsystem**   As the chronosystem reminds us, when working with adult clients, counselors must attend to the salient aspects of the clients' microsystem across time. For example, when Marie was situated in the farming community, her initial microsystem consisted of parents, grandparents, siblings, and extended family (e.g., cousins, aunts, uncles), and then school and church teachers and classmates. As Marie entered secondary school, her microsystem expanded to include school and church friends; boyfriend; athletic teammates; choir, band, and orchestra members; and new teachers and coaches. Marie's decision to attend college significantly changed the composition of Marie's microsystem (e.g., new friends, roommate, residence hall personnel and friends, new professors and coaches, other students, first girlfriend). The microsystem continued to evolve as Marie began her teaching career, living with her girlfriend, finding other lesbian friends and couples, and continuing connections (albeit less frequent contact) with her family of origin. Today, Marie's microsystem includes her ex-partner, other lesbian friends, friends in her graduate program, professors, support group members, her counselor, and minimal interactions with her family of origin. In hearing Marie's story, both the counselor and client must notice the significant players and the interactions Marie has had with them.

**Mesosystem**   As mentioned above, the construction of Marie's mesosystem altered over time. Initially, home, grandparents' home, and church interacted, then school, youth group, extracurricular activities, and friends' homes became settings that Marie frequented. The mesosystem became more complex as Marie moved away from home, attended an undergraduate institution, and then began her career and life with a female partner. Initially, when Marie was a young girl, the synergy between and among the components of her mesosystem was complimentary; expectations and messages about her sexuality, religiosity, and her role as a female were similar. However, as Marie advanced in her life and interactions in new settings exposed her to new ideas and experiences, she encountered a developmental impasse when she began to question some of the messages she had received as a child and adolescent. It is at this point Marie began to recognize a socially constructed relationship to power and discovered that power was used to foster or inhibit her development. The role of the counselor then is to help clients like Marie learn how to navigate through the myriad of these enabling and constraining influences that pepper their existence.

**Exosystem**   In her youth, Marie was indirectly affected by her father's need to work long hours at two jobs to support the family. He often came home tired and frustrated, and the pressure and anger he felt was taken out on Marie, her siblings, and their mother. When her father was able to balance this pressured life with periods of involvement with his athletic activities, home was a happier and safer place. Although her father's work situation had inhibiting effects on Marie, the financial support he was able to provide through additional employment afforded Marie the opportunity to attend college. Throughout the next phases of her life, Marie was impacted by new factors in her exosystem (e.g., family illnesses, laws regulating relationships between same sex couples, school board's decisions on curriculum). True to the theory, as people age, they continue to be affected by their exosystem even as the components of the system change with time.

Even today, Marie's exosystem, though different than that of her past, is having a profound effect on her life situation. Within the past three months, Marie's partner (Jennifer), also a graduate student, was diagnosed with a debilitating illness that caused Jennifer to drop out of school and leave her teaching assistantship. Without these resources, Jennifer did not have adequate health insurance to cover the costs of the extensive tests and treatment of her illness. During their relationship, Jennifer had been maintaining an ongoing connection with an ex-boyfriend who continued to offer her marriage. Jennifer's decision to leave the relationship with Marie was shaped by illness, confusion, fear of the future, an offer of a sanctioned relationship, the economic security of marriage, and homophobia. Jennifer was faced with living as an unmarried, unemployed, ill person without health benefits. Without exploring the exosystem and, therefore, missing the more externally constructed influences (e.g., economic security and social approval) and limitations to the relationship, Marie may be left feeling rejected, as if she was simply not a good enough girlfriend because she was not the person ultimately chosen by Jennifer.

**Macrosystem**  In listening to Marie's story, it became clear that in addition to dealing with the grief connected to her father and her partner, she was grieving the loss of a way of life and a belief system she left behind to pursue her education and live her life as a lesbian. Her worldview no longer included the beliefs of her traditional, religious upbringing that held little respect for not only her sexual orientation but also her development of autonomy and personal and professional independence. Everything she was coming to value (e.g., social justice, feminism, liberalism, spirituality, and Eastern philosophies) contradicted the views of her family (e.g., pull yourself up by the bootstraps mentality, patriarchy, social conservatism, religiosity). By accessing alternative cultural messages in the macrosystem, Marie learned that there were competing messages about the nature of reality that were in stark contrast to the messages she had previously been able to tap. These new messages afforded her a perspective that rejected yet contextualized the powerlessness and silencing she experienced. Marie was struggling to reconcile the effects of these two conflicting worlds. By attending to the macrosystem, the counselor was able to facilitate Marie's exploration of the content of the messages that were transmitted to her and how those cultural messages were mediated—intensified, deflected, or minimized—by members of her microsystem.

**Chronosystem**  Viewing Marie's situation through the lens of the chronosystem we see the fluidity of her circumstances. Each of Marie's experiences is time-bound, a snapshot in time so to speak. For example, Marie's experience of realizing her lesbian sexual orientation in 2000 had far different effects than she would have experienced had she come out in 1978 while working as an elementary school teacher. Although openly gay, lesbian, bisexual, and transgendered people face discrimination and violence today, there is a strong, visible gay rights movement that provides a counter narrative about human rights that Marie is able to access for support, strength, and legal protection, if needed. Also consider that in the 1960s there was considerable secrecy around child sexual abuse and even if victims did make claims of abuse often they were not believed. Due in part to the women's movement, today's culture understands violence against women and children as a expression of power and control, and adults abused as children are speaking out for themselves against their abusers to a culture prepared to listen and act on their behalf.

So here we see two situations where Marie, because of the period in which these events occurred, did not have a viable outlet for breaking silence. Had these same situations occurred in the present day, it may have been safer for Marie to have voice and be heard. Likewise, projecting Marie's situation fifty years into the future, universal health care might be in effect, gay marriage might be an option, and society may not structure people's lives in ways that make decisions about relationships based on to availability of health care and social sanctions.

## Summarizing Marie's Case

Operationalizing this theory in practice required first and foremost recognizing the importance of conceptualizing Marie's current situation through an ecological perspective and understanding that her development can most effectively be viewed within a model of interconnected social systems. The model reminds us that Marie brings to counseling a complex history and set of experiences that are influencing her current situation. In using an ecological model, we are asked to unpack this complexity to discover what is most salient to Marie.

In exploring Marie's microsystem and mesosystem throughout her lifetime, we come to know who and what interacted to have facilitating and inhibiting influence in Marie's life and how the messages of the macrosystem were mediated through her microsystem and mesosystem. Once the players, circumstances, and interactions are known, Marie is helped to see the impact the social world has had on her individual experiences (e.g., cultural norms and messages around expression of emotion and grief, power and voice, sexuality). As Marie begins to understand that some of the situations she has experienced are not about her personal failures but that these conditions (e.g., oppression and victimization) were structured around her by larger social forces in her exosystem and macrosystem, her understanding of her situation expands and suffering eases. As Marie's knowledge and systemic awareness increase, her pain, self-blame, and sadness begin to subside. Through the course of counseling, Marie, the once passive, helpless victim, claims her voice. The myopic lens through which she once saw her world now takes on the form of a prism, reflecting multiple new ways of understanding her past and pathways for her future growth.

## The Bereavement Group

Now we ask you to consider how an ecological perspective may inform counseling in a group context. This group is an eight-week, semistructured bereavement group for adults whose partners have died within the last six months. The group is held weekly for one and three-quarter hours. Although our primary focus will be on one member of the group (Beatrice), we provide some background for each of the group members.

### Group Members

Anthony is a thirty-nine-year-old, White male whose thirty-four-year-old wife, Erin, (also White) died six months after she was diagnosed with breast cancer. They had been married for nine years and prior to the diagnosis were planning to become parents. During his wife's illness, he struggled to finish building a house for her. Now he laments that, wishing he had spent less time working on the house and more time with Erin.

Niesha is a forty-nine-year-old African American woman whose fifty-three-year-old African American husband, Michael, died two and one-half years after being diagnosed with lung cancer. They have three children (Rosa, twenty-nine, Michael Jr., twenty-five, and Beverly, nineteen) who live nearby. They also have three grandchildren. Niesha holds much anger toward Michael because he refused to stop smoking cigarettes after his diagnosis.

Martha is a seventy-four-year-old, White female whose seventy-three-year-old, White husband, Nate, committed suicide in the attic of their home. They were married for fifty-two years and had three children (Barbara, fifty-three, Brenda, fifty, and Jeremy, forty-three) and six grandchildren. The children have been taking turns staying with their mother. Martha knew her husband was "feeling down" after his retirement but she does not understand why he would kill himself and leave her alone after so many years of marriage. Also, she is reeling from comments made to her during the viewing/funeral (e.g., a woman told Martha that her husband was going to hell because suicide is a sin).

Brian is a sixty-two-year-old, Asian American male whose sixty-one-year-old, Asian American wife, Sue, was in a car accident and died after she was taken off of life-support. Brian was driving the car and fell asleep at the wheel. He suffered some physical injuries, including a broken arm. He is tormented by the guilt he feels at having caused his wife's death. Brian and Sue have one child (Lee, thirty-eight) who lives 3,000 miles away on the west coast.

Keith is a forty-one-year-old, African American male whose thirty-seven-year-old, White partner, Bill, died from a heroin overdose. They have been together for ten years. Bill, after returning from serving in the Iraq war where he was seriously injured, became addicted to pain killers. Bill also sought other drugs to numb his physical and emotional scars. Although Keith has the support of Bill's parents and Bill's two sisters, Keith's family of origin has never acknowledged his relationship with Bill.

Beatrice is a seventy-five-year-old, White female whose seventy-six-year-old, White husband, George, died after a six-year battle with Alzheimer's and Parkinson's diseases. When George became ill, both Beatrice and George completed living wills because neither wanted to be kept alive through extraordinary means. Although Beatrice had been George's primary caregiver, George was under the care of hospice for his last seven months. Their church was also very supportive, often bringing meals and providing care for George so Beatrice could have some respite. Because of their limited income, they received assistance from their local Office on Aging (e.g., Meals on Wheels, respite care). They were married for fifty-five years and had one daughter who was killed in a car accident when she was sixteen. Neither Beatrice nor George had living siblings; however, they had two nieces and two nephews who visited on occasion. Prior to George's illness both Beatrice and George were active members of their church, participating in the choir, volunteering their services at fund-raisers, and doing home and hospital visits. They also attended weekly Bible study and other social gatherings sponsored by their church. George's progressive deterioration over the last two years prevented them from engaging in their regular activities.

## Ecological Questions to Consider

In an ecological system, what the group members have in common is their interconnectedness through grieving, however many other systemic factors shape their individual experience of grief. In contrast to stages of grieving, as many models suggest, an ecological systems approach suggests the presence of other influences on the grief process. What kinds of questions would an ecological counselor seek to understand in working with this group? How might grief be conceptualized through an ecological perspective, particularly in Beatrice's case?

For example, in addition to each group member's unique microsystem, the group members themselves, as well as the counselor, are now part of each other's microsystem. From reading and imagining each person's experience of grief, how might members affect and be affected by each other within this new aspect of their microsystem?

What effect might sociocultural factors (e.g., age, gender, race, class, sexual orientation, religion) have on the grief process? How are the different cultural roles (e.g., mother, father, sister, employee, members) individuals are expected to enact affect their grief?

What supports are present or lacking in each member's four systems? How are these support structures similar to or different from those of the other members in the group? What role will members' varying emotions (e.g., regret, guilt, remorse, anger, sadness) have in their process of grieving. What effect might these similarities and differences have on the group process?

What are the cultural norms surrounding members' bereavement experience? For example, the fact that a bereavement group exists is a cultural phenomenon. What messages have members received from their culture about the expectations of the appropriate ways one grieves? How much time does their culture permit for bereavement? What stigmas or judgments are associated with some member's experiences of death (e.g., suicide, falling asleep at the wheel, drug overdose) and how might these factors affect the grief process?

How do social and economic policies and legal issues (e.g., health care, laws defining life and death, advances in medical technology, domestic partner benefits) influence aspects of the grief process? Also consider that group members lost their significant others in 2000; what might be different about their losses had the deaths occurred in 1900 or in 2050?

We have raised some ecological considerations to help us understand what the loss of a spouse/partner might mean to our clients. However, there are many factors that influence group members' experience of grief, their interactions with each other, and the healing process. What other considerations are important to address? For example, how would your views about bereavement and your experiences of loss affect the group and its process?

## Summary

Ecological models ask us to view our clients contextually and consider the interconnectedness among the many influences on our clients' lives (e.g., microsystem, mesosystem, exosystem, macrosystem, chronosystem). As our world becomes more complex, the impact on human development will be critically connected to that evolution. Therefore, it is our ethical and professional responsibility to practice from theoretical models (e.g., Bronfenbrenner) that embrace this complexity.

## Annotated Bibliography

Baltes, P. B. (1987). Theoretical propositions of lifespan development: On the dynamics between growth and decline. *Developmental Psychology, 23,* 611–626. Baltes proffers a metatheoretical view on the nature of lifespan development that includes a "family of theoretical propositions." Among these propositions are: (1) development is a lifelong process; (2) change is multidirectional; (3) development includes both aspects of growth (gain) and decline (loss); (4) individual development can take varying forms (plasticity); (5) development is influenced by sociocultural conditions (historical embeddedness); (6) the interaction among age-graded, history-graded, and nonnormative systems influences development; and (7) lifespan development occurs within an interdisciplinary context (multidisciplinary). The propositions of plasticity and gains and losses are given particular emphasis.

Bronfenbrenner, U. (1979). *The ecology of human development: Experiments by nature and design.* Cambridge, MA: Harvard University Press. Bronfenbrenner invites the reader to engage in the exploration of a "new" theoretical perspective for viewing human development. Here Bronfenbrenner introduces an ecological systems approach to development that explores the developing person, the environmental context, and the interaction between the two. He describes this ecological environment as composed of "nested" interconnected structures (e.g., microsystem, mesosystem, exosystem, and macrosystem).

Bronfenbrenner, U. (1988). Interacting systems in human development: Research paradigms: Present and future. In N. Bolger, A. Caspi, G. Doowney, & M. Moorehouse (Eds.), *Persons in context: Developmental processes* (pp. 25–49). New York: Cambridge University Press. Bronfenbrenner examines theoretical models in research on human development such as class-theoretical (e.g., social address, personal attribute, sociological niche) and process paradigms (e.g., microsystem process, process-context, and process-person-context). Chronosystem designs are also introduced. The strengths and limitations of these models are explored and recommendations for the use of more comprehensive conceptual and operational research designs are provided.

Bronfenbrenner, U. (1993). Ecosystems, affordances, transactions, and skills: Theories of person/situation interaction. In R. H. Wozniak & K. W. Fischer (Eds.), *Development in context: Acting and thinking in specific environments.* Hillside, NJ: Erlbaum.

Bronfenbrenner describes his transformation of Lewin's equation (i.e., behavior is a joint function of person and environment) to view development as a joint function of person and environment. He describes an ecological perspective on development in which there is a synergistic interaction between individuals and their context (e.g., microsystem, mesosystem, exosystem, macrosystem, chronosystem). Implications for research on cognitive development are explored.

Bronfenbrenner, U. (1995). Development ecology through space and time: A future perspective. In P. Moen, G. H. Elder, Jr., & K. Luscher (Eds.), *Examining lives in context: Perspectives on the ecology of human development* (pp. 619–647). Washington, DC: APA Books.
Here Bronfenbrenner adds the element of time to his earlier process-person-context model and suggests a bioecological model that addresses development within the context of time and posits that the conditions and events that occur during the historical period of a person's life shape development. Bronfenbrenner identifies this model as PPCT (process-person-context-time). Throughout the chapter, research studies are discussed and critiqued and research designs are theorized.

# References

Baltes, P. B. (1987). Theoretical propositions of lifespan developmental psychology: On the dynamics between growth and decline. *Developmental Psychology, 23*, 611–626.

Bronfenbrenner, U. (1977). Toward an experimental ecology of human development. *American Psychologist, 32*, 513–530.

Bronfenbrenner, U. (1979). *The ecology of human development: Experiments by nature and design.* Cambridge, MA: Harvard University Press.

Bronfenbrenner, U. (1988). Interacting systems in human development: Research paradigms: Present and future. In N. Bolger, A. Caspi, G. Doowney, & M. Moorehouse, *Persons in context: Developmental processes* (pp. 25–49). New York: Cambridge University Press.

Bronfenbrenner, U., & Crouter, A. C. (1983). The evolution of environmental models in developmental research. In P. H. Mussen (Ed.), *Handbook of child psychology, Vol. 1. History, theory, methods* (pp. 357–414). New York: Wiley.

Lemert, C. (1997). *Social things: American introduction to the sociological life.* Lanham, MD: Rowman and Littlefield.

Mills, C. W. (1959). *Sociological imagination.* New York: Oxford University Press.

# CHAPTER FOUR

# Cognition, Culture, and Society: Understanding Cognitive Development in the Tradition of Vygotsky

## Kathryn Douthit

As counselors make their way through the first decade of the twenty-first century, they are increasingly awed by the new understandings of the human mind being generated in neuroscience, genetics, pharmacology, and psychiatry. Often, however, the scientific advancements coming out these fields seem to overshadow concepts that are central to counselors' understanding of human psychology. Multiculturalism, contextualism, developmentalism, humanism, holistic wellness, and prevention—the bedrocks of counseling practice—often seem to lose their saliency in the face of scientific approaches to psychological well-being.

The counseling profession, in its ongoing efforts to maintain a strong voice in the conceptualization of psychological care, has a powerful ally in early twentieth-century interdisciplinary scholar, Lev Vygotsky. Unlike others in his day, Vygotsky was keenly aware of the profound ways in which culture, society, and historical events shape the way human beings think, see, and feel. For students of counseling, understanding Vygotsky's vision of cognitive development provides a strong theoretical base for the uniqueness of the counseling profession's attention to the many ways environment shapes our mental wellness. For practicing counselors, Vygotsky's foresight provides a sound rationale for our attention to multiculturalism, commitment to social justice, and focus on the developmental forces in the lives of individuals.

If genius in the social sciences can be measured by the ability of ideas to endure over time and to become increasingly relevant to our understanding of human existence, then Vygotsky should undoubtedly rank among those we revere as our most exceptional thinkers. As you read through this chapter, consider the following questions and decide for yourself whether Vygotsky has made an invaluable contribution to our understanding of human processes: Is psychological development something that occurs within individuals or between individuals? How is it possible that social and cultural practices can actually shape the course of psychological development? Don't the structures that constitute the human mind have a predictable, biological maturation process that is the same for all human beings? How can our knowledge of human development help to shape a more socially just world? How can societies ensure that development of psychological capacity is maximized for all of its citizens?

Keep in mind as you are studying this chapter that you are one of a small handful of trailblazers attempting to apply Vygotsky's ideas to counseling practice. Until now, his ideas have primarily guided research in teacher education and cultural studies. I hope that you feel as I do that Vygotskian principles can facilitate the practice of socially just counseling by honoring a multiplicity of worldviews and by engaging clients' critical thinking skills, thus empowering them to act on their own behalf.

## ABOUT THE CHAPTER AUTHOR

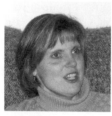

**Kathryn Z. Douthit**

Kathryn Z. Douthit, Ph.D., LMHC, is an associate professor of counseling and human development at the University of Rochester. In her professional work she is interested in the ecology of mental disorders such as dementia and ADHD and attempts to find common ground between contemporary biopsychiatry and the principles and values of counseling practice. Kathryn has practiced as a community college counselor. She currently lives with her family in Rochester, New York, where her interests include singing, gardening, needlecraft, global politics, and alternative medicine.

# An Overview of Vygotsky's Cultural-Historical Activity Theory

Cultural-Historical Activity Theory (CHAT) is a broad and complex theory of cognitive development that depicts cognition, and consciousness more generally, as a product of the natural unfolding of individual physical development (ontogeny), human evolution (phylogeny), and the changing social and cultural conditions that constitute human history. According to Vygotsky, these three basic elements—ontogeny, phylogeny and sociocultural context—intersect in the course of human activity, which acts as a medium through which consciousness is developed (Davydov & Radzikhovskii, 1985; van der Veer & Valsiner, 1991).

These three elements are easily understood by considering them in the context of a young, suburban adult's cognitive development. As the teen's understanding of the world around her develops, that understanding is constrained by the physical limitations of body and brain development (ontogeny) that are part of the individual aging process. A baby girl would not be expected to increase her understanding of human nature in a lecture on Shakespeare as would a seventeen-year-old who has well-developed language skills. Additionally, it is unlikely that an adult chimpanzee would get much out of the lecture on Shakespeare, while an older adolescent has a pretty good chance of assimilating knowledge and understanding. This is because, in the course of human evolution (phylogeny), receptive language skills have developed that allow humans to understand complex, abstract language. Finally, a seventeen-year-old in a wealthy suburban high school would very likely assimilate more understanding of human nature studying Shakespeare than a similarly aged adolescent in the jungles of Peru. This is not because the suburban teen is smarter or wiser. Rather, it is because she has been exposed to abstract logic, is a native English speaker, and is already familiar with Western, European culture (sociocultural context), thereby allowing her to understand the text at a deeper level.

Although Vygotsky worked primarily with children, it will become apparent that his principles can easily be applied across the lifespan. While at first glance, CHAT may appear to be too ambitious and too broad in scope to be of great utility, much of the content in Vygotsky's writing actually reflects remarkable foresight. The echoes of his work in contemporary development theory and the wisdom of his insights in conceptualizing twenty-first-century educational and psychological research are a testimony to the genius of his bold, sweeping vision.

The applicability of Vygotsky's theory to contemporary research and scholarship is even more intriguing in light of the fact that it is informed as much by the social theory of Karl Marx as it is by scholarship in psychology. Marx's understanding of the process of social transformation served as the bedrock for Vygotsky's understanding of individual cognitive development. Vygotsky's personal life history was immersed in the tumult of the Russian Revolution and he, like other scholars of his day, was a witness to the transformative power of Marxist doctrine. As the Russian people in the early twentieth century, energized by the Marxian spirit, expelled the centuries-old Russian Czarist regime, Russian scholars were given the charge of reshaping, according to the principles of Marxian philosophy, entire academic disciplines (Newman & Holzman, 1993; van der Veer & Valsiner, 1991, Wertsch, 1985). Vygotsky and his colleagues in psychology embraced this challenge and it is upon this canvas that CHAT was painted.

## Background to the Theory

In light of the overwhelming influence of Marxist thought on the theory conceived by Vygotsky and his colleagues, I begin this journey to unravel the tenets of CHAT with a brief excursion into the philosophy of Karl Marx. In addition, I consider the thought of Engels and Hegel, because both of these philosophers profoundly influenced Marx and Vygotsky, and are integral to Vygotskian theory. I then review Vygotsky's understanding of the relationship between thought, language, and activity, and end by discussing applications of CHAT that are likely to bolster the developmental process of individuals in contemporary classrooms and counseling settings. Most of Vygotsky's insights were based on his work with young children, but if throughout this review the reader remains mindful of the potential for expanding the concepts of CHAT across the lifespan, together we can create bold new vistas for approaching developmental issues that arise in the context of the counseling relationship. (See Table 4.1 for a summary of CHAT.)

### The Influence of Marx, Engels, and Hegel

Noted neo-Vygotskian scholar, James Wertsch (1985), underscores three salient themes that depict Marx's influence on Vygotsky, namely, (1) the "psychological cell" is the foundation of a psychological method, (2) human psychological functioning represents an embodiment of

TABLE 4.1   Summary of Vygotsky's Cultural-Historical
           Activity Theory (CHAT)

| Theory Dimensions | CHAT Description |
| --- | --- |
| Aspect of development considered | CHAT is narrowly defined as a theory of cognitive development, but is also described more broadly as a theory of consciousness that includes cognition, volition, motivation, need, desire, and affect. |
| Age applicability | Most of Vygotsky's work focused on children, but the theory can be applied across the lifespan. |
| Factors influencing development | Development is under the control of three factors: ontogeny, phylogeny, and sociocultural history. |
| Philosophical foundations | CHAT is influenced by the philosophies of Marx, Engels, and Hegel, including, respectively, the notions of embodiment of social relations, tool use, and dialecticism. |
| Unique features | Cognitive development takes place as an outcome of sociocultural activity involving culture-based tool use, primarily language. Development is best facilitated when a more developed teacher scaffolds learning in the zone of proximal development. |

social relations, and (3) activity is central in uniting the external world
with internal process. I will consider each of these three themes in
some detail.

**The Psychological Cell**   Contemporaries of Vygotsky in the world of
psychology largely aimed to understand psychological phenomena by
examining them at the level of their smallest component parts. Taking
his cue from Marx, Vygotsky resisted this notion of componentiality
and embraced a method of inquiry that would result in what Wertsch
terms a "genetic explanation" of psychological process (Wertsch, 1985,
p. 5). This genetic perspective aims to understand how complete living

units of functioning develop over time. Hence, just as Marx sought the smallest functioning units in the production of human history, Vygotsky attempted to elucidate the smallest functional unit of conscious process, a unit aptly termed the *psychological cell.*

Many examples highlighting the difference between componential and genetic approaches can be taken from biology. For instance, to understand the function of a leaf, looking at the individual carbon, oxygen, hydrogen, and other atoms that make up the leaf would not tell an observer very much about how the leaf works. However, looking at leaf cells in which atoms are joined in a meaningful way would give the observer a window into the operations of the whole leaf because photosynthesis and other processes associated with whole leaves occur on a micro level in individual leaf cells. In this example, the leaf cell represents the genetic view while the atoms comprising the cell represent the componential view.

Vygotsky's understanding of the psychological cell changed over time. In his earlier writing, he largely considered word meaning to be the psychological cell that comprises all of human consciousness. For Vygotsky, words—the building blocks of language—embodied the essence of culture and served as psychological tools in human activity to mediate the constitution of conscious thought. Later, however, in one of his final works, *Thought and Language,* the notion of the psychological cell was expanded. Vygotsky wrote that when considering

> the planes of inner thought [i.e., consciousness] . . . (t)hought is not the superior authority in this process. Thought is not begotten by thought; it is engendered by motivation, i.e., by our desires and needs, our interests and emotions. Behind every thought there is an affective-volitional tendency, which holds the answer to the last "why" in the analysis of thinking. (Vygotsky, 1934/1986, p. 252)

Thus, for Vygotsky, the unit of psychological functioning ultimately involved culturally and historically informed tool use, the most common of which is speech, *as well as desires, needs, interests and emotions* (Zinchenko, 1985). Although his theory is generally associated with cognitive development, Vygotsky clearly understood that cognitive understanding is intimately linked to how we feel about the world around us. Returning to the example of the suburban teen studying Shakespeare, it is easy to see how a young suburban adult with a successful academic history who is aspiring to become an English major at her father's Ivy League alma mater would be more likely to learn the lessons about human nature woven into Shakespearean text than an angry teen coming from a life of poverty and violence who has few hopes for the future and finds school to be a place where curriculum has little relevance to her life.

## Psychological Functioning as an Embodiment of Social Relations

In 1845, at the young age of twenty-seven, Marx summarized his view of human essence: "(H)uman essence is no abstraction inherent in each individual. In its reality it is the ensemble of the social relations" (Marx, 1845/1978b, p. 145). In this succinct statement, he conveys one of the pillars of his philosophy, namely, that human nature is a reflection of embodied social relations. Put more simply, human nature is not something that develops within each individual in isolation. Rather, individuals are constituted through their interaction with the social environment, and the nature of that social environment is undergoing constant transformation in response to changes in history. It follows, therefore, that human nature is ultimately a reflection of the cultural and social practices that are shaped by history and that human consciousness is thus a reflection of material reality.

The actual mechanism involved in mediating the internalization of social and cultural transformations is dependent on dialecticism and tool use, concepts elaborated by Georg Hegel and Frederich Engels respectively. Georg Hegel was a great nineteenth-century German philosopher who, in his youth, was inspired by the French Revolution. Hegel believed that as new ideas emerge in a society, they often conflict with long-held beliefs, and that society ultimately evolves as the new ideas are dialectically reconciled with the old. Dialecticism in this context can be understood as a negotiation process in which individuals adjust to some aspects of the environment while attempting to modify others—the individual and the social environment reciprocally change over time until an equilibrium is reached (cf. Caird, 1883 for an extended biography of Hegel). Marx, borrowing from Hegel, contended that history evolves through a dialectical process in which technological advances devised to foster evolving forms of economic growth, technologies that Marx called "means of production" (e.g., the use of computers in an information-based economy), conflict with older established means of production and are then resolved through social and cultural negotiation (Marx, 1859/1978c).

Frederick Engels, a collaborator of Karl Marx, was born in the year 1820 in the industrial city of Barmen, Germany. Although Engels spent much of his life working in textile mills owned by his father and grand-father, a period of service in the Prussian army brought him to Berlin where he became involved with a young group of scholars interested in the work of Hegel (German, 1994). He later met Karl Marx with whom he formed a lasting and productive intellectual relationship. In light of his many years of exposure to work in textile mills, it is not surprising that Engels became focused on the role of tool use as the material means through which history evolves. According to Engels (1925/1979), the collective human physical and psychological adjustment to existing tool use, such as the use of the computer in the twenty-first century, fuels historical periods of social transformation, including establishing new power relations among individuals in the society. Tools, in essence, mediate the link between means of production and social transforma-tion: human tool use ultimately constitutes history.

Vygotsky, striving to understand the development of human con-sciousness, believed, in the spirit of Marx, Hegel, and Engels, that between the internal psyche and the external cultural-historical context, a dialectical language-dependent developmental process intervenes in which the external structures are transformed to create internal planes of consciousness (Wertsch & Stone, 1985). Language, for Vygotsky, is the quintessential cultural tool and thus plays a major role in the individ-ual's dialectical mediation of new sociocultural input. In his work with children, Vygotsky called this process of dialectical mediation the "gen-eral genetic law of cultural development" (p. 164). According to Vygot-sky's general genetic law, aspects of the child's cultural development appear first on the interpersonal social plane, which uses language as its primary tool, and then on the intrapersonal psychological plane. For example, a child who is learning to share his toys might be introduced to the concept of sharing through a series of verbal exchanges with his mother. It may take several conversations before the child actually gains an understanding about the cultural expectations concerning sharing, incorporates the general principles of sharing into his thought patterns, and applies them to his behaviors. Vygotsky contended that this same general genetic process applies to development of voluntary attention, logical memory, concept formation, and volition (Wertsch & Stone, 1985).

**Activity, Language, and Thought**    A central question that emerged in Vygotsky's depiction of cognitive/consciousness development was: What factor or factors facilitate the translation of external sociocultural practices, constraints, and possibilities into what we understand to be human consciousness? Put more simply, he wanted to grasp the mechanism or process that allows the conditions in the world around us to define how we think and see. Vygotsky came to understand this process by relying, once again, on the philosophy of Karl Marx. Like Marx, Vygotsky believed that human activity is the primary mediating force in the internalization of extant contextual conditions (Marx, 1932/1978a), while he contended that tool use, primarily in the form of language (see above), plays a pivotal role in helping to shape the substance and meaning of activity (Vygotsky, 1978). For example, as an adolescent experiences the daily practices of being in high school, much of what he or she comes to understand about the culture of high school is assimilated through the use of language. While other senses such as sight and smell most certainly play a role in the teen's thoughts about the experience of high school life, much of that information is stored in the form of language.

In Vygotsky's writing, language is a centrally important tool for applying the substance of conscious thought to human activity and, reciprocally, of interpreting human activity and integrating it into consciousness. Thought provides the blueprint for how one engages in activity, and it allows one engaged in activity to process perceptions and reshape thought: ". . . (the) unity of perception, speech and action, which ultimately produces internalization of the visual field, constitutes the central subject matter for any analysis of the origin of uniquely human forms of behavior" (Vygotsky, 1978, p. 26).

Thus, thought imparts an intentionality on human action that is distinct from basic animal instinct. According to van de Veer and Valsiner (1991), Vygotsky believed that instinct, a type of action characterized by automaticity rather than negotiated thought, develops in the biological evolution of the species, that is, phylogenetically, as does *the capacity* for human thought. The content of human thought, however, develops in the course of individual lifespan development, that is, ontogeny, and is constituted by cultural, social, and historical forces.

## Practical Applications of CHAT: Scaffolding in the Zone of Proximal Development

### The Zone of Proximal Development (ZPD)

Relative to his well-known contemporaries in psychology, Vygotsky had a unique theoretical view concerning the relationship between learning and development. Unlike Piaget, who believed that development occurs independently of learning through a process of biological maturation, or Pavlov, who believed that learning *is* development, Vygotsky believed

that development follows learning and that "learning awakens a variety
of internal developmental processes that are able to operate only when
the child is interacting with people in his environment and in cooperation with his peers" (Vygotsky, 1978, p. 90). This pronouncement by
Vygotsky served to underscore that development is facilitated by social
interaction with peers, teachers, and others who are part of the developing individual's environment. More specifically, he proposed that optimal development exists in a learning context that he termed the *ZPD*.

In one of his most famous collections, *Mind in Society*, Vygotsky
defined the ZPD as "the distance between the actual developmental
level as determined by independent problem solving and the level of
potential development as determined through problem solving under
adult guidance or in collaboration with more capable peers" (Vygotsky,
1978, p. 86). Simply put, Vygotsky believed that teaching is most effective and thus incurs the greatest gains in child development when children engage with individuals who are more developmentally advanced
in activity that is just beyond their current level of development.
Although Vygotsky thought it advantageous to work beyond the existing developmental level of the learner, he clearly understood that the
degree of developmental advancement possible at any given time is limited by potential inherent in the learner. By working within the developmental "zone" that exists between the learner's present level of
functioning and her maximum potential at that moment in time, the
teacher/facilitator is able to incur the greatest possible gains in development. For example, a counselor wishing to help a female client to
depersonalize problematic power dynamics in her workplace could
engage in a dialogue that might incorporate concepts concerning gender identity and Western ideals of autonomy, individualism, meritoc-
racy, and personal power. At first the counselor might walk the client
through these concepts so that she is better able to understand the
impetus behind much of the offensive behavior in her workplace environment. Over time, as the client processes behaviors in her office using
the counselor's insights, she is able, on her own, to think differently
about the offensive acts committed by colleagues and is thus able to
respond in a manner that goes directly to the heart of the problem.

Jerome Bruner (1985), a distinguished contemporary neo-Vygotskian
scholar, emphasizes that the teacher/facilitator working in the zone
will have greater success if they have a knowledge of instruments or
props that will advance development when working within the ZPD
and a qualitative understanding of the types of activities that will
make children *receptive* to developmental changes and practices. In any

case, the ZPD has utility in both formal and informal educational settings, and is particularly germane to our understanding of client development in the counseling relationship. To truly understand how the notion of the ZPD can be applied in counseling, we need to introduce two additional CHAT-related concepts: scaffolding and metacognition.

**Metacognition and Scaffolding**   At the core of CHAT is the notion that development is mediated through activity, and that the type of activity that optimizes ZPD development occurs between the learner and a more developmentally advanced facilitator. Vygotsky is clear in stating that the educative interaction between learner and facilitator, what he called transactional learning, is not a simple transfer of information from facilitator to learner resulting in what we know as consciousness, this is, how an individual thinks about a particular topic. Rather than assimilating a perfect likeness of information as it is received from the facilitator, the learner steps back and through spontaneous, unconscious processing of the new information, eventually develops consciousness by viewing his or her own thoughts in a new way. When the mind thinks about how it is thinking, it is engaged in a phenomenon called *metacognition* (Bruner, 1985; Vygotsky, 1934/1986). This suggests that "consciousness . . . is a way of buffering immediate response so that the situation can be better appraised from higher ground" (Bruner, 1985, p. 24). The mind essentially engages in its own internal debate between old and new information and when the debate is resolved, new understanding emerges. As this new understanding surfaces, the mind, through the process of metacognition, is able to consciously discern how its own thinking has changed. It is at this point that development has been achieved.

How, then, does learning in the ZPD facilitate the metacognition that is so crucial to the assimilative process? Bruner (1985) contends that the teacher/facilitator working with a learner in the ZPD provides structure that in essence functions as an external consciousness. The process of making this external consciousness available to the learner is called *scaffolding* and is a pivotal component in maximizing transactional learning in the ZPD. The teacher/facilitator is not merely transmitting information; rather, she is modeling, through the use of meaningful activity, how to think about the information being transmitted. *It is the assimilation of the metacognitive process by the learner that truly completes the transactional learning process.* Thus, for the client struggling with a developmental issue, the Vygotskian perspective provides: (1) an empowering new understanding of how to think about a specific developmental issue and (2) the ability to think about one's developmental process more generally.

Both of these possibilities will become clearer in the case study later in this chapter, but for now, briefly reconsider the child learning how to share his toys. As the child enters the ZPD, he is determined to keep all of his toys to himself. His mother, acting as a facilitator, aims to change how the child thinks about the notion of sharing. Acting as an external consciousness, the mother models how the child might think about sharing. She may emphasize the importance of generosity in promoting the common good, evoke feelings of empathy by having the child realize how badly a friend might feel if there is no sharing, or perhaps appeal to the notion of reciprocity by explaining how other children share with him so that there is an inherent fairness in reciprocation. In any event, the child not only learns to share, but his mother provides a metacognitive scaffolding that allows the child to think about *how* to think about sharing and he thus completes an important step in his own moral development trajectory.

## Development of Self-Regulation

Before ending our overview of CHAT, we will briefly consider one additional application of the theory that is of particular interest to counselors. Vygotsky (1932/1987) understood that much of the mechanism that he conceptualized for consciousness development, that is, internalization of speech to constitute planes of consciousness, can also be applied to the development of self-regulatory processes such as volition, will, and values. It was his contention that through the assimilation of social, cultural, and historical norms, children develop a self-guiding set of maxims that they use to negotiate the decisions in their lives. Thus much of what we might define as basic "character," an important component of self-regulation, is actually a reflection of the same type of language-mediated contextual internalization process typical of cognitive development in general. Values, ethics, and morals—the basic building blocks of character—are internally negotiated just as in the case of the boy learning to share through his mother's metacognitive scaffolding.

Vygotsky (1932/1987) tells us that when individuals are engaged in decisions that require value-laden judgments, for example, a decision to act in a certain way, they utilize inner speech, a reflection of their consciousness, to internally negotiate a course of action. Thus, a child engaged in a moral dilemma such as whether or not to lie to a parent will consider assimilated cultural and social norms concerning the practice of lying, the possible social benefits of telling the lie, and socially or culturally sanctioned repercussions that might arise if the lie is revealed. In thinking about each of these dimensions of her decision, the child will not only be applying the logic of inner speech, she will also be influenced by the emotional responses that each incurs. Applying CHAT in this way expands the possibilities for conceptualizing clients' decision-making process in a more ecologically and culturally cognizant framework.

## Vygotsky's Vision

Vygotsky was a great thinker for his time, and had it not been for his untimely death at the age of thirty-seven, we can only imagine where his theorizing might have taken him. Still, even in his short lifetime, Vygotsky left us with a sweeping vision of human development that addresses many of the basic principles fundamental to counselors' vision of psychological wellness. Centrally important concepts such as race, class, gender, sexual orientation, religion, and other dimensions of the sociocultural milieu are understood as embodied. Although Vygotsky did not clearly articulate how these collective sociocultural phenomena infiltrate individual activity, his predecessors have understood that for CHAT to fulfill the vision set in motion by Vygotsky, the relationship between the individual and the collective must be clarified and operationalized (see, for example, Engström, 1987; Leont'ev, 1959/1981). Still, Vygotsky was steadfast in his belief that sociocultural forces constitute consciousness and dictate how we think, feel, and act—a notion that must inform any attempt by counselors to facilitate growth or change.

## The Importance of Cultural-Historical Activity Theory

### The Central Role of Context

Contextualism has long been the bedrock of the counseling profession. Whether it is framed as multiculturalism, developmentalism, ecological counseling, advocacy, or social justice counseling, the role of context, that is, the numerous interrelated social and cultural forces that constitute "environment" in shaping clients lives and as a key consideration in intervention strategy is of central importance in promoting dignity, diversity, and justice in counseling practice. With the sociocultural milieu having such a fundamental place in conceptualization

## ABOUT VYGOTSKI, COLE, AND WERTSCH
### Key Cultural-Historical Activity Theorists

Cultural-Historical Activity Theory (CHAT) was conceived in Russia in the early years of the twentieth century due largely to the work of psychologist Lev Semenovich Vygotsky. While Vygotsky is widely recognized as a key figure in the development of CHAT, the devotion of many scholars to his work and the durability of his ideas over time have led numerous contemporary psychologists, anthropologists, and educators to devote their careers to applying and expanding the fundamental principles of CHAT.

In an attempt to familiarize the reader with the lineage of Vygotskian scholars, we begin with a biographical sketch of the life of Vygotsky, underscoring the pivotal role of his close collaborators Alexander Luria and Alexei Leont'ev in disseminating his ideas following his early death. We then turn to two contemporary scholars James Wertsch and Michael Cole, both of whom have been instrumental in keeping Vygotsky's work alive in late twentieth- and early twenty-first-century academic literature.

Lev Semenovich Vygotsky, a Russian Jew, was born in 1896 and lived most of his early years with his seven brothers and sisters in the western Russian port city of Gomel (Vygodskaya, 1995). As a young scholar, Vygotsky simultaneously completed a law degree at the University of Moscow and took courses at Shanyavskii People's University, a haven for professors expelled from the University of Moscow because of their opposition to the Czarist regime. His time at the People's University would prove to be quite influential in Vygotsky's intellectual development (Blanck, 1992; Kozulin, 1987; Wertsch, 1985).

After receiving his law degree, Vygotsky became a literature and psychology teacher at a local school in Gomel. Wertsch (1985) describes how at this time Vygotsky was surrounded by the tumult of the Russian Revolution and was able to observe first hand a society attempting to embrace socialist principles. The ideology of Karl Marx was becoming an organizing principle, not only around issues of economy and government, but it had also entered the halls of the academy and was informing disciplinary theory. It was in this environment of Marxian foment that Vygotsky, in spite of an increasingly challenging battle with tuberculosis, moved to Moscow in the autumn of 1924 and assumed a position in the famous Institute of Psychology (Wertsch, 1985). It was in Moscow that he was first joined by two colleagues, Alexei Leont'ev and Alexander Luria, who were to become his chief collaborators and play a major role in expanding Vygotsky's work after his early death from tuberculosis at the age of 37 (Vygodskaya, 1995; Wertsch, 1985).

Leont'ev's distinguished career in psychology was primarily affiliated with the Moscow State Lomonosov University and his Activity Theory, an integral part of CHAT, made the significant contribution of systematically looking at human activity as a unit of analysis when studying human sciences (Cole, n.d.). Luria, a member of the Institute of Psychology in Moscow, is widely regarded as a seminal scholar in the field of neuropsychology. Although he had great interest in the neurological basis of psychological abnormality, much of his work involved research that attempted to show the relationship between physical maturation and cultural milieu (Cole, 1997).

With the rise of Stalin after the Russian Revolution came the suppression of much of Marxist Soviet psychology. Vygotsky's work, banned by the Stalinist regime, did not reappear until the 1960s, and it then gained considerable stature in the 1980s. Two contemporary scholars who were instrumental in the resurgence of Vygotsky's ideas are Michael Cole and James Wertsch.

Cole, a professor of psychology at University of California, San Diego, has devoted considerable attention to developing a theory of the mind that combines Russian activity theory psychology with American traditions in psychology that favor more positivist and experimental methods. In an attempt to integrate these two traditions, early in his career Cole launched a series of studies that attempted to show how cognitive development varies across cultures (University of California, San Diego, 1996). More recently Cole's research has been focused on his so-called Fifth Dimension afterschool programs promoting literacy through collaborative learning in the context of model cultures that operate under their own norms, rules, and artifacts. The Fifth Dimension model is used to study learning in many countries around the world.

James Wertsch is a professor in the Department of Anthropology at Washington University in St. Louis and holds joint
*continued*

appointments in the departments of education, Russian studies, philosophy, neuroscience, and psychology. He is particularly interested in the interconnections among language, thought, and culture, applying much of his work to understanding the relationship between history, collective memory, and national identity. Wertsch has projects underway in Russia, Estonia, and the Republic of Georgia. (Washington University, St. Louis, 2006).

Other Vygotskian scholars of note include Sylvia Scribner, Luis Moll, Vera John-Steiner, Jerome Bruner, Jaan Valsiner, René van der Veer, and Yrjo Engeström.

of counseling practice, counselors need a theory of human development that adequately captures the complex relationship between context and human thought, emotion, and action. Although some aspects of this complex relationship are addressed by popular theories of development, few speak to the full range of complexity as thoroughly as Cultural-Historical Activity Theory.

Because of CHAT's focus on the central dynamic role of contextual issues in constitution of the human psyche, its potential utility for counselors, although largely untapped, is considerable. Most theories of human development acknowledge to some degree the role of context in shaping human lives, but characterize environmental variables in a rather passive light relative to unfolding ontogeny. This is particularly true of developmental theorists like Piaget, Bowlby, and Lorenz, who with their orientation to internal process assume that individual development follows a biologically prescribed pathway on which the environment may impose some variation. Such theory does not adequately capture counselors' understanding of the active role that environment plays in shaping how we think, feel, and act.

In stark contrast to the more biologically oriented theorists, behavioral theorists like Pavlov, Skinner, and Bandura see the individual as a passive recipient of environmental input whose thought and action is largely controlled by external variables. These theorists place considerable importance on context, but they offer little understanding of the complex sociocultural and political nature of environment, the role of human agency, and the importance of individual biology. As is true of biological theory, behavioral theory is of limited use to counselors because it fails to capture the active role of the self in relation to issues of cultural diversity, social and political challenge, and significant events in the unfolding of human history.

CHAT addresses the conceptual shortfalls of both biological and learning models of development by providing counselors with an anchoring in contextualism while preserving the notion of human agency and acknowledging the importance of a healthy biological foundation. While maintaining the integrity of the autonomous individual, CHAT underscores the interactive multisystemic nature of human development, ranging from proximal family and community systems to larger social, cultural, and historical considerations. It will become apparent as the next part of this chapter unfolds that Vygotsky's proposed mechanism for transforming human consciousness can provide counselors with new and exciting ways to think about helping their clients to change in the face of painful systemic challenges. More specifically, the case study that follows demonstrates how integrating Vygotsky's vision into existing counseling theory could help counselors to facilitate human change in a manner that is consistent with the broad scope and vision of the profession.

## The Validity of CHAT

Unlike other theories of human development such as Erikson's theory of psychosocial development or Piaget's theory of cognitive development, CHAT does not have a long history of empirical studies that attest to the validity of Vygotsky's vision. It is important to note that testing the validity of a theory like CHAT is more complicated than testing structured theories like those of Erikson and Piaget. These more structured theories, which you will undoubtedly study as you work through the other chapters in this text, have clearly defined stages and elements of behavior or observable change at each stage of development that can easily be measured. Vygotsky's theory is much broader is scope, more abstract, and is more concerned with providing a framework for thinking about development than providing a specific road map that precisely articulates each incremental step in the developmental process. In present day research, CHAT most commonly provides a theoretical framework for qualitative studies tackling complex questions that focus on individuals in context. Thus the context and its reciprocal interplay with individual development is the primary aim of inquiry rather than an internal developmental mechanism. In such studies, development cannot be understood as a self-contained process that is stable over time but is viewed instead as a dynamic unfolding whose nature changes along with course of human history.

## The Utility of Vygotsky's Broad Vision

In spite of its lack of strict empirical validation, based on what we know about counseling theory and process, it is easy to see how Vygotsky's vision broadens the range of practice possibilities. In particular, Vygotsky provides us with a window into the change process and through techniques that stimulate metacognitive activity and target the ZPD, gives us a framework to build holistic knowledge of self-in-relation. The case illustration that follows actually scaffolds a client's journey through his ZPD while he attempts to resolve a shattering identity crisis and shows how the notion of metacognition can be used to augment the therapeutic process. In fact, as the case demonstrates the use of metacognition in counseling, it shows how knowledge of other developmental theories can be integrated into counseling sessions to help the clients step back and think metacognitively about their own developmental processes.

Although the practice of making strict developmental predictions is outside the purview of CHAT, it is this more general framework that broadens the general utility of the theory. The case here deals with an identity crisis in an adolescent boy, but the techniques used could just as easily have been utilized with a seventy-year-old woman or an eight-year-old girl. The usefulness of the CHAT approach extends across the lifespan, across cultures, and across the range of counseling venues. Thus, a mental health counselor could use CHAT to help a client work through her concerns about racism in the workplace, while a school counselor could help a child struggling with his family's responses to sexual identity issues. Likewise, a college counselor could use a Vygotskian approach to work a student through a vocational identity crisis.

An aspect of the broad, sweeping nature of CHAT that is particularly germane to the counseling profession is its effectiveness in bringing a wide range of contextual issues into the counseling arena. CHAT, for example, encourages clients to engage in critical analyses of contextual issues related to race, socioeconomic status, sexual identity, age, and ability. Additionally, Vygotsky's broad framework invites the integration of counseling techniques that encourage clients to process the feelings that they experience as they work through their therapeutic journey. It is my hope that you will embrace the challenge of this pioneering excursion into the use of Vygotsky's work in the counseling setting and that you will seize the opportunity to forge new ways of helping clients transcend painful life circumstances.

# Russell Jackson: A Painful Crisis of Identity

"I am so sick of you people! I am going to live my life the way I want to whether you like it or not! I am seventeen years old and if you don't get off my back I am out of here—I would rather live on the street than listen to your crap all day!" The door slams so hard that the china in the dish drain sends a rattling noise through the kitchen as Russell, the bane of his parents' current existence, screeches out of the driveway in his car.

It is another typical evening in the Jackson household. Russell, an enraged seventeen-year-old, is going through a stormy rebellious period where he seems to loathe everything associated with his parents and their way of life. Mr. and Mrs. Jackson are dismayed that their son, "who has gotten everything he has ever wanted without having to work for it," could be so ungrateful and hurtful. The growing rift between them is sad and distressing for everyone, and it is clear that without some intervention the damage to the relationship between Russell and his parents may become irreparable.

The problems in the Jackson household between the parents and their adolescent son will be used to illustrate how Vygotsky's understanding of consciousness development can be used to inform counseling practice. As a theorist associated with cognitive development, Vygotsky's insights are not commonly applied to counseling theory or process. But in spite of the fact that the name Vygotsky does not typically emerge in counseling discourse, there is considerable potential for application of the basic tenets of CHAT to a counseling practice that involves developmental issues. The case here illustrates how Vygotsky's work can be used to conceptualize developmental counseling theory and how these new iterations of theory can be used to construct a powerful counseling intervention strategy that we will call *Developmental Cultural-Historical Theory (DCHAT) Counseling*.

The case begins with a background sketch of the client, Russell, an adolescent boy entering his junior year of high school. The background is narrated from an "objective" third person perspective and describes the conditions that lead Russell to seek counseling. On the heels of this background information is an exposition of the case from Russell's perspective, followed by an analysis that is informed by Vygotsky's understanding of the relationship between context, language, activity, and consciousness. Particular emphasis will be placed on Vygotsky's understanding of the relationship between cognition, emotion, motivation, volition, and need, thus maximizing the potential for the use of his theory in conceptualizing developmental counseling case studies (Vygotsky, 1934/1986).

## Background Information

Russell is a seventeen-year-old boy who is persuaded by his track coach, Mr. Edwards, to seek counseling. It is apparent to Coach Edwards that Russell is just "not himself." During his freshman and sophomore years, Russell was a rising star on the track team. He was one of the most promising distance runners that the coach had trained in years. A combination of talent, dedication, and psychological "steadiness" provided Russell with the potential to be a top-notch contender. But junior year brought out a side of Russell that Coach Edwards found quite disturbing.

Russell, up to that point, exemplified the prototypical above-average, suburban kid—thick brown hair that neatly brushed the top of his ears, a slim but athletic build that could model the latest Abercrombie fashions, bright hazel eyes that reflected both compassion and intellect, a slim chiseled nose that was the perfect complement to a quick warm smile reflecting orthodontically-engineered perfection, and a plethora of social skills, good nature, and intellectual sophistication that made him a pleasure to have in class, a great candidate for student council president, and the kind of friend that any kid could confidently bring home to mom and dad.

Now the image has dramatically changed. The crown of rich brown hair now looks more like a shroud as it hangs limply below his chin line and the slender athletic body now looks gaunt. The bright hazel eyes reflect a dark sadness, and the warm smile seems both anxious and angry. Russell, who was once a remarkably good-natured, model student and friend now is a loner who displays an air of hostile disregard toward many of his former friends. The competitive drive that once propelled Russell, both on the track and in the classroom, had mysteriously vanished, replaced by long hours of escape through "alternative" music, experimentation with marijuana and alcohol, and video games.

When Coach Edwards first suggested that Russell should consider seeking the help of a counselor, his former star athlete viewed the suggestion as judgmental and meddling: "There is nothing wrong with me. People think that just because they can't control me that there is something wrong. I just want to live my life the way I want to live it!" Still, the palpable tension between Russell and those who had previously had a central role in his life was taking its toll on him. Although he felt that seeking counseling was tantamount to "caving in" and that it somehow exonerated those around him from assuming any responsibility for the growing rift, general unhappiness finally drove him to initiate counseling with Peter, a counselor with a private practice in the community.

## Russell's Personal Narrative

Russell has felt a growing discontent since he entered high school. Ever since he can remember, he has felt an intense pressure to succeed, but only now has he become aware of the degree to which this dominates every corner of his life:

> Everyone expects me to always be the best at everything all of the time. I never feel like I have a break from the pressure; I am "on" twenty-four/seven. Even things that are supposed to be fun, like sports, become this huge competition. Why can't I just relax and kick a ball around like everybody else?

According to Russell, he feels "indoctrinated" with a definition of success that translates into excelling in competitive sports, maintaining superlative grades, having leadership roles in extracurricular activities, bringing home the "right girl," and the "right friends," and maintaining a visual image that reflects his upper middle-class roots.

Russell firmly believes that most of what he has been taught about success and image has been dictated by his father who for twenty years has been what Russell calls "a slave to corporate America." For Russell this has translated into clothing with designer labels, a brand new Jeep Wrangler when he turned sixteen, many years of rejecting peers who did not fit the model of the White suburban ideal, expensive vacations, a plethora of enrichment activities, and a 3,200-square-foot house in a wealthy suburb with a top-notch school district. In both tacit and explicit ways, Russell has gotten the clear message that his life of privilege was a product of his father's achievement and that he is expected to keep the legacy alive: "I feel like if I don't strive toward a job that earns huge bucks that I will be considered a total failure . . . like I will be less of a person if I earn less than my father."

Russell feels that Coach Edwards, the man who first suggested that he talk to a counselor, is just like everyone else toward whom he is feeling a growing sense of hostility. Rather than valuing him for who he "really is," Coach Edwards is viewing him as an exploitable commodity and is "pushing" the idea of counseling in the hopes of preserving his star athlete:

> I don't think that he would really care if I dropped dead tomorrow as long as I ran a good race for him before I died. As far as

he is concerned, I am nothing more than a pair of legs that bring status to the team and lots of kudos for him.

Russell also feels that his parents are primarily interested in using him to "massage their own egos." Through his eyes, he sees that they are seeking their own affirmation through his stellar academic and athletic performances:

> They are just using me to make themselves look good. They really don't care what I want or how I want to live my life. They just want to be able to show their friends my name in the paper and then act like it is something that they actually achieved themselves.

Russell believes that his old friends, like the adults in his life, are not interested in the person that he "really is," but in the image of success, attractiveness, and popularity that he once projected and the status that was gained from having an association with him:

> I knew that if I stopped being so good at sports and wasn't getting super high grades that most of my friends would just drop me. There is a lot of pressure to fit into the mold and if you don't, it is like you don't exist. No one talks to you or includes you in anything unless you wear the right clothes and drive the right car.

## Counseling Strategy

With considerable reluctance, Russell agrees to some sessions with Peter. As a graduate student, Peter had encountered a human development professor with a strong background in CHAT, and this innovative counselor now seized the opportunity to integrate Vygotskian principles into his practice. Peter, in fact, finds a number of CHAT principles to be quite useful in the way he thinks about intervention. The first principle is that changes in consciousness (i.e., changes in how we think about things) come about as a consequence of activity that involves tool use, the most important of which is language. Peter understands that the primary tool used in counseling is language and that the types of activities that counselors facilitate are ideally suited to bring about desired changes in consciousness. Even in cases where counselors do not use language, such as in sand-play or drawing, Peter still recognizes that activities are rife with the potential for helping to change how people think about things.

The second principle that Peter deems useful in a counseling setting is the notion that consciousness and changes in consciousness are reflections of socioculturally and historically defined social relations that become internalized primarily through language-based activity. For Peter, it follows that consciousness becomes more developed when knowledge of cultural and historical roots of that consciousness are understood. Put in terms of the Vygotskian concept of metacognition (i.e., thinking about thinking), Peter sees that the clients' understanding of how social structure, culture, and history shape their own thought adds a sophisticated and useful dimension to metacognition.

The third CHAT principle embraced by Peter is that scaffolding in the ZPD facilitates changes in consciousness. He sees that the counselor, as facilitator, can act as an external form of consciousness and by helping the client to restructure their thoughts within the zone, create optimal conditions for development in the form of changes in consciousness. Peter knows that if the counselor is interested in working with the client in the ZPD, he or she must ascertain the client's current level of development in relation to a particular developmental trajectory, determine how much additional growth is possible in the course of the counseling relationship, and build a scaffolding in the course of the therapy that will facilitate the aspect of development in question.

The fourth principle that Peter utilizes is that development occurs as the result of a dialectical process that resolves disequilibrium (i.e., conflict) between old and new forms of consciousness. He knows that it is rarely the case that one mode of thought is completely eclipsed by a new and more developed one. Rather, the old is reconciled with the new through a dialectical mechanism that generates a consonant alternative. Peter is mindful of the notion that disequilibrium can be cognitive, affective, motivational, and/or volitional.

After listening to Russell tell his story, together Russell and Peter decide to pursue three key areas of exploration. First, they will attempt to expand the notion of what Russell means when he makes references to "who he really is." Second, they will try to understand the key developmental activities that precipitated the dramatic changes and intense feelings experienced by Russell. Third, they will attempt to get a handle on what Russell needs to do so that he can resolve the overwhelming conflict that is driving him into isolation and reestablish meaningful and productive close relationships with family and friends. These three areas of exploration will provide the target for client change and will be managed within the general guidelines of a Developmental Cultural-Historical Activity Theory (DCHAT) counseling framework. The general steps comprising this framework are listed below and each is followed by a more detailed understanding of how Russell and Peter are able to work through these four steps.

## Four-Step DCHAT Counseling Framework

*Step 1:* In dialogue with the client, identify the specific aspect or aspects of development that is/are most germane to her or his current concerns.

Russell and Peter spend considerable time thoughtfully and collaboratively elaborating Russell's story and making sense of the powerful emotions and dramatic changes that have swept through his life in recent months. In the course of their conversations, it becomes clear to both of them, that in his day-to-day life, Russell is both implicitly and explicitly expressing deep distress around the issue of "who I really am." Russell feels that much of his social and academic disengagement is a reflection of his disenchantment with "the realities of his old life." He feels "uncomfortable in his own skin," and close relationships that at one time gave him a sense of security and belonging are often unsatisfying, laborious, and engender feeling of sadness, loneliness, and anger.

Over the course of their conversation, it is apparent to Peter that Russell is undergoing a major developmental shift in self-identity, and that this shift has thrown him into a distressful state of affective and cognitive disequilibrium. Peter recognizes that to reach a new state of equilibrium, his client would likely benefit from a deep exploration of identity development. Although Russell has some insight into his emotional turmoil, he is unable to articulate the exact nature of the changes, how they have come about, why they are causing problems in relationships, and why he has turned to behaviors that are sometimes self-sabotaging.

*Step 2:* Using a scaffolding activity, bolster the client's metacognitive insight into how development unfolds in relation to their identified developmental concern(s).

Peter provides a general scaffolded structure that allows Russell to "think about how to think about" self-identity development within a multidimensional framework. Because Peter is attempting to use Vygotskian principles in his work, he wants to ensure that sociocultural and historical dimensions of self-identity development are included in how

Russell thinks about his concept of "self." Prior to his work with Russell, Peter, as the counselor, would need to integrate his own understanding of identity development into a coherent, multidimensional model to successfully facilitate this type of dialogue with his client.

By combining his understanding of human development and the principles of CHAT, Peter compiles the following list of concepts to help him structure his discussion with Russell concerning self-identity: Self-identity is formed by a multiplicity of dimensions, including the need for relatedness; expressions of identity coming from parents, other relatives, and close friends; biological factors such as temperament and capacity for thought; social norms transmitted through relationships, educational institutions, media, and community; and role expectations dictated by multicultural factors such as race, class, gender, ability, appearance, age, and religion. Self-identity is plastic and thus changes over time in relation to sociocultural factors and personal history. Changes in self-identity are likely to come about due to changes that include major life events, new relationships that are emotionally or intellectually provocative, and other shifting conditions in the social environment that might cause individuals to question their basic assumptions. Self-identity in the Vygotskian tradition is not merely a cognitive construct, but one that also involves motivation, volition, and affect—emotional wants and needs that will impact how one thinks and sees and what one chooses to assimilate.

Through conversation, Peter is able to determine Russell's current level of development in relation to how he thinks about identity or, in Vygoskian terms, the degree to which Russell has developed his metacognitive capacities concerning issues of self-identity. Peter then walks Russell through a series of scaffolded conversations that will allow his client to build a thorough understanding of how identity is constituted. A small segment of this scaffolded conversation dealing with how social class values become a part of self-identity might resemble the following:

*Peter:* "What do you think makes you who you are?"

*Russell:* "I guess that I was mostly born this way and the rest I picked up because my parents made me become certain things."

*P:* "Do you think that your parents got together and decided that they would impose certain things on you? If not, how did they decide what things were important enough to try to make them a part of your identity?"

*R:* "That's a good question. Maybe they didn't have big discussions but just let everything happen sort of naturally."

*P:* "Are you saying that you think that maybe they didn't make conscious decisions—that maybe they acted in ways that are just normal for them?"

*R:* "I guess so, but they are always telling me I have to take responsibility for my actions so how come they don't have to take responsibility for theirs?"

*P:* "That is a very important question. Would it be okay with you if we came back to it a bit later after we try to figure out the answer to the question of how you became who you are?"

*R:* "Sure, as long as we don't let them get by without having to be accountable."

*P:* "That's a deal. So, back to the things that your parents would like you to be. What things do you think your parents would most like you to incorporate into your identity?"

*R:* "They want me to have the drive to be successful and to want all of the material things that they have. They also want me to be competitive about everything from school to sports to music to whatever. They want me to like girls who look like models and who come from families that have money . . . I could go on with this forever!"

*P:* "How do you think that they came to want these things? Were they born with these ideas? Did they just stumble on them naturally?"

*R:* "I think that it is just what you do to get ahead, which is what everyone wants to do. I guess that is what everyone wants although I think I heard somewhere that Native Americans were not competitive and were not that interested in accumulating a lot of material things."

*P:* "So perhaps this is not a natural thing?"

*R:* "No, I guess that we must learn it from the people around us who learn it from the people around them, who learn it from TV, magazines, movies, and who knows where else. I guess it is all part of the middle-class dream."

*P:* "So a part of your identity has to do with middle-class values that are reinforced in many corners of our daily existence and that become what appears to be a natural way of life?"

At first glance, Step 2 may appear to be a didactic diversion from Russell's intense array of feelings and conflicts. However, the purpose of bolstering Russell's metacognitive insights into identity development is to give him the tools to make sense of his current state of distress and *to help him take charge of resolving his own change process.* This step will give Russell the tools to understand how he arrived at his current thoughts and feelings, how those thoughts and feelings have served him, and how he can best resolve his distress without sacrificing the most important basic values and needs that comprise self-identity. Ideally, Peter will be able to shape the discussion so that Russell is able to understand the breadth of sources of identity and how they are transmitted.

*Step 3:* Using newly acquired metacognitive insight, explore the client's personal developmental trajectory including beginning and end points of the current developmental crisis and sources of disequilibrium (i.e., conflict).

According to Vygotsky, developmental processes are triggered when new circumstances arise that disrupt an individual's current state of developmental equilibrium. Consciousness cannot accommodate the new set of circumstances, and a state of disequilibrium is thus created. Through a dialectical process, generally involving language-related activity, a new level of development emerges that is characterized by an alteration in consciousness and reestablished equilibrium. By utilizing this understanding of the developmental process, Peter acts as an external form of consciousness, and in doing so provides Russell with the cognitive scaffolding that he needs to reach a new developmental equilibrium in relation to his current disequilibrated state of self-identity development.

Using the scaffolding that Peter provides as a way of thinking about his identity development, Russell is able to trace the roots of his current state of disequilibrium to a relationship that began when he joined the staff of the school newspaper during his freshman year. It was at this time that Russell met Manny, a cerebral, artistic, and somewhat unconventional junior. Manny, who was greatly influenced by his "alternative" parents, had decided that he was not going to become part of the "frenetic, cut-throat, high-achievement culture of suburban high schools." Manny spent much of his time writing fiction and poetry, working with an urban organization devoted to social justice issues, and backpacking.

Although Russell and Manny were "very different people," Russell was drawn to Manny's critical eye. Over the two years in high school that their paths crossed, Russell increasingly questioned his own direction and values, which, when he met Manny, were undeniably consonant with his new friend's portrait of the typical suburban high school student. Initially, their interactions were limited to the afterschool time spent working on the newspaper, but slowly the time expanded into weekends and summers. During this time, Russell's old circle of friends remained his primary contact. His parents' and friends' discomfort with Manny was palpable, so that most of his time with his new friend was limited to one-on-one activities and encounters outside the home. By the end of his sophomore year, Russell was feeling like he was leading a double life. Not only was he questioning his role as the "model high school student," Manny's influence spurred him to think differently about his place in the world, his commitment to a socially responsible life, and the personal growth he sacrificed by "clinging to the suburban dream." These thoughts left Russell confused about the direction his life was taking, angry that he had been "brainwashed" by his parents, resentful that they did not extend the same cordiality to Manny that they offered to his more conventional friends, and feeling empty, sad, and "incomplete" from trying to live in "two different worlds." By all counts, Russell had entered a Vygotskian state of disequilibrium.

In the summer prior to Russell's junior year, before Manny prepared to leave for college, the two shared an extended backpacking experience that marked a significant turning point in their relationship and "made going back impossible." Russell realized that being out in the woods with Manny and "looking at the world through different eyes" he felt closer to his unique friend than to anyone else he had ever known, and for the first time since he could remember, "living felt completely natural." The encounter was bittersweet, however, in that Manny would be moving out of state in a few short weeks leaving Russell to find his way among parents, teachers, and old friends who would "never understand" his changing priorities. Russell experienced feelings of alienation, loneliness, loss, and anger as he began his school year.

Now that Russell was able to articulate the factors that catalyzed his developmental identity changes, he and Peter focused on areas of Russell's emergent identity that created serious personal conflicts in his day-to-day life. Using his understanding of identity as socioculturally, relationally, and biologically constructed, Russell described his primary area of concern. In his pursuit of a superlative academic, athletic, and extracurricular profile, he was "living someone else's dream of success." He understood that his parents had worked hard to create the conditions for their family to live the "twenty-first-century American dream" and that up to this point he had successfully "carried on the tradition." But Manny had changed the way he saw the world, and along with that came a change in priorities.

Russell was not sure how this change in priorities would ultimately "play out," but he knew that he would need considerable room to "explore the world outside of AP courses and a house in the burbs." He was quite sure that this exploration would be difficult for his parents, teachers, and friends, and that it would likely cause him considerable social conflict. Peter encouraged Russell to talk about the feelings that his insights created. With some help and encouragement, Russell was able to express the anger he felt toward his parents for, as he stated, "forcing me into a lifestyle that doesn't allow me to really live." He described a similar anger toward his old friends whom he felt were "like sheep," and at the same time felt sad and anxious at having lost important connections with people who had been the center of his life for many years. Interactions with his parents and former circle of friends seemed "empty and distant" and fueled Russell's feelings of loneliness and alienation. Russell admitted that even though it "wasn't a problem," that he would occasionally use marijuana or alcohol to attempt a "brief escape from the emptiness." More often than not, the substance use made him feel more alone and was, therefore, something that he realized was not a solution.

*Step 4:* Consider the conflict (i.e., disequilibrium) generated by the developmental progression and how that conflict can be resolved dialectically. Remember that conflict can arise on a cognitive, affective, motivational, or volitional level.

Peter and Russell spent considerable time exploring Russell's feelings about his parents and former friends, and worked collaboratively to consider how some of these feelings might be resolved. Russell began by focusing on his parents. With his new understanding of self-identity, Russell was able to see that his parents' identity was also constituted through powerful sociocultural forces. He recalled numerous wrenching stories about his grandparents' experience with the Great Depression, making it clear to Peter that this historical event left a deep imprint on his parents. Russell and Peter speculated about how the sudden scarcity in resources might make families feel that material accumulation was a matter of survival. They also talked about how the contemporary world of work had splintered Russell's extended family by moving his father to many different locations around the country. Russell insightfully suggested that his parents perhaps thought that they could "try to buy the safety and security that they lost by having to move far away from home." Russell and Peter also talked about the barrage of media pressure to accumulate material goods and how difficult it is to resist the message that material wealth equates to success.

With Peter's input, Russell was able to reframe his parents' lifestyle and understand it as being partially rooted in security and survival. He was also able to see that his parents were trying to impose life choices on him in an attempt to ensure his future safety and security. Although he still felt some anger that his mother and father could not think more critically about their lifestyle or about what they were tacitly imposing on him, Russell was clearly able to make significant strides toward engaging his parents in a productive dialogue that would hopefully engender mutual respect and allow them to find common understanding.

With Peter, Russell was also able to reframe his view of his old friends. Russell became more cognizant of the pressures imposed by contemporary youth culture and was thus able to make sense of his friends' focus on appearance, consumption, and success. He also understood that like his mother and father, his friends' parents were attempting to ensure security and safety for their children's future and were thus imposing pressure on them to emulate a "successful" lifestyle. Russell came to terms with the fact that it was unlikely that his friends would change significantly during their remaining time in high school. Together, he and Peter brainstormed strategies to make certain that he would have a rich and satisfying social life during his junior and senior years. Russell decided that he would pursue several new social venues in the hopes of finding more like-minded friends. He decided that he would join some organizations in school that attracted less popular and more politically active students, and that he would also pursue activities with socially active groups in the city. Russell would still maintain contact with his old friends, but his expectations were changed and he would not anticipate that they would be his sole social outlet.

Peter also thought that it was important that he and Russell try to find "a new state of equilibrium" regarding his client's long-standing interest in distance running. After considerable introspection, Russell was able to think beyond his aversion to competition, and became more mindful of the rewards that his sport offered. He began to think of the running as a foundation for a healthy mind and body, and recalled the mental clarity, inner peace, high energy level, and feelings of harmony with the natural surroundings that he felt before he became consumed with resentment. He decided to rededicate himself to the running for the purposes of maximizing his physical and mental potential for the service of self and other. The combination of his recommitment to running and his hope for building new relationships eliminated Russell's interest in substance use.

## Conclusion

Developmental crises comprise a regular part of counseling practice. The work of Vygotsky, with its focus on cognitive development, and more specifically on development of consciousness, is quite germane to a wide array of developmental issues including moral development, cultural identity development, gender identity development, and career development. The case of Russell, a clear example of an adolescent identity development crisis, illustrates several key principles espoused by Vygotsky that are useful in conceptualization of the counseling process.

Peter, using Vygotskian principles, was able to ascertain that Russell was experiencing disequilibrium precipitated by a disparity between his newly emerging self-identity and the beliefs of those with whom he has had close relationships. Russell had not yet developed his consciousness to the point were he was able to reconcile the differences that he had with the people in his life. Peter, working in Russell's ZPD, gave him the metacognitive tools that he needed to resolve much of this disequilibrium and thus facilitated this chapter in Russell's identity development.

# Summary

Although Vygotsky did not attempt to use his theory to address problems and questions in counseling, the utility of his work in this setting is clear. By incorporating Vygotsky's understanding of various dimensions of consciousness—such as cognition, volition, motivation, need, and affect—into his work on the ZPD, scaffolding, language-based activity, and metacognition, counselors dealing with developmental issues can construct activities, based primarily on language, that can assist clients attempting to resolve developmental conflicts or crises. Unlike other theories of cognitive development that conceptualize cognition simply as a function of knowledge capacity, Vygotsky's notion that feeling, need, and motivation are important components in knowledge assimilation is more in line with counselors' holistic understanding of growth and change. Hence CHAT is compatible with a wide range of counseling orientations and can comfortably be used across a variety of counseling settings to conceptualize client transformation.

A key benefit, for counselors, of Vygotsky's theoretical vision is its capacity to help clients think critically about the complex circumstances of their lives. As an adjunct to counseling theory, CHAT attends to the larger systemic forces that contribute to the client's sense of self. For example, the college student who is experiencing a career decision crisis can understand that crisis not only in the context of talents, abilities, and interest, but also in arenas such as ethnic/racial identity, social class experiences, Western values, and parental identity. Helping clients to understand their "multidimensional selves" allows them to work toward multidimensional transformations. Not only can clients attend to personal thoughts and feelings, they are able to look outside of themselves for solutions. Awareness of the power of the larger social, cultural, and historical milieu in shaping human beings gives clients the impetus to act as change agents on their own and others behalf. This awareness also makes race, ethnicity, sexual orientation, age, and ability central considerations in psychological wellness and self-understanding. Hence CHAT is consistent with the social activism and social justice themes that characterize the counseling mission and is aligned with the multicultural foundations of counseling practice.

Although the complexity of CHAT can be quite daunting, it is this same complexity that makes it so valuable for the counseling profession and for development scholars more generally. As counselors, we are in the practice of studying human nature; and if anything is clear, it is that humans are very complex beings. Vygotsky, rather than attempting to capture human nature in a capsulated, controlled theory, chose to embrace the complex, multidimensional nature of development. As counselors, it is our job to follow in the footsteps of Vygotsky by embracing the complex, multidimensional nature of our clients and to know that we will spend our lives trying to unravel the depth of human nature. It is my hope that the spirit of CHAT provides inspiration for us in "knowing that we do not know."

## Annotated Bibliography

Lev Vygotsky Archive. (n.d.). Retrieved January 28, 2005, from http://www2 .cddc.vt.edu/marxists/archive/vygotsky/index.htm
  The Lev Vygotsky Archive provides an engaging biographical sketch of Vygotsky's life and contains links to excerpts of key Vygotsky works. Vygotsky's close collaborators Luria and Leont'ev, as well as other scholars from the "Vygotsky School," are also represented with biographical material and links to important samples of their scholarship. This site provides direct access to a treasure trove of literature and is of particular interest for those wanting to understand how Vygotsky influenced some of his most renowned students and colleagues.

Meyer, D. K. (1993). What is scaffolded instruction? Definitions, distinguishing features, and misnomers. In D. J. Leu & C. K. Kinzer (Eds.), *Examining central issues in literacy research, theory, and practice: Forty-second yearbook of The National Reading Conference* (pp. 41–53). Washington, DC: National Reading Conference.

Meyer offers an in-depth view of scaffolding theory and describes the elements of effective scaffolding, many of which have direct application to counselor–client co-constructive processes. Elements include student/client support, shared dialogue, nonjudgmental collaboration, and choosing an appropriate level of instruction.

Tucker, R. C. (Ed.). (1978). *The Marx-Engels Reader*. New York: Norton.

This sweeping anthology of Marxist thought includes translations of many of the original works of Marx and Engels that had direct influence on the young Vygotsky. Arranged to reflect the chronological and topical progression of Marx's thought throughout his lifetime, the text provides a comprehensive introduction to the range of Marxist philosophy. This compendium edited by Tucker is of particular use to counselors interested in deconstruction of Vygotsky's thought as well as the work of other counseling theorists.

University of Helsinki, Center for Developmental Activity and Research Work. (2003–2004). Retrieved on January 28, 2005, from achttp://www.edu .helsinki.fi/activity/pages/chatanddwr/chat/.

This site offers a window into contemporary iterations of CHAT. For the counseling researcher interested in establishing a research project based on Vygotskian principles, this website provides an excellent springboard for exploration of the complex and compelling expansions of CHAT that have occurred in contemporary development scholarship.

Vygotsky and Cultural-Historical Activity Theory. (n.d.). Retrieved January 28, 2005, from http://129.171.53.1/blantonw/5dClhse/publications/ bibliography/bib_vycult.html

This web page, part of a larger site from the University of Miami, contains a sizable compilation of key texts related to Vygotsky and CHAT. The page contains links to the remainder of the website, which provides readers with the details of a CHAT-based university–community afterschool action research project. Although this project deals primarily with issues in education, it may be of particular relevance to counselors interested in applying CHAT in the context of larger systemic intervention strategies or community-based action research.

Vygotsky, L. S. (1978). *Mind in society: The development of higher psychological processes* (M. Cole, V. John-Steiner, S. Scribner, & S. Souberman, Eds.). Cambridge, MA: Harvard University Press.

*Mind in Society* is a collection of important Vygotsky essays edited by a group of distinguished Vygotsky scholars. The text includes works pertaining to theory, methodological considerations, and educational implementation. Vygoskian concepts germane to counseling practice including scaffolding, the ZPD, and the internalization of social and historical meaning are presented in translations of the original works. This very popular Vygotsky text, widely used in cognitive development classrooms, addresses core issues in his thinking.

Vygotsky, L. S. (1986). *Thought and language* (A. Kozulin, Rev. Trans.). Cambridge, MA: MIT Press. (Original work published in 1934)
*Thought and Language*, one of Vygotsky's later works, contains compelling insights into the complex multidimensional mechanisms that constitute thought. Diverging far from the notion that thought is essentially a reflection of speech, Vygotsky elaborates a view of consciousness that integrates biology, individual experience, and sociocultural activity. This text is particularly useful for counselors wanting a more detailed understanding of some of the basic principles of CHAT germane to counseling practice.

Wertsch, J. V. (Ed.). (1985). *Culture, communication, and cognition: Vygotskian perspectives*. Cambridge: Cambridge University Press.
Wertsch has gathered an impressive group of Vygotskian scholars to provide an in-depth analysis of an array of centrally important themes in Vygotsky's work. Noted contributors such as Jerome Bruner, Michael Cole, Sylvia Scribner, V. P. Zinchenko, and V. V. Davydov, to name a few, provide insight into the foundations of Vygotskian theory, explore the notion of semiotics in relation to Vygotsky's original writing, and expand applications of his theory to educational and developmental venues. Because of its intense focus on theory fundamentals, this book is particularly useful for counselors interested in considering how Vygotsky's work can be used to augment extant counseling theory.

# References

Blanck, G. (1992). Vygotsky: The man and his cause. In L. C. Moll (Ed.), *Vygotsky and education: Instructional implications and applications of sociohistorical psychology* (pp. 31–58). New York: Cambridge University Press.

Bruner, J. (1985). Vygotsky: A historical and conceptual perspective. In J. V. Wertsch (Ed.), *Culture and communication: Vygotskian perspectives* (pp. 21–34). New York: Cambridge University Press.

Caird, E. (1883). *Hegel*. Edinburgh and London: William Blackwood. Retrieved June 29, 2006 from: http://www.gwfhegel.org/Books/CAIRD.html #Pref

Cole, M. (n.d.). *A Brief Overview of Luria's Life and Work*. Retrieved August 2, 2006, From Marxists Internet Archive website: http://www.marxists.org/archive/luria/ comments/bio.htm.

Cole, M. (1997). *Alexander Luria, Cultural Psychology and the Resolution of the Crisis in Psychology*. Retrieved August 2, 2006, from University of

California, San Diego, Department of Communication website: http://lchc
.ucsd.edu/People/Localz/MCole/luria.html

Davydov, V. V., & Radzikhovskii, L. A. (1985). Vygotsky and activity-oriented
psychology. In J. V. Wertsch (Ed.), *Culture and communication: Vygotskian perspectives* (pp. 35–65). New York: Cambridge University Press.

Engels, F. (1979). *Dialectics of Nature* (C. Dutt, Trans.). New York: International Publishers. (Original work published in 1925)

Engström, Y. (1987). *Learning by expanding: An activity-theoretical approach to
developmental research.* Helsinki: Orienta-Konsultit.

German, L. (1994). Frederick Engels: Life of a revolutionary. *International
Socialism Journal, 64.* Retrieved June 29, 2006, from http://pubs.socialist
reviewindex.org.uk/isj65/contents.htm

Kozulin, A. (1987). Vygotsky in context. In L. Vygotsky, *Thought and language*
(A. Kozulin, Rev. Trans.). Cambridge, MA: MIT Press. (Original work published in 1934)

Leont'ev, A. N. (1981). *Problems of the development of the mind.* Moscow: Progress
Publishers. (Original work published in 1959)

Marx, K. (1978a). Economic and philosophic manuscripts of 1844. In R. C. Tucker
(Ed.), *The Marx-Engels Reader* (pp. 3–6). New York: Norton. (Original work
published in 1932)

Marx, K. (1978b). Theses on Feuerbach. In R. C. Tucker (Ed.), *The Marx-Engels
Reader* (pp. 143–145). New York: Norton. (Original work published in 1845)

Marx, K. (1978c). Marx on the history of his opinions. In R. C. Tucker (Ed.),
*The Marx-Engels Reader* (pp. 3–6). New York: Norton. (Original work published in 1859)

Newman, F., & Holzman, L. (1993). *Lev Vygotsky: Revolutionary scientist.* New
York: Routledge.

University of California, San Diego (n.d.). *Department of Communication Faculty.*
Retrieved June 29, 2006, from http://communication.ucsd.edu/people/
f_cole.html.

van der Veer, R., & Valsiner, J. (1991). *Understanding Vygotsky: A quest for synthesis.* Cambridge, MA: Blackwell.

Vygodskaya, G. L. (1995). His life. *School Psychology International, 16,* 105–116.

Vygotsky, L. S. (1978). *Mind in society: The development of higher psychological
processes* (M. Cole, V. John-Steiner, S. Scribner, & S. Souberman, Eds.). Cambridge, MA: Harvard University Press.

Vygotsky, L. S. (1986). *Thought and language* (A. Kozulin, Rev. Trans.). Cambridge, MA: MIT Press. (Original work published in 1934)

Vygotsky, L. S. (1987). The problem of will and its development in childhood.
In R. W. Reiber & A. S. Carton (Eds.), *The collected works of L. S. Vygotsky*
(pp. 351–358). (Vol. I, N. Minick, Trans.). New York: Plenum Press. (Original work published in 1932)

Washington University St. Louis (2006). *James V. Wertsch.* Retrieved from
http://artsci.wustl.edu/~anthro/blurb/b_wertsch.htm

Wertsch, J. V. (1985). Introduction. In J. V. Wertsch (Ed.), *Culture and communication: Vygotskian perspectives* (pp. 1–18). New York: Cambridge University Press.

Wertsch, J. V., & Stone, C. A. (1985). The concept of internalization. In J. V. Wertsch (Ed.), *Culture and communication: Vygotskian perspectives* (pp. 162–179). New York: Cambridge University Press.

Zinchenko, V. P. (1985). Vygotsky and units for the analysis of mind. In J. V. Wertsch (Ed.), *Culture and communication: Vygotskian perspectives* (pp. 94–118). New York: Cambridge University Press.

# CHAPTER FIVE

# Robert Kegan's Subject-Object Theory of Development

## Karen Eriksen

R obert Kegan's work was introduced to me in my last year of doctoral work. I had nearly eighteen years of clinical work and twelve of supervisory work. I was primarily a structural family therapist, with competency and contextual flavors added to the usual mix, and had been struck by how little explanation we often had for the failures in our work. Kegan and other adult developmentalists' theories finally gave me, my students, and my supervisees a perspective on these failures, that is, we were using therapeutic strategies for creating change that were "over the heads" of our clients (Kegan, 1994). We were choosing a theory that we preferred, as we had been urged to do in graduate school, and assuming that it should work with all of our clients. From a developmental perspective (and perhaps from other perspectives), this approach was doomed to fail with some clients. Kegan's developmental theory offered us suggestions for successful strategies when our previous strategies had failed.[1]

Robert Kegan's constructive developmental theory is a stage theory that extends Piagetian thinking (Piaget, 1963) into adulthood. It has been largely absent in counselor training programs, although when presented students show great enthusiasm for the theory. This is no doubt because it offers a powerful guide for personal and professional development.

---

[1]This chapter includes some reorganized material from the following articles in the *Family Journal* and is included with permission from Sage Publications: Counseling the Imperial Client, by K. P. Eriksen (2007), *The Family Journal,* 15, 174–182; The Constructive Developmental Theory of Robert Kegan, by K. P. Eriksen (2006), *The Family Journal,* 14(3), 290–298.

## ABOUT THE CHAPTER AUTHOR

Constructive developmental theory has changed my life, personally and professionally. My teaching, supervision, research, writing, and clinical work have been profoundly affected by the hopefulness of this theory and by its ability to explain failures that emerge from practicing traditionally. The theory is rarely presented in counseling programs (except student affairs counseling), but students have universally felt as excited as I when learning about the theory. I hope my passion for this theory will be "caught" by you as you realize how positively it can affect your work as well.

I received my doctorate from George Mason University and my master's degree from California State University, Fullerton. My

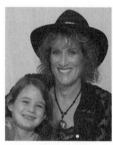

**Karen Eriksen and daughter**

doctoral study emphasized family therapy, counselor education, supervision, and counselor advocacy. I practiced most recently in Virginia while licensed as a Professional Counselor and Marriage and Family Counselor. I spent eighteen years as a mental health and community agency counselor, gaining specialties in family therapy, addictions, survivors of sexual abuse, and the intersection of spirituality and counseling. I then re-careered and began teaching counseling in 1993. I am a Nationally Certified Counselor, an AAMFT Clinical Member, and an AAMFT Approved Supervisor. I wrote the first book on the counselor advocacy, *Making an Impact: A Handbook on Counselor Advocacy*. I have also co-authored three books on counselor education: *Preparing Counselors and Therapists: Creating Constructivist and Developmental Programs, Teaching Counselors and Therapists: Constructivist and Developmental Course Design,* and *Teaching Strategies for Constructivist and Developmental Counselor Education.* My most recent book is *Beyond the DSM Story: Challenges, Quandaries, and Solutions.* My research areas are counselor preparation, constructive development, multicul-turalism, and spirituality. I have been active in leadership of several state and national professional associations and regularly present workshops on advocacy, counselor preparation, and constructive development at local, state, and national conferences.

Personally, students find in Kegan's theory an explanation for their own life experiences at different ages, which leads to the relief of self-understanding about the "whys" of those experiences and to an awareness of how they might progress developmentally. Familiarity with the theory brings about developmental growth, and growth leads to a kinder, gentler, more growth enhancing attitude toward those in one's surround. That is, the escape from a pathologizing, mental illness perspective reduces blaming and anger, and empowers the theory's user to strategically and intentionally support and challenge friends, partners, and family members toward further growth and capacities.

Professionally, students find that Kegan's theory offers a developmental grid for assessing clients so as to determine the therapies that are most likely to be effective and the ways to implement those therapies in optimally supportive and challenging ways. The theory also explains why counseling strategies from certain theoretical perspectives are not helpful for particular clients. This chapter, of course, primarily focuses on ways to apply the theory professionally.

Finally, for those who move beyond counseling practice into counselor education, supervision, or administration, Kegan's theory offers a guide to counselor educators, supervisors, and other leaders for promoting the development of counselors-in-training and others under their purview.

## Subject Object Theory

In *The Evolving Self* (1982) and *In Over Our Heads* (1994), Robert Kegan introduced his version of constructive developmental theory. His model extends Piagetian-style stages of development into adulthood, and concerns itself with regular and progressive changes in how individuals make meaning or "know" epistemologically. Each stage, way of knowing, position, domain, balance, or order of consciousness represents the set of common organizing principles that individuals use in constructing experience. With helpful environments, people's epistemological growth can continue throughout the lifespan; only in childhood are the stages associated with particular ages. Table 5.1 offers information on characteristics of each stage, along with guidelines for counselors, teachers, parents, and others about how to optimally support and challenge people in particular stages. Some terminology in the table may be unfamiliar to readers, but will be further explained as the chapter progresses.

TABLE 5.1  Kegan's Subject-Object Theory

| Stages or Balances | Characteristics | Support or Match | Challenge or Mismatch |
|---|---|---|---|
| **Incorporative** (Infancy to 2) | • Aware of own immediate needs<br>• Unaware of the "other"<br>• Dependent upon and merged with caretaker<br>• Surround is extension of self<br>• *Subject to:* reflexes, sensing, and moving | • Caregivers need to hold them; to offer them close physical contact, comfort, protection, and eye contact | • Provide timely differentiation<br>• Reduce carrying and meeting every need<br>• Acknowledge independence and willful refusal |
| **Impulsive** (2–7 years old) | • Short attention span, particularly related to others' needs or desires<br>• Hard time sitting still<br>• Unpredictable movement<br>• Fantasies predominate<br>• Aware of others, but confuse their impulses with caregiver's<br>• Language only one means of communication<br>• *Make object:* reflexes<br>• *Subject to:* impulses & perceptions | • Be able to receive child's love<br>• Appreciate spontaneity<br>• Hold child securely when not loved<br>• Encourage fantasy, intense attachment, and rivalry | • Set limits clearly to teach boundaries between parents and child and to encourage self-regulation<br>• Parents who have not grown beyond interpersonal stage will have trouble setting limits |
| **Imperial** (8–11 + years old) | • Interests, hobbies, "enduring dispositions," self-concept all develop<br>• Commitment to competence in these areas develops<br>• More self-sufficient<br>• Movement into "peer gang" that helps socialization<br>• Full awareness of others' differences from self | • Give clear behavioral directions<br>• Spell out consequences for following or not following<br>• Offer incentives for socially acceptable behavior<br>• Support developing competence in hobbies, interests, peer relationships | • Challenge to attend to social norms or rules of right and wrong behavior<br>• Urge attention to others' feelings and needs<br>• Suggest ways to reconcile their needs with the need to maintain relationships |

| Stage | Characteristics | | Encourage |
|---|---|---|---|
| *(continued)* | • Others exist to meet own needs<br>• Worry about consequences, but no real guilt<br>• Need authorities to direct them<br>• *Make object:* impulses & perceptions<br>• *Subject to:* needs, wishes, interests | | Encourage:<br>• Thinking about why they are doing what they are doing<br>• Examining inner urges<br>• Deciding whether preserving relationships at all costs is helpful<br>• Self definition<br>• Self reflection |
| **Interpersonal**<br>(after age 20) | • Good, productive, rule following citizens with meaningful lives<br>• Fully socialized into (and determined by) values, ideals, beliefs of their surround<br>• Trustworthy, employable<br>• Have insight & consciousness<br>• Think of future consequences before acting<br>• Have friends/family with whom relationships are ultimate<br>• Determined by others; need to be approved of and not rock boat<br>• No intimacy, only fusion<br>• Able to tolerate those who are different only from a distance<br>• *Make Object:* needs<br>• *Subject to:* relationships & rules | • Express appreciation of and encourage all of the advances of the interpersonal stage (maintaining relationships, expressing feelings, behaving responsibly, tuning in to others' needs, etc.)<br>• Give clear direction and provide structure | |
| **Institutional**<br>(reached by 20%–30% of adults) | • Well-defined and protected boundaries; competing roles well balanced<br>• Self-controlled, self-defining, self-initiating, self-directing, self-evaluating | Encourage & validate institutional characteristics:<br>• Developing own ideas, thoughts, & projects<br>• Making own decisions | Encourage:<br>• Exploring higher principles behind institutions, systems, theories |

(*Continued*)

**TABLE 5.1** (Continued)

| | | | |
|---|---|---|---|
| **Institutional** (continued) | • Leaders with vision that they induct others into; masters in their work<br>• Live out self-determined theory, ideology, or values<br>• Able to think systemically, seeing their relationship to the whole<br>• Stand their ground in conflict, while also hearing others' position; able to compromise<br>• Closeness & distinctness possible in relationships<br>• *Make object:* relationships & roles<br>• *Subject to:* institutions, career positions, systems within which they operate | • Carefully weighing choices among values or ideologies<br>• Choosing and acting on the basis of own ideology<br>• Setting clear limits to allow pursuit of own life projects<br>• Differentiation in relationships<br>• Independence | • Hearing negative reports as valuable input<br>• Pursuing connections as well as independence, particularly with those who are different<br>• Perceiving each interpersonal encounter as an opportunity to create something bigger than what is possible alone |
| **Interindividual** (not earlier than age 40) | • Understand interdependence in which distinctiveness is preserved while creating a context for connections<br>• Oriented toward tension, dynamism, or relationships between systems of deciding<br>• Perceive movement, process, and change as irreducible features of reality, and focus on these, rather than products<br>• Have no need to resolve contradictions or paradoxes<br>• Become less certain, more tentative<br>• *Make object:* institutions, systems, theories—so can stand back and see, and negotiate relationships among them | • Attend to and encourage each of the interindividual characteristics<br>• Attend to one's own development in order to understand and be able to encourage these characteristics | |

Kegan's (1982, 1994) model incorporates all emotional, relational, and cognitive functioning into each stage. The stages, which are described in more detail below, are: the Incorporative Balance, in which reflexes are primary (Stage 0); the Impulsive Balance, in which knowing is only about one's own immediate impulses (Stage 1); the Imperial Balance, in which the individual is aware of his or her own experiences as well as another's experiences (Stage 2); the Interpersonal Balance, Romanticism, or Cross-Categorical Knowing, in which abstractions and more mutual relationships become possible (Stage 3); the Institutional Balance or Modernism, in which understanding of systems, greater autonomy, and self-authorship become possible (Stage 4); and the Interindividual Balance or Postmodernism, in which people become the directors and creators of systems, understanding how systems fit together meaningfully (Stage 5).

Kegan proposed that the "deep structure of any principle of mental organization is the subject-object relationship" (Kegan, 1994, p. 32). Development requires shifts in what is subject and what is object, thus necessitating a shift in the relationship between what is subject and what is object. Some definitions may be necessary here. Kegan defined those things as *object* that people could "reflect on, handle, look at, be responsible for, relate to each other, take control of, internalize, assimilate, or otherwise operate on" (p. 32). He defined those things as *subject* that people are "identified with, tied to, fused with, or embedded in" (p. 32). People lack awareness of those entities that they are subject to. They behave automatically in relationship to what they are subject to. Thus, these things become unconsciously absolute or ultimate in their lives (examples to follow).

Change in stage is progressive in that it represents individuals' taking increased responsibility for the sense that they make of their lives and choices and relationships (Kegan, 1994). As meaning-making evolves, thinking becomes less rigid, exclusive, simple, and dogmatic, and more flexible, open, complex, and tolerant of differences. Therefore, stage theory assumes that increased constructive capacity is generally more adaptive and incorporates more meaning-making options—including the prior stage capacities—at least in contemporary "schooled" societies (McAuliffe & Eriksen, 1999).

Rather than focusing on the stages themselves, Kegan (1982, 1994) focused primarily on the transformation from one stage to another. This transformation results from those in the individual's environment acknowledging the person's currently dominant way of knowing (*matching* or supporting) *and* relating to them from the next potential way of knowing (*mismatching* or challenging; McAuliffe & Eriksen, 1999).

(Examples of how this might be done are given in the next sections.) From Kegan's (1982, 1994) perspective, life or interpersonal problems may emerge from a mismatch between external demands or cultural expectations and a person's epistemological capacity.

## Incorporative Balance

During the incorporative balance of the first eighteen months of life, babies are embedded in reflexes, sensing, and moving (Kegan, 1982). Newborns exist in an "objectless world" (p. 78) in which everything around them is merely an extension of themselves and in which anything that leaves their immediate surround no longer exists. They are only aware of their own immediate needs and are unaware of the "other." They are dependent upon and merged with the mother or caretaker.

In order to *support* or *match* infants developmentally, caregivers need to hold them, to offer them close physical contact, comfort, protection, and eye contact. Infants are "endowed with a host of abilities that seduce the mother" (Kegan, 1982, p. 122) to behave in this way. In order to *challenge* or *mismatch* infants developmentally, particularly as infants develop the ability to physically move on their own and to stand up and walk away, caretakers provide "timely differentiation" (p. 127), that is, they gradually become less a part of the infant. They end the practice of meeting every need of the child, reduce carrying, and acknowledge displays of independence and willful refusal. Infants' success at letting go depends not only on their own physical maturation but also upon the parents' abilities to grant their children the opportunity to differentiate.

The culmination of the first eighteen months is the creation of the object of "object relations" (Kegan, 1982, p. 78). From a Piagetian perspective, the infant emerges from embeddedness and differentiates her- or himself from the world. The child "brings into being that which is independent of its own sensing and moving" (p. 78). As soon as the infant can make reflexes object, that is, understand self as distinct from reflexes, she or he creates a world separate from her- or himself. It is from this point that subject-object relations can exist, and here begins "preserving or renegotiating the balance between what is taken as subject or self and what is taken as object or other" (p. 81).

Counselors, teachers, nurses, or other mental health providers working in infant mental health, with women with postpartum depression, or with quite dysfunctional new mothers (mentally ill, homeless, drug addicted) may need to provide new mothers with education about these developmental needs of infants. Helpers may need to assess the level of attachment mothers have with their infants and determine whether the mothers' developmental capacities enable them to invest in their children's needs. Helpers may need to show willing mothers how to connect with their babies. Helpers may further need to help mothers to resolve their own early traumas in order to move ahead developmentally, particularly if traumas have left the mothers unable to connect effectively with their infants. Finally, helpers may need to influence policy or institutional procedures to ensure that babies who have been abandoned or removed from their parents' care receive the substitute connection with *one* dependable caretaker or foster parent who can consistently care for the baby over a long period of time.

## Impulsive Balance

Children between ages two and seven operate primarily from the impulsive order of consciousness. From Kegan's (1982) perspective, they are subject to their impulses and perceptions, but can make their reflexes object. As a result, they may have a hard time sitting still for any length of time, may continually move around with little predictability, and will display a short attention span, particularly related to others' needs or desires. Their use of language will be only one, and perhaps a tangential, means of communication, and life will be filled "with fantasy and fantasy about the fantastic (being Spiderman)" (p. 136). They make decisions about right and wrong based on what the authority figures in their lives deem to be right and wrong. Although impulsive children realize that there is a world separate from themselves, they confuse their impulses with their family's impulses, needs, and desires. The feeling of the child toward the parent—usually the same sex parent—is of "unmediated, unqualified, and unbounded yearning to be completely cared for in the company of this other person who is distinct from her and yet knows her completely—body, mind, heart, and soul" (p. 141). As a result of these powerful yearnings, impulsive children are enormously appealing, physically as well as psychologically, to the parent(s).

In order to adequately *support* or *match* the child at this age, the parent–recipient of this yearning needs to be able to receive this love, and the unfavored parent needs to be able to be sympathetic to the child's need and to continue to hold the child securely. The unfavored parent provides a balance, a protection against overholding, and a support for the emerging ability of the child to parent him or herself. Parents and other caregivers need to acknowledge and encourage exercises of fantasy, intense attachments, and rivalries (Kegan, 1982).

In order to adequately *challenge* or *mismatch* the child at this age, parents need to be able to set limits on children's behavior so that children (1) can gradually recognize appropriate boundaries between themselves and their parents, (2) can eventually know the boundaries between their impulses and themselves, and (3) can become self-regulating.

Parents or other caregivers who have not themselves evolved beyond the interpersonal stage will not be able to limit the child's demands, which may result in the child exploiting the parents' subservience, sometimes resulting in a sort of tyranny by the child (Kegan, 1982). Therefore, counselors, teachers, nurses, or other mental health providers who address difficulties in children from this stage generally intervene with parents or with care-taking institutions. Such helpers might, in order to assist parents and other caretakers in setting appropriate limits on children's behavior without anger or in enhancing fantasy or play activities, teach workshops on the developmental needs of children of this age, on parenting skills, or on behavior management. As mentioned in the "incorporative balance" section, helpers might also work to promote growth in parents or caretakers who have not acquired the developmental capacities to fully enjoy the enthusiasms and playfulness of children this age, or work to develop the capacities to set boundaries on overexuberance or unsafe/undesirable behaviors.

## Imperial Balance

The transformation from the impulsive to the imperial balance during preadolescence is about the birth of the role, that is, the ability to "take the role of the other, to see that others have a perspective of their own" (Kegan, 1982, p. 137). The children are now able to make their impulses and perceptions object, which allows them to make choices among impulses. However, they are subject to their needs, wishes, and interests. Their needs and interests become "enduring dispositions" or notions about themselves that persist through time (self-concept). They develop and commit to interests and hobbies, sharing these with both friends and family. Children during this stage seem to become more self-sufficient, cognitively, affectively, and behaviorally.

Imperial children move beyond the structures of the family into the "peer gang" (Kegan, 1982, p. 157), which further supports the development of interests and hobbies. For the first time, they have "developmental contemporaries" (p. 166), which allows for a debut of behaviors and attitudes necessary to survive in society, a debut that will fully blossom in adolescence. In the imperial balance, parents and peers share this socializing role, while by adolescence, peers serve the major socializing role.

In order to succeed in the tasks of this stage, children must be able take the role of another and envision another as a separate person with separate intentions and purposes. However, during this balance, they will gain only an awareness of others' needs; they will not gain a sense of responsibility to others. Instead, they become aware of others primarily as providers of their own needs. They make deals with others in order to "purchase" what they need. They worry about consequences or punishment, without experiencing real guilt. They aim to control the world so as to get their needs met. And they need authorities to direct them (Kegan, 1982, 1994).

**Transition**    Transition to the next—interpersonal—stage takes place between ages twelve to twenty. Transition implies a period during which some imperial and some interpersonal capacities are present. Thus, a mistake that is sometimes made by those in a teen's environment is expecting the teen to be fully interpersonal before they are capable of being so (e.g., expecting them to think about how their parents will worry if they stay out beyond curfew without calling, without having set up consequences for failing to call). Such expectations are "over their heads," but may result in inappropriately labeling a teen's behavior as "misbehavior" or "emotional disturbance" (Kegan, 1982, 1994).

**Clinical Problems**    When people emerge from adolescence without having progressed developmentally to the interpersonal balance, the mental demands of society outstrip their mental capacity, that is, they are incapable of operating as adults are expected to act. They cannot subordinate their present urges to their future goals, and are, as a result, considered sociopathic in some way. Adults who remain imperial act on their own needs and interests with little comprehension of how these ought to be balanced with the needs of others or the broader society (Kegan, 1982, 1994). If one imagines the self-focused and present-oriented behavior of young childhood extending into adulthood, one might imagine various forms of irresponsibility, such as a grown up (1) working at a job as long as it was fun, but quitting as soon as demands became unpleasant; (2) using a credit card to purchase items, without attending to the funds necessary to pay off the credit card; (3) pursuing their own pleasure sexually without anticipating that the partner's pleasure should also be considered. Examples of imperial adults in the clinical population seem relatively easy to find. Often prisoners, substance abusers, the unemployed or unemployable, or others with various addictions or school or work problems have not emerged beyond the imperial balance.

In order to *match* or *support* people in the imperial balance, whether normally developing children or clinically impaired adults, counselors, parents, or teachers give clear behavioral instructions and spell out the consequences of following or not following these instructions. They offer incentives for socially acceptable behavior. For instance, helpers might create a behavioral chart of expected behaviors, preferably behaviors that cancel out less desirable behaviors; they might then negotiate rewards for performing the desirable behaviors and more negative consequences for failing to perform expected behaviors or for engaging in harmful behaviors. In order to *mismatch* imperial people and thus promote forward progress, a counselor, teacher, or parent challenges them to attend to social norms of right and wrong behavior, to others' feelings and needs, and to reconciling their individual needs with the need to maintain relationships (Kegan, 1982, 1994). For instance, imperial adults who quit work when the demands became unpleasant might be challenged to consider what would happen if everyone did that; to think about why many people choose to persevere at their jobs; or to examine what their coworkers or boss might be experiencing as a result of their behavior. Those imperial adults who overcharge their credit cards might be asked not only about the consequences for doing so (matching), but also about (1) how their spouse or parents will feel when they find out about the increased financial challenges or (2) what responsible behavior is with regard to spending.

## Interpersonal Balance

Counselors will likely encounter many clients operating primarily out of Stage 3, or *interpersonal balance, romanticism,* or *conventionalism,* or the transition between stages 3 and 4, because research indicates that only between 20% to 30% of adults reach Stage 4 (Allison, 1988; Alvarez, 1985; Bar-Yam, 1991; Beukema, 1990; Binner, 1991; Dixon, 1986; Goodman, 1983; Greenwald, 1991; Jacobs, 1984; Lahey, 1986; Osgood, 1991; Roy, 1993; Sonnenschein, 1990). People operating from Stage 3 are able to see needs as object, but are embedded in or subject to their relationships and to rules. This means that they have moved ahead from the imperial balance in that they are good and productive citizens, are trustworthy and employable, take others into account, have the capacity for insight and consciousness, think before acting, exercise common sense, consider the long-term consequences of their choices, have friends, and develop a meaningful life based on clear ideals. They are fully socialized; that is, they have internalized the values of society or their surround (Kegan, 1982, 1994).

Those operating from the interpersonal order of consciousness understand another's point of view, even when it might be different from their own. They can empathize with the other's point of view, often subordinating their own perspective in favor of preserving the relationship. Interpersonal knowers can identify inner motivations, emotions, and emotional conflict. They possess the capacity for insight. They operate on the basis of values, ideals, and beliefs. They have thus moved beyond allegiance to immediate impulses to a future-orientedness (Kegan, 1994, 1982).

The limitations of the interpersonal balance parallel its strengths. That is, although a relational focus and capacities are more advantageous to people, relationships, and society than the more narcissistic and impulsive imperial balance; being defined by relationships may leave one being determined by others; needing to maintain relationships, be approved of, and not rock the boat at any cost; being unable to experience intimacy (the full sharing of two different people), that is, experiencing only fusion in relationships (the sharing only of samenesses); and subjectivist knowing, that is, the intuitive, unexamined following of inner urges, sometimes reactively (Kegan, 1982, 1994).

Further, interpersonal people unthinkingly adopt ideals and values "inherited" from their families or heritage, which makes it difficult for interpersonal people to emerge beyond a "that's the way I was brought up" or "that's the way it has always been done" mentality. They will, as a result, most likely distance themselves from others who are different or allow themselves to be defined by others' ways, subjugating their own needs and feelings to others so as not to cause problems. They may consider those who make different choices to be "trouble makers" (Kegan, 1982, 1994).

In order to *match* or *support* people at the interpersonal balance, counselors and others in the person's environment express appreciation of and attention to clients' abilities to form relationships, express feelings, and operate out of intuitive knowledge. They punctuate all of the beneficial characteristics/behaviors/attitudes of the interpersonal balance. Counselors and others in the interpersonal person's environment would also give clear direction and offer plenty of structure, given that those operating interpersonally still need an authority-based experience (Kegan, 1982, 1994).

In order to *mismatch* or *challenge* people at the interpersonal balance, counselors, teachers, and parents urge people in this balance to think about why they are doing what they are doing, to examine their inner urges, to decide whether preserving relationships at all costs is helpful to them, to establish a separateness from others' definitions, and to be self-reflective (Kegan, 1982, 1994).

## Institutional Balance

Stage 4, or *institutional balance, systemic,* or *procedural knowers,* have their relationships and values, making them object. They are embedded in or subject to their roles in institutions, to their career positions, and to the organizing frameworks of these institutions. They have well-defined boundaries that they protect very carefully. They are very well-controlled and self-possessed (Kegan, 1982, p. 242).

Family and work are two central institutions that require institutional capacities (Kegan, 1994). For instance, parents need to be able to be leaders of the family; institute a vision and induct family members into it; live out some theory, ideology, or values; manage boundaries effectively; set limits on children and on themselves in the process of instituting a vision for the family (Kegan, 1994).

Members of a couple need to be able to (1) define a sense of self or separate identity, so that the other does not organize or define them; (2) navigate closeness and distinctness simultaneously; (3) set limits to preserve the couple as a separate subsystem; (4) support their partner's development and accomplishment of goals; (5) communicate directly, standing their ground, and making known unhappy feelings in a productive way; and (6) be aware of how their own history impacts the current relationship. If one partner is upset, an institutional partner can provide company for her or him in the upset, can fully care about her or his feelings, can work with the other to discover solutions, and will expect both partners to feel free to create and choose solutions (Kegan, 1994).

Workers operating from an institutional order of consciousness invent their own work, and are guided by their own visions, rather than merely responding to management's demands. They are self-initiating, self-correcting, and self-evaluating. They take responsibility for what happens to them at work externally and internally. They become accomplished masters of their particular work roles, jobs, or careers. And they conceive of the organization from the "outside in," as a whole, understanding their relationship to the whole, and envisioning the relationships of the parts to the whole (Kegan, 1994, p. 153). They seek "mastery, promotion, recognition, credentials, and confidence; crystallizing work identity; [and]

readjusting career goals to realign with changing expectations of self and significant others" (p. 180).

Institutional knowers are not bound by the current surround. One can see how the work and family capacities noted here require remaining conscious of systems beyond here and now dyadic relationships. Institutional knowers take responsibility for balancing their different roles, rather than merely being responsible to their roles, as was evident in interpersonal knowers (Kegan, 1994).

In order to *match* or *support* clients at the institutional order of consciousness, counselors, teachers, and leaders encourage and validate (1) developing individual ideas and thoughts (self-authoring), (2) making decisions for oneself, (3) reflectively weighing choices among various values or ideologies, (4) choosing and operating from an ideology based on one's own careful evaluation, (5) setting clear limits so as to allow pursuit of one's own life projects, (6) differentiating in relationships, (7) designing one's own projects, and (8) being independent. In order to *challenge* clients at this stage, counselors, teachers, and leaders help clients or others explore the "higher" principles behind the roles and institutions (e.g., "justice" as the principle behind the law; "love" as a principle behind the church); hear negative reports as important input and feedback, something to learn from, rather than as destructive of the self; maintain, and in fact, pursue connections with others, particularly those who are different from themselves; and see each interpersonal encounter as the opportunity to construct something bigger than the individual can create him- or herself (e.g., a group of faculty members bring different strengths to the table and use and value conflict as a means to challenge themselves individually and as a group to create a better program than any of them could conceive of by themselves— the higher principle here would be the development of student potential, and in turn, client potential (Kegan, 1982, 1994)).

## Interindividual Balance

Stage 5, or *postmodernism* or the *interindividual balance*, is difficult to understand, probably because few people we know ever reach this stage. However, those *moving toward* interindividualism recognize that they have "not been with others" or been truly intimate with others and find themselves becoming more available to relational intimacy (Kegan, 1982, p. 242). They find themselves questioning their previously held ways of making decisions (e.g., perhaps they used the scientific method or the Bible or some other specific principles), even wondering whether it is possible to construct rules for making these decisions because any rule would necessarily require ignoring certain particulars. Those moving toward interindividualism begin to realize that contradiction and paradox do not threaten the system or urgently require resolution. Instead, interindividual people find themselves examining relationships between ideological poles, believing it to be less necessary to choose between poles. For instance, rather than espousing the values of conservative Christianity *or* liberal Christianity (or substitute politics or another construct for Christianity), the interindividual person might recognize the benefit of the conversations between the poles, that neither pole is really complete or inspired without the other. The person might then pursue and value literal conversations between people representing different poles, or might engage the poles within her- or himself in conversation, with the aim of creating something better, of learning, of growing.

In the movement from institutional knower to interindividual knower, people may experience a philosophical crisis. Their urge to move ahead developmentally and the promise of what lies ahead may feel at battle with what they have previously held to be ethical; and thus, their new choices may initially feel like an underground activity. Kegan (1982) indicates that forward progress requires giving their developmental urges some play and going "with the flow" (p. 237).

In summary, interindividual people (1) accept and focus on relationship/dynamism/tension between systems of deciding; (2) see "motion, process, and change . . . as the irreducible and primary feature of reality" (Basseches, 1980, p. 406); (3) orient to movement through forms; (4) stand back from decision-making systems and see them in relationship to one another, see the movement from form to form, and see how the systems are constructed; (5) find nourishment in contradiction rather than trying to escape it; (6) become responsible for systems, rather than to systems; (7) become more tentative and less certain because of seeing that any form is temporary, preliminary, and self-constructed; (8) transcend allegiance to the product "in favor of an orientation to the process that creates the product" (Kegan, 1982, p. 248); and (9) mutually preserve each other's distinctiveness simultaneously with creating a context in which these separate identities "interpenetrate" (Kegan, 1982, p. 253). Limited space precludes further explanation of each of these characteristics. However, readers who are close to the interindividual stage may find some benefit from merely reflecting on the list. Others are directed to Kegan's works for a fuller understanding of each concept.

Creating an optimal holding environment for interindividual people or those moving toward this stage may be impossible for most

## ABOUT ROBERT KEGAN

Robert Kegan was born in Minnesota, a Jew in the middle of Scandinavian Protestants, and always found himself living "out on the edge." (Biographical information taken from an interview that can be viewed at http://www.dialogonledership.org/Kegan-1999cp.html.) One of his most formative experiences was coming of age during the protests against the Vietnam War and during the first stages of the civil rights movement. These social revolutions provided holding environments for youth to break out of the traditional frames of reference provided by their parents.

After finishing Dartmouth, he was drafted, and because he found himself determined not to fight in a war that he didn't believe in, he chose a deferment option in which he taught children. While teaching these children, he became very interested in the minds and hearts of children, and in the ways in which they developed. However, because he couldn't pursue graduate education without losing his deferment, he began conversations at a distance with Harvard University as it developed an interdepartmental, self-designed doctoral program.

Kegan attributes his movement from the third to the fourth order of consciousness to the holding nature of each of the above contexts, that is, they were each social experiences that challenged the dominant social discourse and challenged the perspective with which he had grown up, while offering a supportive community of others on a similar journey.

When Kegan was finally able to attend Harvard, his participation in a self-designed program also took him outside of conventional educational patterns and offered him freedom to grow and develop without devoting himself to any of the current leaders in psychological or philosophical thought or to any of the traditional structures of academia. From this place, he began exploring a dream that had been percolating through his years of living outside of convention: to bring lifespan and internal phenomenological and existential dimensions together with "what was otherwise, at some level, a very dry cognitive psychology," in order to "create a richer developmental psychology that was both powerfully descriptive from the outside, but also powerfully descriptive from the inside—the internal experience of being a growing person and thinking about the context and support of development" (www.dialogonledership.org/Kegan-1999cp).

Kegan earned a Ph.D. from Harvard University, where he currently holds a faculty appointment. In addition to this faculty position, he serves as the educational chair of the Harvard Graduate School of Education Institute for Management and Leadership in Education; as co-director of a joint program with the Harvard Medical School that brings principles of adult learning to the reform of medical education; and as co-director of a Gates Foundation–funded project at the Harvard Graduate School of Education that aims to train change leadership coaches for schools and school district leaders.

Kegan's principal publications are *How the Way We Talk Can Change the Way We Work: Seven Languages for Transformation* (with L. Lahey) (2000); *In Over Our Heads: the Mental Demands of Modern Life* (1994); and *The Evolving Self* (1982). Kegan is a licensed clinical psychologist and practicing therapist, lectures widely to professional and lay audiences, and consults in the area of professional development. "I have been told," he says, "it may help to know that I am also a husband and a father; influenced by Hasidism; an airplane pilot; a poker player; and the unheralded inventor of the 'Base Average,' a more comprehensive way of gauging a baseball player's offensive contributions."

counselors, teachers, or leaders, because most of these professionals will not have reached the interindividual balance themselves. It is more likely that the interindividual people will themselves be the counselors, teachers, or leaders. In fact, should an interindividual person pursue counseling with someone who has not reached such a balance themselves, it is likely that both will experience a disconnect. Interindividual people may, however, attract others at similar developmental levels, and may thus find more frequent opportunities to be "held" in their social and professional environments rather than in a counseling office.

## Assessing Stage

Both formal and informal methods might be used to assess a client's general stage tendency (McAuliffe & Eriksen, 1999). During a session, a practitioner might informally ask, "How did you come to decide or know . . . (e.g., that this gender role in necessary, or that a person cannot marry someone of another ethnic group, or that you must follow the career path that your parents prefer)?" or "What lets you know that something is (good, right, important)?" (Lahey, Souvaine, Kegan, Goodman, & Felix; 1985; McAuliffe & Eriksen, 1999; Vacc & Juhnke, 1997). An inexact cue to epistemology might be the brevity of a client's response: Those who generally rely on "outside" sources of knowing (e.g., conventions, parents, religious tradition, peers, or authorities) seem to provide brief, minimal responses to such epistemology-evoking probes (Lahey et al., 1985). More "internal" or "self-authoring" knowers tend to offer a method of considering pros and cons to come to a decision (McAuliffe & Eriksen, 1999). However, the most powerful method of assessing stage, from my perspective and experience, is to proceed with a typical assessment interview or classroom exercise and to determine how the content of the person's conversation and the way in which the person communicates or comes across matches the stage characteristics listed in Table 5.1 and discussed here.

McAuliffe and Eriksen (1999) also enumerate some of the more formal ways in which stage might be assessed. For instance, stage-evoking interview methods are elaborated in the *Ways of Knowing Interview Schedule* (Belenky, Clinchy, Goldberger, & Tarule, 1986) and the *Subject-Object Interview* (Lahey et al., 1985). Recognition tasks, in which the client must choose responses from options on an inventory, also help to identify stage (e.g., Erwin, 1983; Kitchener & King, 1981; Moore, 1989). A more intensive and time-consuming measure of Perry's theory (1970) is Baxter-Magolda and Porterfield's *Measure of Epistemological Reflection* (1988). Rest's *Defining Issues Test* (1979; see also Rest, Narvaez, Bebeau, & Thoma, 1999) determines moral reasoning via the Kohlberg (1981, 1984) scheme. Loevinger's stage theory of ego development can be measured by the *Sentence Completion Test* (1976). However, as helpful as these assessment tools are for research and for accurate pre- and posttesting, the less formal approach is often sufficient for counselor, teacher, and parent decisions about matching and mismatching clients, students, and children.

## Concluding Thoughts

Challenges do exist to conceiving of people from a developmental stage perspective. For instance, feminist and narrative theorists view the hierarchies of stage models of development as "patriarchal" and consider the notion of an "expert" evaluation of supervisees' or clients' needs to be patronizing and egotistical (Gilligan, 1982). However, feminist and

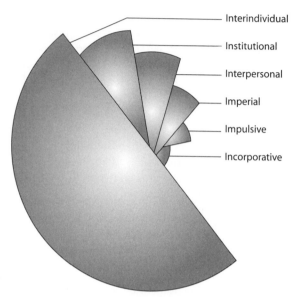

Interindividual

Institutional

Interpersonal

Imperial

Impulsive

Incorporative

FIGURE 5.1    Domains of Knowing as Concentric Spheres

narrative theories, often grounded in social constructionism, seem to fail to recognize the developmental demands of the "co-construction" that they advocate (according to cognitive developmental theorists). It is my contention that social constructionism is beyond the meaning-making capacity of many supervisors and therapists. Social constructionism postulates that meaning is inevitably made within an interpersonal and cultural context (Olson, 1989) and relativizes meanings as socially derived creations, rather than references to already-existing essences (Anderson, 1990). As a result, social constructivists tend to eschew theories, and develop points of reference during counseling or supervision through dialogue (e.g., supervisors and counselors would, for instance, decide together how supervision ought to be conducted and what a counselor should learn). I contend that such activities require institutional capacities and that those functioning below that level would not be full participants in creating mutual meanings.

I have made an effort, however, to move beyond the negative consequences of hierarchical models with the notion of *domains of knowing*, pictured as concentric spheres (see Figure 5.1; Eriksen & McAuliffe, 2006). In such a conceptualization, people expand their capacities to function in the world as they emerge from one sphere or domain outward to another, becoming less limited as they expand their abilities, but never leaving behind the capacities of the incorporated domains. Such a conceptualization avoids the notion that some people are "above" or better than others, and instead promotes development with the enticement of fewer limitations and expanded capacities.

Another limitation of the stage construct is the risk of rigidly stereotyping and "totalizing" a person's constructive tendencies. Practitioners must remind themselves that the notion of "stage" is itself an artifact or a construction and it cannot represent any individual's total way of making meaning. It is likely that much meaning-making is situational and contextual and that stage refers to a "more or less" tendency to use certain constructive capacities in specific situations. This fluid notion has been called the "soft stage" approach to constructive development (McAuliffe & Eriksen, 1999).

Despite these challenges, my experiences, as noted elsewhere in this chapter, indicate that Kegan's constructive developmental theory offers great richness in understanding people and in understanding how to effectively promote development as a counselor, teacher, and leader. Such work is still in its infancy. However, other developmental educators and I have experienced great success in creating developmentally targeted programs and in conducting developmentally relevant counseling sessions. I hope that as you read on, you will also discover ways to apply such principles to your own life and work.

## Relevance of Theory to Counseling Practice

As mentioned above, part of my excitement about constructive developmental theory began with its explanations for our clinical failures. Therefore, some examples of how one might find relevance for the theories in clinical practice, psychoeducation and program development, and counselor education are offered here.

### Private Practice and Supervision

The wife in a couple that I was seeing was complaining about her husband's failures, and I was trying to understand what the husband thought about these complaints and what ideas he had about addressing them. This was a middle-class family seeking counseling in a private practice setting. He was a career military man and she worked as a teacher. They had three children, one of whom was severely developmentally disabled. The husband had aspirations to become an officer in the military, although his individual therapist did not think his particular plans to do so would succeed. The wife had fairly typical female complaints about having to do everything around the house and with the children, about his watching sports on TV too frequently, and about his failing to approach her romantically or sexually.

As I asked the husband about his thoughts and what solutions he had in mind, he merely agreed with what his wife said and committed to try harder. When I asked him what he would do to try harder, he could contribute little in the way of practical or specific ideas. When I continued to try to help him to create a picture of what his trying harder would look like, believing that it would help his relationship if his wife could hear clear commitments from him, he became confused. It was as though there was nothing in his head or heart to share with her. As long as he could merely do as she told him to do, he was fine. If she yelled louder, he knew that her requests needed more immediate attention. She, however, did not want to continue these methods of defining his behavior for him. She believed that if he did not generate ideas himself, they were not really "him," that he did not really "mean them," and that he was merely conforming to her demands rather than truly loving her.

His individual therapist revealed that he had been an enlisted person in the military for his entire career (nearly 20 years). He found himself "in trouble" when given assignments that required him to think for himself. When the individual counselor asked questions about what he would do to pursue career advancement, he could identify very few activities in which he could take initiative. It seemed that he believed that if he followed orders, he should be rewarded with advancement to the officers' corp.

From Kegan's perspective, my usual therapeutic approach—that is, to help him take more responsibility in the home and to help his wife to let go of some responsibilities—was defeated by the husband's developmental order of consciousness. That is, he operated primarily out of an imperial order of consciousness in which his natural inclinations to do what he wanted were only curbed by others' demands, and in particular by the rewards and punishments doled out by others. He was able to make deals, but unable to generate notions of "good behavior" from within. This worked fairly well in his position as enlisted person in the military, where structure, hierarchy, and clear consequences are often the norm for enlisted personnel. However, his wife was ready to move ahead from an interpersonal order of consciousness into a more self-authorizing place, and she was no longer satisfied with doling out the orders.

Two similar situations were experienced by supervisees who were participating in my supervision group. In both of these situations, adult clients were operating primarily from an imperial order of consciousness. One supervisee's primary referral source was a psychiatrist who referred her people who had just been released from psychiatric hospitals. Most of her clients, despite being beyond their twenties, had never succeeded in adult life, for instance, they had never held jobs, never had love relationships, and were still living with parents or family members. The supervisee preferred to work psychoanalytically and was extremely frustrated by her clients' failure to respond to her interventions. Another supervisee was working in prisons, and was trying to run Yalom-style groups with male prison inmates, because this was the only type of group that had been taught during her master's program. This model stresses, among other things, (1) interpersonal communication in the "here and now" as a means for assessing clients' ways of behaving interpersonally; (2) offering honest feedback to the group member who is "working" about they are experienced by other group members, including how successful the working member is in communicating congruently, addressing conflict, and working on issues; and (3) asking group members to reflect on their own as well as the group process—or success in "working." It is assumed that group members re-create their family dynamics in the group and that "work" in the group may help them to heal outside relationships (Yalom, 1995). The supervisee in question couldn't understand how the prison inmates could talk for hours and seemingly make no forward progress. After our discussions, it became clear that the developmental levels and capacities were the same for these two groups of clients.

In supervision related to these supervisees' concerns and based on Kegan's perspective, we concluded that these clients would not benefit cathartically from therapy that focused on their internal thinking, feeling, or behaving. Instead, if the counselors were to adequately support and challenge these clients, they would have to match the clients' imperial levels of development and challenge them to operate from the interpersonal order of consciousness. In order to *support* them or *match* their developmental level, the supervision group developed various behavioral strategies with relevance for each of the clients, strategies that had clear consequences attached. The therapist for the prison inmates developed skills training groups on topics such as anger management, conflict resolution, and employment strategies. She worked with the prison system on reward systems for group members. The therapist for those clients who had been recently released from psychiatric hospitals began asking other members of the patients' families to attend the sessions so as to set up similar behavioral systems. She also began referring the clients to more intensive treatments than the one-hour-per-week outpatient therapy that she offered (e.g., intensive substance abuse treatment, partial hospitalization), treatments in which they would have regular and dependable consequences applied.

But because we wanted the clients to move ahead developmentally, we could not merely stop with behavioral strategies. We needed to *challenge* or *mismatch* clients toward behavior more suited to the interpersonal order of consciousness. So, in addition to skills training about how to resolve conflicts with one's wife or significant other, we asked the clients to think about how the wife might feel when the client shoved her up against the wall (or went to prison, or ended up in the hospital, or hung around the house watching TV all weekend). However, we were cautious to pose such questions only infrequently in the midst of the behavioral strategies. Not only did clients experience forward movement when we did not use strategies that were over their heads, we were less frustrated with the clients, and did a great deal less "client bashing" as a result of lessened frustration.

## A Developmental Community Agency

Based on these experiences, I began a developmentally grounded afterschool program in an urban, African American, Title I school. I wanted to answer the following question: If we created a community agency that optimally matched and mismatched clients' developmental levels, could we be more successful with the clients and would interns trained in such an agency feel less burned out and more committed to future work in community agencies? (We had observed "agency flight" once supervisees completed the two years of supervised experience required for licensure.) The afterschool program involved parents and children in a behaviorally grounded mentoring program (reading, activities, one-to-one support, incentives). The parents also participated in psychoeducational groups (job skills training, building your child's self-esteem). Counseling services were available to participants as well. The families were primarily operating out of the imperial order of consciousness, and as would be expected for this balance, they were more motivated to fully participate in services that were behavioral and psychoeducational. Further, the service providers found themselves enthused with the work, rather than burned out or reluctant to continue in agency work. Unlike the experiences of most community agencies, we had no trouble with client participation—families showed up and completed the program. School officials, who had known many of these families for years, were very surprised at both the success we experienced and at the consistency of the families' participation. The parents, when participating in a focus group afterwards, tearfully spoke of how the program had changed their lives. What was particularly surprising was that these results were accomplished after a mere three-month program, when we knew that the literature usually reported recalcitrance among these sorts of clients.

## Practitioner Training Programs

A number of counselor educators have also explored the applicability of developmental theory for the education of mental health practitioners (Borders & Fong, 1989; Borders, Fong, & Neimeyer, 1986; Eriksen & McAuliffe, 2006; Haag-Granello & Hazler, 1998; Knefelkamp & Slepitza, 1976; Knefelkamp, Widick, & Parker, 1978; Lovell, 1999; McAuliffe, 2002; McAuliffe & Lovell, 2000). They began with the observation that it seemed as though students who became better counselors demonstrated higher orders of developmental functioning. They then researched whether students in counseling training programs progress developmentally during their programs (Haag-Granello & Hazler, 1998); whether students at higher developmental levels demonstrated more empathy (Neukrug & McAuliffe, 1993); whether students entering graduate programs at higher developmental levels developed better counseling skills (Eriksen & McAuliffe, 2006); and whether developmentally structured pedagogy promoted student's constructive development (e.g., Bebeau & Brabeck, 1987; Haag-Granello & Hazler, 1998; Knefelkamp & Slepitza, 1976; Knefelkamp et al., 1978; Kohlberg & Mayer, 1972; Lovell, 1999; McAuliffe & Eriksen, 2000, 2002; Paisley & Benshoff, 1998; Sprinthall, 1994; Sprinthall & Thies-Sprinthall, 1983).

Initial research, although still in its infancy, supports the correlations between higher developmental levels and both better counseling skills and empathy, and indicates that development can be promoted by educators. That is, some specialties of counselors do progress developmentally during their counseling-training programs (Haag-Granello & Hazler, 1998). Counselors beginning their training programs at higher developmental levels are better able to learn counseling skills (Eriksen & McAuliffe, 2006). And students grouped for classroom activities by developmental level report getting more out of their learning experiences (Lovell, 1999).

## Conclusions

It would seem, then, that Kegan and other adult developmentalists' theories have great potential to contribute to therapeutic, psychoeducational, and training processes. Clients seem to progress more when optimally matched and mismatched developmentally. Counselors who integrate developmental notions seem clearer about what strategies to use with clients. Educators of mental health practitioners seem to be able to predict who will become a quality service provider and seem to be able to promote development through specifically targeted pedagogical practices. And finally, educators and practitioners seem less stressed (burned out) by the apparent failures in their work; instead, they use these apparent failures as evidence of mismatches with client or student developmental functioning, and shift their approaches to more appropriately match and mismatch their clients and students. What seems to be missing is literature that offers educators and practitioners clear, easy to understand guidelines about how to incorporate this theory. Developmental theorists seem to breathe the rarified air of the "ivory tower," which reaches to heights unscaled by most educators and practitioners. This chapter and other articles by the author aim to bring the heights of theory down to the nuts and bolts of practice. It is hoped that the following case, as followed through the lifespan, will successfully illustrate how developmental theory might be used in conceptualizing and treating a client.

## Theory into Action: The Case of Kirsten

Kirsten is a fifty-year-old woman who sought counseling to address some nagging dissatisfactions with her work and relationships. She is a single parent of a young child. She has had a number of satisfying long-term relationships, although she has been married only once, quite unsatisfactorily. She was recently promoted to vice president of research in a pharmaceutical company; prior to this promotion, she worked as a pharmaceutical researcher. She has great clarity about who she is and who she wants to be, but finds herself frustrated—due to the time constraints of being a single professional parent—in bringing her sense of vocation into fruition. She is looking for greater integrity and balance, more congruent living that fully actualizes the principles that she believes in, and greater awareness of these higher principles as she moves through her daily life. She anticipates that reaching these goals will reduce her currently high stress level.

In order to illustrate Kegan and other adult developmentalists' theories, I will briefly outline the early stages of Kirsten's life, identifying issues and intervention strategies. I will more fully conceptualize the later stages of her life. I will, somewhat artificially, streamline the presentation to more clearly illustrate Kegan's theory. Each childhood stage is presented as though parents have not, in fact, pursued counseling.

## Early Childhood

Kirsten was born the first of three children into a close-knit professional, middle-class, Midwestern, White family. Her parents had advanced degrees in the medical fields. When Kirsten was born, her mother did as many women did at that time: quit work to become a stay-at-home mother, taking on most of the childcare and household responsibilities. Her father did as many men did at that time: invested in working hard, getting promoted, and providing well for his family. The family did many family activities together as a nuclear family but engaged in few activities with other families. For instance, they regularly shared a sit-down dinner in the evenings, did various outdoor activities on weekends, and took a sailing or skiing vacation each year. The parents were committed to Catholicism and involved the family in the church very consistently and actively. They were also committed to education, reading every night to the children and pursuing other educationally enriching activities. When the children became old enough, the parents participated actively with them in sporting, church, and school events (see Table 5.2).

## Later Childhood

As Kirsten grew older and began elementary school, the parents continued their involvement with the children. Now, there were school activities, sports, the city choir, and 4H. Kirsten did well in school, although she was not a star. She remembers clear expressions of rules and expectations from her parents, and clear, though not unreasonable, punishments for failing to abide by them. She remembers being helped with homework and coached in sports. She was a cooperative and compliant child. Most importantly, she remembers a clear switch in her way of operating that occurred after a family move to a different part of the country (see Table 5.3).

TABLE 5.2  Early Childhood: Incorporative and Impulsive Balances—
Parents at Interpersonal Balance

### Issues

- Family of "doers" rather than "feelers" or "relaters."
- Parents have little knowledge of, and therefore ability to attend to, Kirsten's developmental needs, particularly her emotional needs.
- Kirsten left to figure out own social and sibling relationships and what to do with her day while mother takes care of household responsibilities.
- Mother stressed by isolation of being at home with 2 young children, 18 months apart.

### Goals

- Parents will move ahead developmentally.
- Parents will respond developmentally and appropriately to children's needs.

### Interventions

*Support for Parents*
- Assign a book on children's developmental needs and on parenting; review book's ideas and instructions during counseling sessions; and punctuate the social and emotional needs of children and how to meet them.
- Role-play possible responses to children's behaviors or expression of needs.
- Punctuate parents' successes in responding appropriately to the children's physical and intellectual needs, urging them to attend to emotional needs similarly.
- Urge the parents to structure Kirsten's time and to give her simple directives when they are spending time with her.

*Challenge for Parents*
- Urge the parents to negotiate a division of responsibilities that prevents either parent from became overloaded, helping them to hear one another and learn conflict resolution skills.
- Help the parents to resolve any historical or relationship issues that might preclude their ability to think about Kirsten's needs and feelings, or intentionally and developmentally respond to these.
- Help parents to carefully reflect on why they do what they do as parents and partners, to compare what they have been doing with what the book suggests, and to choose what fits best for them.

## Teenage Years

Kirsten used the junior high school years to transform herself. So by the time she reached high school, she knew how to accomplish. She played every sport, was on student council, joined multiple clubs, was

TABLE 5.3    Later Childhood: Imperial Balance—
Parents at Interpersonal Balance

## Issues

- Unhappiness following move, sense of not fitting in, difficulty making friends.
- Parents don't respond to emotional needs, so Kirsten chooses their strategy of "doing"—buckling down and trying hard to accomplish.
- Left alone to figure out solutions.
- Successful at accomplishing, but this doesn't meet emotional needs.
- So develops somatic symptoms: headaches, back aches, leg aches (parents' medical inclinations lead them to attend to these problems).

## Goals

- Parents will continue what is working—involvement with children, clear structure, clear boundaries, good role modeling.
- Similar to previous stage: Parents will move ahead developmentally, and will respond developmentally and appropriately to children's needs.

## Interventions

### Support for Parents

- Punctuate the parents' successes with directives, structure, and systems of consequences.
- Recommend a book on child development that clearly articulates social and emotional needs of children Kirsten's age.
- Pose questions about how they might extend their current successes into the additional domain of meeting the children's emotional and social needs. For instance, in shifting to being very involved in problem solving rather than "hands off," the parents might give Kirsten directions about how to be a good friend and to make good friends.
- Support the parents in "hanging out," talking, and playing with the children, while expecting no "productive" or structured activity or accomplishments.
- Help the parents to model helpful social behavior by planning social events that include other children; making these relaxed, fun events, rather than "productions"; intervening to encourage play and fun and conversations among the children.
- Suggest that the parents "read" some of Kirsten's minor physical complaints as signs that a problem needs to be solved or that Kirsten needs more emotional or social attention.
- In family therapy, use age appropriate means of assisting Kirsten and family members to express feelings (e.g., congruent words, family murals with emotional content, using colors to express feelings), and assign family to continue such at home.

*(Continued)*

TABLE 5.3   (*Continued*)

*Challenge for Parents*

- In assisting family to communicate together, assist parents to listen to feelings Kirsten might have that are contrary to their own.
- Help the parents to resolve any historical or relationship issues that might preclude their ability to think about Kirsten's needs and feelings, or interfere with their intentionally and developmentally responding to these.
- Help parents to carefully reflect on why they do what they do as parents and partners, to compare what they have been doing with what the book and therapist suggest, and to choose what fits best for them.

active in leadership in her church, and managed to organize her life well enough that her grades were stellar. She won awards, and was used as a role model for others. She had fully incorporated her parents' model of being an "overfunctioning doer."

Kirsten had also finally achieved her aspirations to become "popular." Everyone knew her, and she was elected to offices. She considered herself to have many friends. She seemed to have fully incorporated the notion that her success with relationships depended on her "doing all of the work."

During Kirsten's high school years, her middle sister was acting out. The parents' focus on her sister's drug usage, running away, and school failures left Kirsten in the familiar place of figuring out her life and problems without their help. She instead transferred her dependence to her religion, centering her life around prayer, Bible study, and church activities. Further, Kirsten's engagement in socially acceptable activities and school successes fooled most people into believing that she was doing well, was more than adequately socialized, and needed little attention (see Table 5.4).

## The College to Early Thirties

The limitations of the interpersonal order of consciousness became abundantly clear as Kirsten left home to go away to college. Kirsten found herself without parents or church or peer group to define who she was, and found her new freedom both frightening and enlivening. She experimented with new sorts of relationships and with letting go and being "crazy" with her peers. She encountered different faiths, which forced her to become clearer about her own. She found her initial declaration of a major to be merely an empty attempt to say she was somebody, but found herself increasingly unclear about her life's direction.

During the initial semester of college, she developed worrying and serious headaches. So she withdrew from the "away" college, returned home, and attended to a large local college where she succeeded academically. However, she floundered emotionally and relationally, becoming depressed about her lack of life direction and lack of a boyfriend or other friends. She wished for a "handsome prince" to come and carry her away, to rescue her from her plight of loneliness and lack of direction.

In the midst of her angst, she had a religious epiphany, decided to join a religious order to explore life as a nun, and transferred to a small Catholic college associated with the religious order. Her family was quite dismayed by this move, considering the college too limiting and her choice overly hasty. However, when it became clear that Kirsten

TABLE 5.4    Teenage Years: Interpersonal Balance
for Kirsten and her Parents

**Issues**

- Feels lonely; no one to "hang out" with outside of structured activities; boys don't ask her out; no best buddy; not invited to social events.
- Results in sadness and depression; still no assistance from parents; she has no language to express her emotional struggles so as to get help.
- Decides social difficulties are because she isn't thin like the other girls; starts dieting cycle that develops into 10 years of bulimia, in which self-definition revolves around whether she is feeling thin or not.
- Eating disorder remains invisible because of her accomplishments.
- Parents engage in power struggles with Kirsten around eating problems; she strikes out on a more extreme path (eating & religion) than might otherwise have been chosen.

**Goals**

- Similar goals to previous stages: Parents will move ahead developmentally; they need to move beyond interpersonal knowing in order to assist Kirsten.
- Parents will developmentally and appropriately respond to children's emotional needs, approaching eating disorder as "stuffed" emotions.
- Parents will promote Kirsten's development.

**Interventions**

*Support*
- Punctuate family and child's achievements: parents as good role models, displays of socially acceptable behavior, abilities to focus on and care for others' needs.

*(Continued)*

TABLE 5.4 *(Continued)*

- Urge the family to translate their successes into solutions for the current problems.
- Use typical family therapy or communication building skills (or psychodynamic, existential, or other humanistic strategies) to encourage family members to discover and express their views and to encourage others to fully listen to, honor, and reflect those views, directively preventing interruptions, blaming, or other destructive ways of interacting.
- Be directive authority.

*Challenge*

- Particularly utilize strategies that assist family to connect emotionally, helping them to recognize and express emotions that need attention, rather than "doing" or eating. Emphasize that this connection and awareness requires stillness and reflection.
- When views conflict, teach conflict resolution skills in the attempt to develop solutions that recognize that different people have different and valid stances that often need to exist side by side. Assist the family in establishing ground rules for continuing good communication at home.
- Validate the ways in which Kirsten chooses differently from the rest of the family, and explore the ways that the family might honor those of Kirsten's choices that are different-but-not-harmful, while constraining those that may be harmful.
- Validate this period as a developmental turning point that requires new skills and abilities.
- Assist all family members to think about why they have always done the things they do, to evaluate what works, to risk thinking about self-chosen alternatives.

was determined, her parents financially supported her choice. Kirsten found herself quite comfortable in this environment, felt that she grew spiritually and personally, and was challenged academically. By the end of her four years of study, she was clear that she did not have a calling to a religious order, and decided to pursue graduate studies in the sciences.

After graduation, in a city far from home, she found herself in a job in which she was to expected to "follow on the coattails" of a charismatic leader. She was lonely, financially strapped, and received little supervision or assistance in her work. So when she began doubting the leadership of the man with charisma, she felt rudderless and without the confidence that she was doing what she needed to do. As a result, she soon lost her job. After a year of taking menial jobs outside of her profession, she again found herself seriously depressed. She chose to go back to graduate school and found herself a "cloister" of Catholic women to live with. She obtained jobs over the next few years in which she progressively "initiated" her profession as a pharmaceutical researcher.

During the initial semester of graduate school, she met her husband, a man who was willing to "rescue" her from her depressed state and provide her with enough of a holding environment to move into a better place emotionally. After several years, they were married. The relationship deteriorated almost immediately.

## Early Thirties to Early Forties

As a result of counseling, Kirsten, in fact, accomplishes many of the goals listed in Table 5.5. However, because her accomplishments are still fairly new and stand on wobbly legs, she unconsciously chooses a new relationship with someone who will not challenge her newfound ways of operating in the world. This gives her newfound meaning-making strategies time to solidify and stabilize. Her new partner operates primarily out of the interpersonal order of consciousness and therefore accommodates Kirsten's desires most of the time. She feels relaxed with him. Life is peaceful. The battles are over. They enjoy a long-term partnership that is fun and reassuring, walking beside each other on life's journey. She pursues personal and professional growth opportunities and feels fully supported by him in whatever endeavors she chooses. She is happy and feels successful in this new relationship.

She also reaches out relationally, again, in limited ways, but with more courage in acting on who she knows herself to be. She chooses friends who are like her in intelligence, interests, and passions. She chooses people who will be good to her, rather than a drain on her. She sets boundaries for herself and ends relationships with people who are not healthy for her. She joins some organizations that will allow her to connect with people and who will encourage her to fully actualize her dreams and abilities, which match, she has discovered, with who she is becoming vocationally. She works at communicating honestly and at listening to others. She finds that her relationships are more satisfying and fun, and that people seem to enjoy being with her more than they did in previous eras. However, her primary relationship and interactions are with her partner. She rarely depends on friends other than him. She "contains" her energies and gifts so that she will avoid the overfunctioning that was such a big part of her former "stage" of life.

TABLE 5.5    College to Early Thirties: Transition
             from Interpersonal Balance

## Issues

- Unclear direction in life choices without authority figure guiding.
- Continuing lack of interpersonal connections and resultant loneliness, depression, and somatic complaints.
- Continuing eating disorder.
- Continuing accomplishments and dieting as "solutions" to emotional discomfort.
- Perception of "savior" being a man; leads to problematic marriage: overfunctioning in marriage with underfunctioning man.
- Premature expectations of independence push her prematurely out into a world whose demands exceed what someone at her developmental level could handle.
- Repeated retreats to "support" environments; concurrent with sense that this was failure.

## Goals

- Kirsten will advance developmentally.
- Kirsten will get emotional needs met in healthy relationships, approaching eating disorder as "stuffed" emotions.

## Interventions

### Support
- Punctuate all of Kirsten's hard work at her job, in her relationship, and in other areas of her life, and her efforts to do the right thing.
- Be directive authority during the sessions.

### Challenge
- Challenge Kirsten with her failure to expect others to perform at the high levels she expects of herself.
- Direct Kirsten to do activities associated with the institutional order of consciousness, e.g., through self-reflection, becoming fully conscious of her own feelings, thoughts, values, and desires; and taking responsible action to express these and to get her needs met.
- Make an event of all of the areas in which Kirsten is striking out on her own, discovering her own ideas, deciding for herself, becoming clear on her OWN values while questioning what happens to that confidence when she is in certain situations or with those who may not share her newfound place.
- Assist Kirsten to become aware of her neglected feeling states, to feel comfortable with them rather than denying them, and to consider them

worthy of being honored by another, rather than not expecting others to care about these feelings.

- Challenge her, in the midst of gaining confidence in who she is becoming, to be able to fully hear others that she is in relationship with, and to work on conflict resolution skills that both honor others and allow her to declare herself.

---

She also chooses work that supports rather than challenges her new-found meaning-making capacities, that is, she goes into business for herself as a pharmaceutical sales rep. This allows her to make her own choices, stand on her own, create a strong business based on her own instincts, and yet deal with clients in limited ways. Although she finds herself having to "sell" her products and "make nice" with clients, she doesn't have to have an office next door to them, which might challenge her new abilities to be herself fully. She succeeds over a long period of time at this new business endeavor and gains respect within her profession (See Table 5.6.).

At some point near the end of her thirties, however, she begins to meet people who relate to her differently. They ask her questions about herself, reaching out to really know her. They are not, as so many she has been involved with before, either listening to her declare herself, declaring themselves, or taking turns as they and she declare themselves. Instead, they seem to put as much value on developing a quality relationship and on deepening it as on the task that she and they might be working on together. In addition, they share themselves deeply. And when they do, they communicate a sense that they are in the process of growth rather than "already there" at some final destination.

Initially, Kirsten considers these people irresponsible and disorganized, figuring that accomplished and successful people present a polished and finished image of themselves at all times. Certainly, she would expect that of herself. But as she relates more to these people, she realizes that their freedom to be "in process" also allows her to share areas of herself that are not "finished." She finds herself more accepted by these new friends. She realizes that they are growing through being in relationship with her—they are learning through the process of dialogue with her. She finds a level of intimacy that is not only very new to her, but very desirable. That is, she is able to fully share herself and have others fully share themselves, able to participate as they share "real selves in process," able to grow in the presence of another human being, able to reflect while with someone rather than only afterward alone at home.

Initially, she believes that these people are simply a "higher" order of human beings than she is, that they have been born with gifts and

TABLE 5.6   Early Thirties to Early Forties: Institutional Balance
             and Transition to Interindividual Balance

## Issues

- Relationship problems due to others' insecurity in the fact of her newly
  found SELF—their difficulty with conflict or with full self-expression—some
  loneliness results at times.
- Partnered with a man who does not share her developmental capacities
  begins to feel empty, boring, lonely. Search for greater intimacy and connections, for community, for creating "more" than what an individual can create
  by her- or himself.
- Sense that current "support" environments are too restrictive and something
  more awaits her.
- Anxiousness about leaving previous way of being without having firm
  ground to stand on wherever she is emerging to; lack of "guidelines" to follow in her search.

## Goals

- Kirsten will advance developmentally by finding adequate supports and challenges for growth.
- Kirsten will explore the range of possibilities in her marriage.
- Kirsten will find a community in which she can "be in process" as she develops, a community in which people are not threatened by this amorphousness.
- Kirsten will explore the "higher principles" behind her usual choices in her
  efforts to discover more fulfilling behavior that is in harmony with "what
  really matters."

## Interventions

### Support
- Punctuate what Kirsten has discovered about herself, her fidelity to her life
  callings, and her ongoing efforts at further development.
- Punctuate all of the successes Kirsten has created for herself, in work and
  relationships, and how she has freed herself from the various hindrances of
  her upbringing.
- Allow Kirsten to be her own authority during the sessions.
- Couples counseling will require supporting both Kirsten and her husband,
  despite their different developmental levels.

### Challenge
- When conflicts emerge during sessions, encourage Kirsten to stay with the
  conflict long enough for both parties to grow into something more than they
  could have been on their own.

- Use empty chair strategies to encourage Kirsten to have conversations among different parts of herself, different ideologies she has advocated, etc.
- Support Kirsten's peace with being in process, with not drawing or coming to conclusions.
- Help Kirsten to focus on the "between" in relationships, the process of decision making, the intersections and interactions among the various systems of which she is a part.
- Support Kirsten's efforts to create working and relationship systems—a community of learners—that honor individuals at the same time as honoring the process of relating and creating together, intentionally relating to others in a way that supports and challenges where they are.
- Encourage Kirsten to seek out relationships with people with views different than her own, engage in conversations and tasks together, and observe and stay in a process that can create "more," with greater fidelity to higher principles, and/or making ideologies object.

---

temperaments and spirits that are qualitatively different from her own. However, through a variety of circumstances, she becomes familiar with developmental theory and with the notion that she, too, might achieve what she considers to be their "advanced" way of living life.

Thus, despite her previous work and relationship satisfaction, she begins to see something more "out there" that she wants and needs and isn't willing to do without. Her current partnership begins to feel "less"—less intimate, more lonely, less satisfying. She begins to realize the limitations of having her own business and working by herself, that perhaps she and her work could actually become "more" if done in relationship, in community. Because neither her relational or work environments can provide her with directions about how to move ahead, she finds a group of people to associate with and to be accountable to who are "seekers," who seem to have this "more" that she wants. She also joins a team of researchers at a mid-size pharmaceutical company. She enters counseling with her partner to figure out a way for their partnership to grow into something more satisfying.

## Early Forties to Early Fifties

Kirsten is fortunate that her new employment site is a supportive one. Her superiors seem to have ways of working with people that exemplify the ways in which she wants to work with people. They are willing to support her developmental efforts as she moves into the vice president position. As a result of their support and of her participation in the Zen center groups, Kirsten finds herself moving ahead developmentally. For instance, she finds when she is talking with people, that she no longer has to present herself as polished and finished, as "a defined and contained" person whose responsibility is to congruently and strongly express herself. Instead, she sees herself as in process and comfortable enough to express that incompleteness. In fact, not only does she experience incompleteness, she experiences the sense that her SELF has deserted her—as though she is many selves, and that these many selves are in constant negotiation. She becomes persuaded that the chaos of too many challenges and responsibilities, chaos that she previously tried to control or eliminate, is really a permanent state—that there is not one firm ground to stand on.

Probably as a result, she also finds herself accepting others as in process, as always emerging, rather than as *selves* that *are* a particular way, sometimes a particular way that might threaten her way. She can therefore proactively create a safe place for others to express their incompleteness— by modeling her own, and by being accepting when others express theirs.

Kirsten no longer sees conflict with others as differences between two different people or positions that need to be resolved into a compromise position, but as opportunities to know others as they are emerging, to make one's own forward process known, and to discover how to blend those processes together to build an environment that encourages forward progress for both parties. In fact, it is only in the expression of differences or conflicts that any of the participants can know how to create such an environment and therefore can continue a mutual growth process. She now recognizes her previous tendency to draw lines in the sand and how that strategy resulted in either compliance or reactiveness on the part of those with whom she was having conflicts, neither of which worked very well for the relationships or for the working environment.

Further, Kirsten finds herself evaluating how her own position of power may affect her relationships with others and works at creating a more egalitarian work environment in which all voices are heard and honored. She regularly considers how to be intentional about creating a developmentally supportive and healthy environment. She realizes that there is no fixed way of doing this, that it will always depend on who is in the research group at the time, and that her perceptions about how to do this will always be emerging. Thus, she sees herself in a growth process around "knowing" and that this "knowing" is a process, rather than a state.

When parenting her child, she finds herself pulling back from definite "right" statements, instead expressing more tentative statements, being willing to change her mind or consider her daughter's input fully. She is able to admit when she is wrong or when there might be several "correct" ways of looking at things or behaving. She assesses her daughter's developmental readiness for certain discussions and activities, and intentionally responds accordingly. Because her daughter is in elementary school, Kirsten tends to use clear structure and direction and behavioral strategies as ways to support her daughter's developmental progress. At the same time, she challenges her daughter developmentally by spending a great deal of time discussing decisions and "rules" with her daughter, explaining the reasons behind them, and considering the relationship between "right" and "wrong" in certain decisions and behaviors.

In personal relationships, she finds herself enjoying people at different developmental levels, reaching out more fully, and needing to be less protective of her time and energy. She finds herself more open to difference in people, learning from it, enjoying it, and taking the opportunity to have these differences challenge her own developing self. She realizes that life would be boring and her child's life education very limited were she the only input into it. When hearing from others, she finds herself able to fully hear them and get into their shoes, without needing to assert her own position. In conflicts, she moves beyond the notion of each person asserting their own position to being more able and less fearful of honoring who the other person is, recognizing the value of their choices and ways of being, commending them on what works well for them. She is able to empathize with their position, rather than considering hers the only right one and their differing perspective inferior in some way. She finds herself able to say, "This isn't working for me right now, even though I can see that it serves you well in other situations. I am wondering how we can learn from these differences, honor them, and still find something that works better for me. Perhaps I will change to a different place in time, but this is where I am now." She also finds herself more conscious of when other people are drawing lines in the sand; she still experiences some difficulty in responding to these people in a helpful or positive way.

Of course, Kirsten is not consistent in her interindividual capacities because they, too, are always emerging, and she is consistently discovering new characteristics within the interindividual order of consciousness. Further, her self-reflectiveness in an environment of support allows her to recognize the ways in which the difficulties in her upbringing sometimes interfere with her interindividual capacities. However, the ability to stand back from them allows her to hold competing tendencies until she discovers ways for them to "solve her."

Intervention, other than her currently supporting environments, would probably be unnecessary for Kirsten. However, because she requested counseling, a highly developed counselor might provide a holding environment during her initial fears about her *self* "flying away," leaving her with no ground to stand on. It is more likely, though, that she would proactively engage in intervening developmentally with others. I think it is only reasonable to admit here that my own lack of interindividual capacities and experiences with interindividual people, may be hindering my conceptions of what might be possible through counseling or other interventions.

## Summary

Writing this chapter has been a developmental challenge and quite enlightening as a reminder about situations within my own life, including my own way of handling relationships at home and at work. My hope is that readers will be able to immediately use this material to think differently about their own challenges, life choices, relationships, and work life. In particular, my hope is that readers will find practical applications for personal life and professional work emerging from this chapter, because its aim has been to expand current developmental literature from what has generally been theoretical into the realm of daily practice. From my mind to yours—may there be transformation.

## Annotated Bibliography

Belenky, M., Clinchy, B., Goldberger, N., & Tarule, J. (1986). *Women's ways of knowing*. New York: Basic Books.

Using interviews with women from many demographic groups about their search for truth and knowledge, the authors determine five learning "perspectives" that characterize "women's way of knowing": silence, received knowing, subjective knowing, procedural knowing, and constructivist knowing. The book skillfully blends narration, documentation, and excerpts from interviews, and aptly illustrates women's developmental process as different in some ways from men's.

Kegan, R. (1982). *The evolving self*. Cambridge, MA: Harvard.

Kegan introduces his theory of development—one that integrates social development and meaning-making into a scheme that can be used to derive testable generalizations and simultaneously inform the practice of therapy. He describes the growth and loss of the incorporative self, the impulsive self, the imperial self, the interpersonal self, and the institutional self.

Kegan, R. (1994). *In over our heads.* Cambridge, MA: Harvard.
Kegan clarifies the theory presented in *The Evolving Self,* while convincingly illustrating that "modern life" demands functioning at the fourth order of consciousness—institutional knowing. The book describes in his developmental terms (1) the demands placed upon adolescents, parents, partners, workers, leaders, counselees, and learners, and (2) the ways in which people's environments might optimally support and challenge them toward the next order of consciousness.

Kegan, R., & Lahey, L. L. (2001). *How the way we talk can change the way we work: Seven languages for transformation.* San Francisco: Jossey-Bass.
Kegan and Lahey apply constructive developmental theory to fostering growth and transformation in both individuals and organizations. They indicate that most individuals and organizations are actually immune to deep and lasting change in spite of their best intentions because they do not understand people's powerful inclinations *not* to change. Kegan and Lahey introduce a new complement of language forms that people can use to overcome this immunity to change.

Loevinger, J. (1976). *Ego development.* San Francisco: Jossey-Bass.
Loevinger describes people's progression through the following stages: presocial, self-protective, conformist, conscientious-conformist, conscientious, individualistic, autonomous, and integrated. She supports her theory with research that has used her *Sentence Completion Test.*

Perry, W. G. (1999). *Forms of intellectual and ethical development in the college years: A scheme.* New York: Holt, Rinehart, and Winston.
In his nine-stage model, Perry describes the steps that move students from a simplistic, categorical view of knowledge to a more complex, contextual view of the world and of themselves. Perry indicates that the most significant changes occur in the forms from which people perceive their world rather than in the particulars of their attitudes and concerns.

Rest, J., Narvaez, D., Bebeau, M. J., Thoma, S. J. (1999). *Postconventional moral thinking: A neo-Kohlbergian approach.* Mahway, NJ: Erlbaum.
Rest and his associates present their and others' research on Kohlberg's moral developmental stages, as assessed using their *Defining Issues Test.* The book convincingly draws correlations between people's moral developmental abilities, their degree of postconventional reasoning abilities, and many areas of adult functioning. Of interest to counselors are the connections drawn between such abilities and optimal functioning in professions similar to counseling.

# References

Allison, S. (1988). *Meaning-making in marriage: An exploratory study.* Unpublished doctoral dissertation, Massachusetts School of Professional Psychology.

Alvarez, M. (1985). *The construing of friendship in adulthood: A structural-developmental approach.* Unpublished doctoral dissertation, Massachusetts School of Professional Psychology.

Anderson, W. T. (1990). *Reality isn't what it used to be.* New York: Harper Collins.

Bar-Yam, M. (1991). Do men and women speak in different voices? A comparative study of self-evolvement. *International Journal of Aging and Human Development, 32,* 247–259.

Basseches, M. (1980). Dialectical schemata: A framework for the empirical study of the development of dialectical thinking. *Human Development, 23,* 400–421.

Baxter-Magolda, M., & Porterfield, W. D. (1988). *Assessing intellectual development: The link between theory and practice.* Alexandria, VA: American College Personnel Association.

Bebeau, M. J., & Brabeck, M. M. (1987). Integrating care and justice issues in professional moral education: A gender perspective. *Journal of Moral Education, 22,*189–203.

Belenky, M., Clinchy, B., Goldberger, N., & Tarule, J. (1986). *Women's ways of knowing.* New York: Basic Books.

Beukema, S. (1990). *Women's best friendships: Their meaning and meaningfulness.* Unpublished doctoral dissertation, Harvard University.

Binner, V. F. (1991). *A study of Minnesota entrepreneurship: Balancing personal, business, and community demands.* Unpublished doctoral dissertation, Graduate School of The Union Institute.

Borders, L. D., & Fong, M. L. (1989). Ego development and counseling ability during training. *Counselor Education and Supervision, 29,*71–83.

Borders, L. D., Fong, M. L., & Neimeyer, G. J. (1986). Counseling students' level of ego development and perceptions of clients. *Counselor Education and Supervision, 26,* 36–49.

Dixon, J. W. (1986). *The relation of social perspective stages to Kegan's stages of ego development.* Unpublished doctoral dissertation, University of Toledo.

Eriksen, K. P. (2006). The constructive developmental theory of Robert Kegan. *The Family Journal, 14*(3), 290–298.

Eriksen, K. P. (2007). Counseling the imperial client. *The Family Journal. 15,* 174–182.

Eriksen, K., & McAuliffe, G. (2006). Adult development as a predictor of counseling competence. *Counselor Education and Supervision, 45,*180–192.

Erwin, T. D. (1983). The Scale on Intellectual Development: Measuring Perry's scheme. *Journal of College Student Personnel, 24,* 6–12.

Gilligan, C. (1982). *In a different voice.* Cambridge, MA: Harvard University Press.

Goodman, R. (1983). *A developmental and systems analysis of marital and family communication in clinic and non-clinic families.* Unpublished doctoral dissertation, Harvard University.

Greenwald, J. M. (1991). *Environmental attitudes: A structural developmental model.* Unpublished doctoral dissertation, University of Massachusetts.

Haag-Granello, D., & Hazler, R. J. (1998). A developmental rationale for curriculum order and teaching styles in counselor education programs. *Counselor Education and Supervision, 38,* 89–105.

Jacobs, J. (1984). *Holding environment and developmental stages: A study of marriage.* Unpublished doctoral dissertation, Harvard University.

Kegan, R. (1982). *The evolving self.* Cambridge, MA: Harvard.

Kegan, R. (1994). *In over our heads.* Cambridge, MA: Harvard.

Kitchener, K. S., & King, P. M. (1981). Reflective judgment: Concepts of justification and their relationship to age and education. *Journal of Applied Developmental Psychology, 2,* 89–116.

Knefelkamp, L., & Slepitza, R. (1976). A cognitive-developmental model of career development: An adaptation of the Perry Scheme. *The Counseling Psychologist, 6,* 53–58.

Knefelkamp, L., Widick, C., & Parker, C. A. (1978). *Applying new developmental findings.* San Francisco: Jossey-Bass.

Kohlberg, L. (1981). *The philosophy of moral development.* San Francisco: Harper & Row.

Kohlberg, L. (1984). *The psychology of moral development: The nature and validity of moral stages.* San Francisco: Harper & Row.

Kohlberg, L., & Mayer, R. (1972). Development as the aim of education. *Harvard Education Review, 42,* 449–496.

Lahey, L., (1986). *Males' and females' construction of conflict in work and love.* Unpublished doctoral dissertation, Harvard University.

Lahey, L., Souvaine, E., Kegan, R., Goodman, R., & Felix, S. (1985). *A guide to the Subject-Object Interview.* Cambridge, MA: The Subject-Object Research Group.

Loevinger, J. (1976). *Ego Development.* San Francisco: Jossey-Bass.

Lovell, C. W. (1999). Empathic-cognitive development in students of counseling. *Journal of Adult Development, 6,* 195–203.

McAuliffe, G. J. (2002, January). *The impact of counselor epistemology on clinical competence: Comparing relativists' and dualists' counseling interviews.* Paper presented at the meeting of the Perry Network, Fullerton, CA.

McAuliffe, G. J., & Eriksen, K. P. (1999). Toward a constructivist and developmental identity for the counseling profession: The Context-Phase-Stage-Style Model. *Journal of Counseling and Development, 77*(3), 267–280.

McAuliffe, G. J., & Eriksen, K. P. (2000). *Preparing counselors and therapists: Creating constructivist and developmental programs.* Alexandria, VA: Association for Counselor Education and Supervision.

McAuliffe, G. J., & Eriksen, K. P. (2002). *Teaching strategies for constructivist and developmental counselor education.* Westport, CT: Bergin & Garvey.

McAuliffe, G. J., & Lovell, C. W. (2000). Encouraging transformation: Guidelines for constructivist and developmental counselor education. In G. McAuliffe, K. Eriksen, and Associates, *Preparing counselors and therapists: Creating constructivist and developmental programs* (pp. 14–41). Alexandria, VA: Association for Counselor Education and Supervision.

Moore, W. S. (1989). The Learning Environment Preferences: Exploring the construct validity of an objective measure of the Perry scheme of intellectual development. *Journal of College Student Development, 30,* 504–514.

Neukrug, E. S., & McAuliffe, G. J. (1993). Cognitive development and human service education. *Human Service Education, 13,* 13–26.

Olson, G. A. (1989). Social construction and composition theory: A conversation with Richard Rorty. *Journal of Advanced Composition, 9,* 1–9.

Osgood, C. N. (1991). *Readiness for parenting teenagers: A structural developmental approach.* Unpublished doctoral dissertation, University of Massachusetts.

Paisley, P. O., & Benshoff, J. M. (1998). A developmental focus: Implications for Counselor education. *Canadian Journal of Counselling, 32,* 27–36.

Perry, W. G. (1970). Forms of intellectual and ethical development in the college years: A scheme. New York: Holt, Rinehart, and Winston.

Piaget, J. (1963). *The origins of intelligence in children.* New York: Norton.

Rest, J. (1979). *Development in judging moral issues.* Minneapolis: University of Minnesota Press.

Rest, J., Narvaez, D., Bebeau, M. J., & Thoma, S. J. (1999). *Postconventional moral thinking: A neo-Kohlbergian approach.* Mahway, NJ: Erlbaum.

Roy, N. S. (1993). *Toward an understanding of family functioning: An analysis of the relationship between family and individual organizing principles.* Unpublished doctoral dissertation. Harvard University.

Sonnenschein, P. C. (1990). *The development of mutually satisfying relationships between adult daughters and their mothers.* Unpublished doctoral dissertation, Harvard University.

Sprinthall, N. A. (1994). Counseling and social role-taking: Promoting moral and ego development. In J. Rest & D. Narvaez (Eds.), *Moral development in the professions: Psychology and applied ethics* (pp. 85–100). Hillsdale, NJ: Erlbaum.

Sprinthall, N. A., & Thies-Sprinthall, L. (1983). The teacher as an adult learner: A cognitive-developmental view. In G. Griffin (Ed.), *Staff development: Eighty-second yearbook of the National Society for the Study of Education* (pp. 13–35). Chicago: University of Chicago Press.

Vacc, N. A., & Juhnke, G. A. (1997). The use of structured clinical interviews for assessment in counseling. *Journal of Counseling and Development, 75,* 470–480.

Yalom, I. D. (1995). *The theory and practice of group psychotherapy* (3rd ed.). New York: Basic Books.

# CHAPTER SIX

# Psychoanalytic Theory in Action

## John Sommers-Flanagan and Aida Hutz

When teaching about psychoanalytic theory, we often begin with a word association game. We ask students to quickly say the first words that come into their mind when they think of the word *Freud*. Students almost always immediately shout out a list of words that could easily be construed as disparaging. They typically say things like, *sex, cocaine, anal*, and of course, *pervert*. We usually try to laugh right along with the students as they generate their popular and negative conceptions of Freud. Then, we ask them to let go of their preconceived ideas and to realistically consider the value and limits of Freud's theories in context and practice. We hope you can do the same as you read this chapter.

Studying psychoanalytic theories is important for many more reasons than can be addressed in this brief section. Consequently, we limit our discussion to a review of Freud as a talk therapy pioneer who introduced a particular and unique therapeutic approach to the medical and scientific community. We also focus on some of the many developmental theories of counseling that were developed as either a transformation or reaction to his work.

Although Freud's ideas are controversial, especially those related to women's development, his impact is undeniable. Freud's early professional influences and his innate curiosity about human motivation propelled him to introduce an innovative theory whereby unconscious mental processes drive behavior. In our Western, linear, scientifically oriented culture, this was the first time that people were referenced as nonrational beings, that is, beings who were not always in control of their behaviors. This lack of rationality and complete control over one's thoughts and feelings was characterized by Hergenhahn (1994, p. 20) as a "blow to human's self-esteem." However, as a result of acknowledging these unconscious processes, Freud was able to develop a therapeutic approach that was based on more than what can be observed, measured, and controlled. He called this approach *psycho-analysis* and claimed it as an effective treatment modality for patients presenting with mental disorders (i.e., hysteria). Freud described this innovative and controversial approach as

> an interchange of words between the patient and the analyst. The patient talks, tells of his [sic] past experiences and present impressions, complains, confesses to his wishes and his emotional impulses. The doctor listens, tries to direct the patient's processes of thought, exhorts, forces his attention in certain directions, gives him explanations and observes the reactions of understanding or rejection which he in this way provokes in him.   (Freud, 1966, pp. 19–20)

One might disagree with Freud's methods of structuring and giving meaning to the therapeutic process, but he did something remarkable: He deeply engaged and listened to his patients. This simple, but profound deportment became the foundation for the future of counseling. Furthermore, it is important to point out that this took place during a period when individuals with mental and emotional disorders were dismissed and degraded. Moreover, physicians who treated these patients were shunned by the medical community (Hergenhahn, 1994). Today, many transformations of the process described above are recognized and respected not only within the mental health field, but also within medicine.

In addition to laying a foundation for talk therapy as a valid form of treatment, Freud also influenced many significant theories and theorists. For example, Carl Jung, Alfred Adler, Erik Erikson, Karen Horney, and many others worked directly with Freud. Ego-psychology has direct roots from Sigmund Freud's and Anna Freud's work (Sommers-Flanagan & Sommers-Flanagan, 2004). Also, object-relations theory and therapy developed in response to traditional psychoanalytic theory, and more contemporary reformulations of attachment theory and therapy are distinctly psychoanalytic in nature (Cooper, Hoffman, Powell, & Marvin, 2005). Today, although voices within the psychoanalytic movement are transformed and pluralistic, they continue to be strong and influential not only in the United States but also through-out the world (Wallerstein, 2002). Interestingly, many nonpsychoanalytic theorists (e.g., Ellis, Beck, Perls) discovered their approaches while using psychoanalytic methods. This historical fact suggests that the psychoanalytic perspective is an outstanding platform from which new theories and therapies may be discovered and constructed.

Not only does this framework have a strong history and tradition, several psychoanalytic concepts are often utilized by virtually all mental health professionals. For example, addressing issues related to countertransference is ubiquitous in the counseling field (Mohr, Gelso, & Hill, 2005; Rosenberger & Hayes, 2002). Counselors-in-training are encouraged to scrutinize themselves to ascertain how their thoughts, feelings, and assumptions affect clients and guide, lead, or impact the therapeutic relationship. This is a frequent focus of supervision, regardless of theoretical orientation (Dass-Brailsford, 2003; Hamburg, 2004). Other widely accepted practices such as talking about past experiences, especially those from childhood, and how they affect clients today also originated with Freud. Moreover, a frequently adopted and often considered necessary therapeutic condition is building a relationship between the client and the counselor. This relationship is to be constructed as one of a safe and trusting environment, where clients can talk about their deepest thoughts and feelings without feeling judged by their therapist. This idea was also first introduced by Freud through his psychoanalytic approach.

In sum, Freud introduced a solid foundation for counseling and psychotherapy. Concepts such as countertransference, talking about childhood past experiences, and even listening and developing a safe and trusting therapeutic environment are rooted in psychoanalysis. Although from its beginning psychoanalysis has been laden with controversy, it is a building block for what is still valued by most counselors today.

## Theoretical Overview

In her developmental psychology text, Patricia Miller refers to Freud's traditional psychoanalytic theory as one of the "Giant" theories of psychological development (Miller, 2002). This is because Freud tried to construct one theory to explain everything about human personality development, psychopathology, and methods for resolving developmental problems.

## ABOUT THE CHAPTER AUTHORS

### John Sommers-Flanagan

Writing this chapter stimulated my thinking on where I am in my lifespan development. There was good news and less good news about this. The less good news for my mature adult friends was the realization that I remain proudly adolescent. The photo of me performing rap is testimony to my adolescent-ness. At the same time, I am now more aware than ever of my oldness. I can now look back in my life farther than I can look forward. This fact provides both joy and sorrow. I embrace and resist it daily.

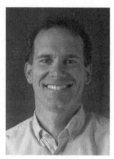

**John Sommers-Flanagan**

This is the second time I've written something with Aida Hutz, a Brazilian woman with great cultural clarity. I appreciate her perspective and hope it shines through to readers. Her push toward counselor self-awareness inspires me to reclaim my culture and my ignorance.

In the end, I'm left with many developmental contradictions about myself. I am young and old, White and not White, insightful and ignorant. I am also an assistant professor of counselor education at the University of Montana, father, step-father, husband, man, and person whose contradictions continue beyond the pages of this book.

### Aida Hutz

Writing this chapter, Psychoanalytic Theory in Action, was an enlightening experience. It gave me an opportunity to read many of Freud's original writings, which was an interesting process because it allowed me to develop a deep appreciation for him. Like many counselors and counselors-in-training, I had many biases and misconceptions about Freud's work. Often, I immediately associated the psychoanalytic framework with something negative, antiquated, and certainly to be avoided. However, as result of learning about this approach in greater depth, I realize that Freud is not only a pioneer but also a courageous, hard-working man who was not afraid to share his perspective with the world.

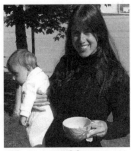

**Aida Hutz and her son**

*Aida Hutz*, Ed.D., LCPC, was born and raised in Brazil. She is currently an assistant professor of counseling at The University of Montana. Her professional interests include teaching and practicing multicultural awareness, learning about transcultural issues particularly related to Brazil, and conducting psychotherapy research. She lives in Missoula with her family, and she enjoys hiking and caring for her newborn son.

The benefit of using a giant, all-encompassing theory like Freud's as a tool for conceptualizing psychotherapeutic or counseling dynamics is that the theory can almost always provide an explanation for even the most puzzling client behaviors. For example, in *The Psychoanalytic Theory of Neurosis* (1945), Otto Fenichel, a disciple of Freud, outlines psychoanalytic explanations for every human ailment from asthma to fetishism to suicide (and many more). Of course, most psychoanalytic explanations for behavioral psychopathology boil down to sex or aggression, but theorists have found no limit to the creative ways these most basic of human issues might cause human problems.

The downside of Freud's all-encompassing theory is that in his prolific effort to explain everything, he wrote extensively about aspects of human behavior with which he had little, if any, firsthand experience. Consequently, many of his theoretical conclusions, particularly those focusing on women, have been strongly criticized and in many cases, scientifically disproved (Fisher & Greenberg, 1985). In contrast to Freud's tendency to play the role of a dogmatic authority, throughout this chapter we employ general principles of psychoanalytic thinking to gently and tentatively provide a guide for working with young clients, ages ten to sixteen.

It is currently inappropriate, if not impossible, to blithely use the term *psychoanalytic* when referring to any counseling approach. This is because psychoanalytic theory, much like Christianity and feminism, has fragmented and taken on so much contemporary baggage that we must identify exactly what sort of psychoanalytic theory to which we are referring. For example, one might ask, Does this chapter adhere to Freud's original or classical drive or instinct-based psychoanalytic theory (S. Freud, 1949)? Does it emphasize the psychoanalytic ego psychology as articulated and practiced by Anna Freud, Erik Erikson, and others (Erikson, 1963; A. Freud, 1966)? Does the chapter consider later analytic thinking, such as object relations or self psychology as foundational (Fairbairn, 1952; Kohut, 1984)? Will we be discussing even more recent developments in psychoanalytic thinking, such as intersubjectivity and two-person psychoanalysis (Ringstrom, 2001)? Or in the following pages, do we emphasize time-limited or short-term psychoanalytic modifications (Luborsky, 1984; Strupp & Binder, 1984)?

Our answer to these important theoretical questions is a hearty yes. To the extent possible, in this chapter we present an eclectic psychoanalytic perspective. We do this despite the fact that in so doing we will undoubtedly anger many proponents of specific psychoanalytic perspectives. Our rationale is that we believe the most practical application of psychoanalytic thinking is, once again in contrast to Freud, a loose (rather than rigid) approach that emphasizes the particular psychoanalytic approach that is the best fit for the client, rather than the counselor's favored approach. This eclectic psychoanalytic perspective has the advantage of acknowledging and potentially integrating the diverse range of developmental discoveries, including attachment research, that have occurred after Freud's death and that have further fueled the evolution of psychoanalytic theory and practice (Ainsworth, Blehar, Waters, & Wall, 1978; Bowlby, 1969; Cooper, et al., 2005; Mahler, 1968).

## General Theoretical Assumptions

The underlying theoretical assumptions guiding our loose, eclectic psychoanalytic model must be discussed. Just keep in mind that the following assumptions are general. And in the spirit of more recent two-person psychoanalytic formulations, they need to be applied to specific therapeutic encounters in ways that provide the greatest potential benefit for both client and counselor (Renik, 1993).

*Human behavior is fueled by pleasure seeking or relationship dynamics.* Early Freudian theory held that human behavior was driven primarily, if not exclusively, by pleasure seeking. Later, Fairbairn (1952) distinguished object relations theory from drive theory by stating "libido is object seeking, not pleasure seeking" (p. 82). Fairbairn's statement emphasizes the object relations perspective that infants orient toward relationship connection rather than pleasure. More recent attachment research also

## ABOUT SIGMUND FREUD

Sigmund Freud was born in Freiberg, Austria, on May 6, 1856, to a Jewish family. When Sigmund's father, Jacob, married his mother, Amalia, he already had two grown sons from a previous marriage. Sigmund's oldest half-brother was about the same age as Freud's mother, who was twenty years junior to her husband, Jacob. Sigmund was the first born of eight siblings; however, one died at seven months when Freud was two years old. When Sigmund was four, his family moved to Vienna where he was to spend most of his life. Amalia died at age ninety-five, only nine years prior to her son, Sigmund Freud, who died in 1939 at the age of eighty-three.

Freud's parents recognized that he was intellectually gifted, and had high ambitions for him. Sigmund was always favored by his parents, who ensured their home environment was conducive to his studies. For example, Freud's brothers and sisters were not allowed to play musical instruments because the noise might interfere with Sigmund's studying.

At that time, there were not many promising career choices for a Jewish man. Medicine seemed to be one of the few. Thus, at age seventeen Freud began studying medicine at the University of Vienna. Unlike many medical students, Freud took eight years to complete his degree. This was due to his interest in diverse academic fields, which led him to take many classes not required for his medical degree. In 1886 after a long engagement, Sigmund finally had the financial means to marry Martha Bernays. They had six children in nine years; Anna Freud, who extended her father's work, was the youngest.

Early influences on Freud's theory stem from his trip to Paris in 1885, where he was introduced to hypnosis by Jean-Martin Charcot. Furthermore, in 1887 an interesting and intimate friendship with Wilhelm Fliess, a nose-and-throat specialist, served as a catalyst to the development of Freud's ideas regarding the connection between sexual drives and mental dysfunctions. Another early influence was Josef Breuer, a fatherly mentor. Breuer's discussions with Freud in 1895, regarding the treatment of Breuer's patient, Anna O., helped bring psychoanalysis to life. That same year, Freud's dream of Irma's injection also served as a model for psychoanalysis. This dream is controversial in nature, and has been generally interpreted as

"Freud's ongoing struggle with his misogynist impulses, his unruly homosexuality" (Lotto, 2001). For detailed information about another controversial part of Freud's legacy, Jeffrey Masson's recounting of Freud's discovery and eventual recanting of the seduction hypothesis is excellent (Masson, 1984).

Four years later in 1899, Freud published what many consider his most influential book, *Interpretation of Dreams*. In his following book, *Psychopathology of Everyday Life*, Freud wrote about unconscious drives also motivating nonpathological, "normal," people. During the next decade, Freud remained very active in his writing and the development of psychoanalytic theory. At the same time, he developed and ended intense relationships with Carl Jung and Alfred Adler. In 1917, while on his only visit to the United States, Freud delivered lectures at Clark University that resulted in the publication of the *Introductory Lectures on Psycho-Analysis*. In 1923 Freud published *The Ego and the Id*, and introduced his "structural theory of the mind." As the psychoanalytic movement continued to grow, Freud gained popularity and became well known throughout the world.

After being diagnosed with cancer of the jaw, Freud endured 33 operations; however, he did not stop thinking and writing until his death. In 1938, due to the invasion of the Nazis and a frightening anti-Semitic movement in Germany, Freud and his family immigrated to London, where he "died in freedom," on September 23, 1939.

---

underlines the survival-based priority of very early caretaker–infant bonding. For example, in a variety of research studies, infants have been shown to prefer their caretaker's face, smell, and voice over all other visual, olfactory, and auditory stimuli (Cernoch & Potter, 1985; Russell, Mendelson, & Peeke, 1983).

In a practical sense, pleasure and relationship seeking frequently overlap in time and space. Therefore, the general model we follow is that humans orient toward and seek *both* pleasure and relationship (and often seek both at the same time). Further, orientation toward pleasure and relationship is frequently laden with strong emotional intensity, which is one reason why sexual and aggressive impulses are sometimes experienced simultaneously (especially when the pleasurable activity or valued relationship is withheld from an individual).

*Primary or significant past relationship dynamics are often reenacted in the present.* Consistent with psychoanalytic as well as attachment theory, we believe early childhood relationship patterns produce an internal interpersonal working model within individuals. This internal model generally guides individuals in their interpersonal relationships.

Freud referred to the manifestation of an internal working model during psychoanalysis as *transference.* Our position is that transference is a real and observable phenomenon and will potentially enter into all relationships and all counseling relationships, regardless of the counselor's theoretical orientation. It is common for clients to project relationship assumptions based on an internal working model derived from their past onto the counselor within counseling sessions.

*Countertransference is also a real and observable phenomenon.* Because as counselors we are just as human and fallible as our clients, it is also common for us to project our past relationship assumptions onto our clients within the counseling session. The reality of this phenomenon has been acknowledged by counselors of many divergent theoretical orientations (Goldfried & Davison, 1994). Moreover, strategies for increasing counselor awareness, both of historical relationship dynamics and of current ethnic and cultural issues, form the foundation for many counselor training programs (Corey, 2005). Finally, it should be noted that transference and countertransference tend to be unconscious, automatic, repetitive, and inappropriate.

*It is usually helpful for counseling process and outcome if the counselor recognizes, understands, and deals constructively with transference and countertransference issues.* During counseling sessions when clients repeatedly exhibit inappropriate or maladaptive interpersonal behavior patterns, it is the responsibility of the counselor to gently and constructively bring these patterns to the client's awareness. Freud and other psychoanalysts use the technique of interpretation to help clients gain insight into these problematic patterns (Kivlighan, 2002). However, research has shown that the counselor's manner and timing of providing interpretations to clients is crucial for helping clients use such information constructively. Specifically, in their work with substance abusing clients, Miller and Rollnick (2002) demonstrated that more confrontational interpretive statements increased client resistance, while more gentle and client-centered interpretations were more likely to result in clients exploring their maladaptive substance use. Additionally, contemporary intersubjective or two-person psychoanalytic models tend to emphasize the importance of being noncritical and mutual when exploring client behavior within or outside of the counseling session (Ringstrom, 2001).

Transference dynamics are usually explored using two different triangles of insight formulations: the conflict-based (or pleasure-based) model and the transference-based (or relationship-based) model. The conflict-based model of insight emphasizes the importance of linking (1) the client's wish, aim, or drive toward pleasure, (2) the threat or imagined threat that makes gratifying the wish unacceptable, and (3) the defensive compromise that the conflict between a client's wish and threat requires. This interpretive model focuses primarily on clients' inner conflicts over pleasurable goals. In contrast, the transference-based triangle of insight emphasizes that maladaptive client interpersonal behavior patterns (which include cognitive and emotional components) can be observed by counselors in three different interpersonal areas: (1) within the in-session or transference domain, (2) within historical reports of early childhood interpersonal dynamics, and (3) within contemporary relationship patterns. It is through the observation and analysis of these maladaptive relationship patterns that the counselor can best help the client to correct his or her misconceptions about how to establish and maintain healthy interpersonal relationships.

*Humans use defense mechanisms to protect themselves from personally threatening information and situations.* For many clients, counseling is a situation in which they feel exposed, vulnerable, and judged. This is especially the case for many teenage and preteen clients who worry and wonder about whether they can trust adults in general and counselors in particular. Consequently, because counseling can feel personally scary or threatening, clients often defend themselves against the counselor's interpretations and feedback. Similarly, clients often resist engaging in the very behaviors that might be positive or growthful for them.

Psychoanalytic theory posits that clients use specific defense mechanisms to protect their vulnerable ego and resist change. These defense mechanisms include denial, repression, sublimation, reaction formation, projection, minimization, and others. Like the concept of transference discussed earlier, defense mechanisms are generally unconscious and automatic, and they distort reality. For example, when a counselor gently suggests to a young teenager that her drug experimentation may be a way for her to express her anger toward her mother who happens to be a probation officer, the teen may initially resist the counselor's interpretation (using the defense mechanism of denial) by shouting, "That's the stupidest thing I've ever heard!"

*During at least part of counseling sessions, it is important to follow Freud's basic rule for psychoanalysis.* The basic rule of psychoanalysis is free association, which involves encouraging clients to "say whatever comes to mind." Following this rule reduces clients' natural defensiveness and thereby allows counselors to observe clients' unconscious conflicts or disturbed relationship patterns more directly. Unfortunately, free association is often contraindicated when working with teenagers because of their tendency to become resistant, defensive, and silent.

The main point of this general free association guideline is to remember that at least from time to time within counseling sessions the counselor should try to help the client take the lead and say whatever he or she wants to say. We believe allowing clients this opportunity is important regardless of your specific theoretical orientation and despite the emphasis by managed care on abbreviated treatment protocols. The simple fact is that sometimes if we just let clients talk freely, we stand to learn a great deal about their repeating personal struggles and potential solutions.

*When prompted with gentle feedback and interpretive statements, clients will often (or at least sometimes) respond with insights about their inner conflicts or problematic relationship patterns.* From the psychoanalytic perspective, the purpose of interpretation is insight. As noted previously, the main focus of the counselors' interpretive statements is on internal conflict and repeating core problematic relationship patterns.

Insight experiences vary for different clients and may or may not involve clear intellectual and emotional components. For some clients, insights into personal conflicts or relationship patterns are sudden, deeply moving, and powerful. For other clients, as in the case described in this chapter, the process of insight seems to slowly dribble into consciousness, almost imperceptibly. We have heard clients refer to their therapeutic insights as having an "ah ha" quality, as being characterized by "Oh no, not again," and as "Hmm. That's interesting."

*Personal insight often leads to increased motivation for positive personal change.* Behaviorists often criticize psychoanalytic approaches by claiming that insight alone is not adequate for behavior change to occur. This criticism is an excellent example of the rhetorical straw man. In fact, psycho-analytically oriented counselors do not claim that insight, in and of itself, is an adequate counseling outcome. Instead, insight is part of the counseling process that enhances client motivation and eventually leads toward working through one's inner conflicts and maladaptive relationship patterns. Alfred Adler was particularly emphatic regarding the motivational properties of insight (Adler, 1956).

*It is possible for counselors to help clients resolve personal problems by providing a corrective emotional experience or corrective relationship experience within counseling sessions.* Alexander and French (1946) were the first to suggest that the corrective emotional experience was the basic healing or therapeutic component in psychotherapy. They said:

> In all forms of . . . psychotherapy, the basic therapeutic principle is the same: To re-expose the patient, under more favorable circumstances, to emotional situations which he [sic] could not handle in the past. The patient, in order to be helped, must undergo a corrective emotional experience suitable to repair the traumatic influence of previous experiences. (p. 66)

Corrective emotional or relational experiences are often viewed as the healing foundation of psychoanalytically oriented counseling. This is especially true for those whose work is informed by object-relations theory. As a consequence, the practical question for the counselor using this approach (and the one used to guide the case discussed later in this chapter) is something like, "How can I provide a secure counseling relationship that will enable my client to face the developmental challenges that have been too threatening or too traumatic to face previously?"

*Much of the work of psychoanalytic counseling involves the remediation of developmental arrests, fixations, or traumas.* Freud, Erikson, Mahler, and other theorists have identified specific ages and issues that form the basis of our understanding of human psychosexual and psychosocial development (Erikson, 1963; S. Freud, 1965; Mahler, 1968). During infancy, childhood, adolescence and beyond, humans face common challenges to their healthy development. Unfortunately, many of our clients have experienced unwieldy challenges during their

TABLE 6.1  Psychoanalytic Developmental Theories

| Years | Theorist | Stage, Crisis, or Challenge and Potential Developmental Problems |
|---|---|---|
| 0–1 | Freud | Oral stage: The infant depends on adults for oral gratification. |
| 0–1 | Erikson | Trust vs. mistrust: Task is to develop trust in others. |
| 0–3 | Mahler | Infants go through many developmental phases including (1) *normal infantile autism* (focus on inner physical sensations during first 3–4 weeks); (2) *symbiosis* (dependency on/attunement with primary caretaker, evident by 3 months); (3) *separation-individuation* (exploration begins at 4–5 months); (4) *emotional object constancy* (begins at 36 months). |
| 1–3 | Freud | Anal stage: The toddler's sense of power, control, and aggression develops. |
| 1–3 | Erikson | Autonomy vs. shame and doubt: Task is to explore and experiment. |
| 3–6 | Freud | Phallic stage: Oedipal desires to be with opposite sex parent emerge. |
| 3–6 | Erikson | Initiative vs. guilt: Task is to develop a sense of achievement. |
| 6–12 | Freud | Latency stage: A relatively quiet period of peer socialization. |
| 6–12 | Erikson | Industry vs. inferiority: Task is to feel productive. |
| 12+ | Freud | Genital stage: The freedom to love and work is achieved. |
| 12–18 | Erikson | Identity vs. role confusion: Task is to achieve sense of self-identity. |
| 18–35 | Erikson | Intimacy vs. isolation: Task is to form lasting intimate relationships. |
| 35–60 | Erikson | Generativity vs. stagnation: Task is to move beyond self to next generation. |
| 60+ | Erikson | Integrity vs. despair: The task is to feel personally worthwhile. |

early development. Consequently, the focus of counseling is to help clients overcome their specific developmental arrests, fixations, or traumas within the context of a secure helping relationship. (See Table 6.1 for more information on psychosexual and psychosocial developmental stages.)

## Psychoanalytic Theory and Diversity

Although psychoanalysts might claim otherwise, psychoanalytic theory is not known for its application to diverse populations. Bankart (1997) casts the limitations in the application of psychoanalytic theory within the context of his time and place in history:

> To fathom Freud's near-obsession with the sexual foundations of emotional distress is also to come to a fuller awareness of the sexual repression and hypocrisy in the lives of the Austrian middle class at the turn of the [nineteenth] century. . . . (p. 8)

Following Bankart's lead, it is important to note that Freud's psychoanalytic theory of the early 1900s is very limited in its direct and narrow application to individuals from other times and places. However, it is also important to remember that although the fine details of Freud's theory may be very culturally limited, the broad strokes based on his detailed and insightful observations of humans in psychological distress may well be more generalizable. For example, as noted earlier, many of his basic principles such as transference, countertransference, developmental fixation, interpretation, and insight may be effectively applied to clients with diverse ethnocultural identities.

# Using the Theory in a Professional Context

## How Psychoanalysis Embraces Diversity

One might not see an immediate connection between psychoanalytic theory and a counseling style that is well suited for working with individuals from diverse ethnocultural backgrounds (i.e., backgrounds other than White, middle-class European American). Although psychoanalytic theory is influential in some parts of the United States, and as such studied in greater depth, many counseling professionals are only exposed to some of the most well-known concepts such as Freud's structural theory of the id, ego, and superego, the psychosexual stages of development (see Table 6.1), and ego defense mechanisms described by Anna Freud.

The common thread among these concepts is the focus *within* the individual. In other words, explanatory hypotheses for clients' distress such as anxiety, depression, or problems of daily living, result from intrapsychic explorations and interpretations, without taking into account external forces that lie within the environment. This framework, focusing only on internal dynamics, provides an immediate disconnect with multicultural theory, which acknowledges the reality of external, sociopolitical forces such as racism, sexism, and social class discrimination that occur not only in our society but also within the context of the client–counselor relationship, because that, too, is a microcosm of the United States (Sue & Sue, 2003).

However, as we more deeply analyze psychoanalytic theory, it becomes apparent that there is space within this framework to work with clients from diverse backgrounds. For instance, from a psychoanalytic perspective, in addition to being aware of the clients' transference, counselors must also be aware of their own countertransference. Therefore, it becomes of paramount importance for counselors-in-training to face their own biases such as racism and homophobia, and embark on the journey of working through them (Wheeler & Izzard, 1997). As Sue and Sue (2003) and many other multicultural theorists recommend, becoming aware of one's personal biases, assumptions, and values, and how they impact the counseling relationship, is a requirement for developing multicultural competence.

If counselors develop a continuous awareness of their inner thoughts and feelings toward those of diverse backgrounds, counselors can also effectively attend to socioracial transference and countertransference as a way to inform the therapeutic process. Hamer (2002) indicates that issues related to race within the counseling relationship serve as "guards at the gate, a place behind which, if you will, all kinds of unspoken materials become hidden" (p. 1225). In part, this suggests that racial difference as well as similarity can become a form of client resistance within the therapeutic relationship (Hamer, 2002). Additionally, unproductive countertransference can also occur. A White, European American counselor working with a client who belongs to socioracial minority group will experience internal processes (e.g., thoughts and feelings) that are related to race, culture, and gender (among others) differently from their client. This is due to the different worldviews of ethnocultural diverse and White individuals, as well as the impact of racism, sexism, classism, and other "isms" that members of ethnocultural minority groups experience on a regular basis. Therefore, from a psychoanytic perspective, counselors must make a conscientious effort to distinguish between experiences that are real (e.g., a Latino's experience of racism on a daily basis) versus those that are transference based (Hamer, 2002). Experiences that are real must be validated, while those that are transference based must be explored and analyzed.

Another difficulty counselors may encounter is client resistance in talking about race-related experiences. However, it is important to point out that this form of resistance is considered a sign of ego-strength, a "healthy paranoia," because people from minority backgrounds have real life experiences that serve as a foundation for not being as open and willing to trust White, European Americans in general, including counselors (Sue & Sue, 2003). At the same time, any differences between the counselor and client could cause anxiety for both of them and become a source of resistance for the counselor as well. Therefore, unless counselors do their own work to uncover racial, ethnic, cultural, and other biases they carry, they may not have the ability to listen to aspects of clients' stories that open the door to deep and meaningful discussions and analyses related to differences (e.g., race, ethnicity, sex, and ability).

In addition to understanding their own biases, assumptions, and values, and how these affect the counseling relationship, it is also important for counselors to understand their diverse clients' worldview (Sue & Sue, 2003). From a psychoanalytic perspective, the therapist is viewed as "a desiring being every step of the way" (Wilson, 2003, p. 73). In other words, counselors as well as clients are driven by unconscious desires that structure, or give form to, the relationship as well as to what is discussed in counseling (Wilson, 2003). As such, to understand a client's worldview and be truly empathic, counselors must work toward removing themselves (i.e., their desires) from getting in the way of their clients' work. Additionally, counselors must not be overly committed to one way of being with clients, but must remain flexible in their therapeutic stance to allow clients to give meaning to their experiences (Wilson, 2003). Remaining flexible requires acknowledging the possibility of external, sociopolitical realities as complementary and/or alternative explanations for psychic conflict.

In sum, many contemporary psychoanalytic authors (e.g., Cohen, 2000; Hamer, 2002; Javier, 1996; Moss, 2003; Okimoto, 2001; Wheeler & Izzard, 1997) acknowledge the need to think about external realities such as racism, homophobia, and class discrimination in working with clients of diverse backgrounds. Overall, psychoanalytic theory, particularly with its emphasis on transference and countertransference analyses and its growing sensitivity toward allowing clients to give meaning to their own experiences, provides a helpful framework for working with clients of diverse backgrounds.

## Practice Considerations

Without hesitation, we recommend that all school counselors and mental health or community counselors obtain at least some education in how to use psychoanalytic theory to understand students and clients on a deeper level. We recognize that not everyone is interested in becoming a psychoanalyst and that many aspects of psychoanalytic theory are out-dated and feel archaic and unrealistic. On the other hand, some of the following examples may help underline the importance of psychoanalytic theory in all forms of counseling practice.

- Like most humans, clients and students will be struggling primarily with issues related to getting pleasure (what they want) and having satisfying relationships. Dealing with sexual issues and anger and aggression will also be challenging. Knowing this can help counselors have deeper empathy right from the start.

- Clients and students will work harder when there is a positive trans-ference, so counselors should be optimistic, supportive, kind, and interested in the clients' or students' welfare.

- When clients or students are negative and angry, there is no need to take it personally. As psychoanalysts like to say, if the person is hys-terical, it is probably historical (i.e., transference).

- Therefore, when clients or students express negative thoughts or feel-ings toward you, your strategy should always involve nondefensive and nonaccusatory, open, and mutual exploration of where these feel-ings come from.

- It is especially important to take a supportive stance with students and clients who have impulse control problems because these prob-lems occur, at least partly, because of weaknesses in ego develop-ment. In some ways, these students and clients need to borrow from the counselor's ego strength to develop self-control.

- Watching and listening for psychoanalytic developmental themes such as oral (food, dependency, and trust), anal (feces, aggression, and control), and phallic (sexual genitalia, power, and achievement) can give counselors ideas about the developmental challenges and remediation needed for a given client.

- If and when the counselor begins having repeated, inappropriate impulses toward the client or student, it is likely that countertransfer-ence is alive and active and that consultation or supervision is needed.

- At times, usually after some level of self-scrutiny and supervision, it may be appropriate for counselors to tactfully share some of their countertransference reactions with the student or client.

Evidence that effective counseling occurs because of the formation and maintenance of a therapeutic or healing relationship has continued to accumulate. In fact, recent research suggests that developing a positive therapeutic relationship with clients is probably the most powerful factor that counselors can contribute to counseling outcomes (Norcross, 2002). Consequently, the overall concept of creating a healing relationship is perhaps the most important guiding psychoanalytic principle for all counselors. Counselors should continually remind themselves of the importance of a positive working relationship and of the fact that high functioning clients will need only small or intermittent doses of such a relationship, while lower functioning clients may need more regular and longer-term contact with the counselor.

## Theoretical Validity and Shortcomings

Based on scientific standards wherein a theory consists of interconnected statements designed to understand, describe, predict, and sometimes control a particular phenomenon, it is likely that there are no formal and complete developmental theories in psychology (P. Miller, 2002). Humans are just too complex to perfectly understand, describe, predict, and control. When it comes to human development, change and variability is the norm.

Rather than focusing on the unattainable goal of theoretical validity, it is probably more important (and much simpler) to discuss the usefulness or utility of psychoanalytic developmental theory in facilitating counseling process and outcome. From our perspective, there are two most crucial and useful contributions of psychoanalytic theory to counseling:

- Deepening the counselor's understanding of the rich and complex subtleties inherent in every individual, and

- Generating tentative hypotheses about the internal conflicts or maladaptive relationship patterns that are causing distress in or around the client or student.

In emphasizing the usefulness of psychoanalytic theory, we do not want to completely avoid the issue of validity. Over the years, psychoanalysts have been strongly and repeatedly criticized for the lack of empirical support for their approach (Eysenck, 1952; Weisz, Weiss, Han, Granger, & Morton, 1995). However, at this point there is substantial evidence supporting the effectiveness of psychoanalytically oriented counseling approaches in general and short-term psychoanalytic counseling in particular (Chambless et al., 1998; Fonagy et al., 1999). Recently, the strongest support for psychoanalytic treatments includes brief dynamic therapy for opiate dependence (Woody, Luborsky, McLellan, & O'Brien, 1990), brief dynamic therapy for depression (Gallagher-Thompson & Steffen, 1994), and insight-oriented marital therapy (Snyder, Wills, & Grady-Fletcher,

1991), all of which have been labeled as "probably efficacious" by the American Psychological Association's Division 12 Task Force on Promotion and Dissemination of Psychological Procedures (American Psychological Association, 2006; Chambless et al., 1998).

# Ben's Case

I (John) initially met with Ben (age ten years, nine months) and his maternal aunt in my private practice office. Ben had briefly seen a highly qualified woman counselor prior to seeing me, but he asked his aunt to see a different therapist because he said he didn't like the female counselor very well. In an effort to identify therapeutic hopes and goals, I met with Ben and his aunt together for about twenty-five minutes during the first session and then met separately with Ben for the last twenty-five minutes of the session.

## Assessment Information: Sessions 1–3

During the initial session, Ben asked if I could "help us get along better" (referring to him, his aunt, and his six-year-old half-brother). Although this is a relatively normal issue, he discussed it in a way that set him apart from most ten-year-old boys. Specifically, he complained that everything would be better if his aunt would be more "strict." He claimed that he and his younger brother needed more "help" making healthy choices. In some ways Ben seemed to be asking for help in controlling his id impulses (including aggressive behaviors such as hitting his brother). He needed his aunt to serve as an extrinsic force or superego that in time he could internalize. He criticized his aunt saying, ". . . she never grounds us and she never takes away our privileges." According to Ben, his aunt would "always" yell, threaten, and disapprove of his behavior, but that she did not exercise any real power or authority over him. His biggest overall complaint was that she would "never follow through" on the threats she made when he and his brother misbehaved.

The fact that Ben blamed his aunt for their family problems was not unusual. Typically, because of both practical and developmental issues, young boys have difficulty taking personal responsibility for their behaviors. However, the fact that Ben blamed his aunt for not being strict enough and for not providing enough adult guidance was more unusual. In psychoanalytic terms, Ben was projecting his own deficits onto his aunt and then rejecting them. He needed and wanted firm limits, but upon referral, Ben was unable to control his impulses or manage his affect on his own. He had particular difficulty with aggressive impulses. For example, his aunt indicated that he regularly hit his brother and that he was impossible to deal with emotionally. One of her reasons or explanations for why she did not follow through with punishments or consequences was because she claimed that Ben "won't be disciplined." As an example, she noted that if he misbehaved and she told him to go to his room, Ben would simply refuse. And so, despite the fact that he craved limits and consequences to shore up his deficient ego strength, at the same time, he rejected his aunt's meager efforts to play a parental role in his life.

Ben was the only child born of the union of his biological parents, James and Donna. His mother Donna reportedly had serious alcohol and drug problems beginning when she was age thirteen and continuing to the time of the initial session and beyond. James and Donna divorced when Ben was three, and Ben has had no contact with his biological father since that time. Further, his biological mother was only intermittently involved in his life after he turned nine years old, and completely dropped out of his life about a year after our initial meeting. Donna's inconsistent involvement and eventual abandonment of her parenting obligations were apparently directly related to her alcohol and drug problems. Donna had a second child, Allen, with a second husband when Ben was four years old.

Ben and his half-brother Allen began living with their maternal aunt when Ben was nine years old and Allen was five years old. According to the aunt and Ben, the two of them (aunt Peggy and Ben) had been "great buddies" before they began living together, but that this amicable relationship quickly deteriorated after Ben and Allen moved in. During the intake session both Ben and his aunt agreed that Ben had a quick and very extreme temper.

During the second session, I met individually with Ben. After initial chit-chat, I used a generative (projective) self-esteem assessment procedure with Ben. The technique is called "What's Good About You?" and its purpose is to provide a structured, interpersonal format for evaluating self-esteem with young clients (Sommers-Flanagan & Sommers-Flanagan, 2007). I introduced the procedure to Ben by saying something like:

> Okay Ben, I'd like to play sort of a game with you. Here's how it goes. I will ask you a question and you just answer it the best you can, with whatever comes to mind. Then, I'll write down your answer and say "Thank you" and then I'll ask you the same question again. I'll do this ten times in a row. The only rule is that you can't use the same answer twice. Okay?

Ben agreed to play the game. I asked him "What's good about you?" ten times. He participated fully. His responses included:

1. My personality.
2. My lifestyle.
3. My friends.
4. My family.
5. All the things I have.
6. My skills in working with my hands.
7. My IQ.
8. The things I can do to help people.
9. All the things I have that some people don't.
10. All the things I have that are special to me, like food and stuff.

During this activity, Ben produced responses that capture both his strengths and weaknesses. Although he has some global sense of his personality and ego strengths, he is very general and nonspecific about these strengths. Perhaps the best example is his seventh response, "My IQ." This response includes the fact that Ben knows he has intellectual potential, but also is informative in that it suggests Ben is quite distant from this laudable attribute and vague about its implications. As I listened to him respond to my questions, I couldn't help but form a picture of a young boy who had been told by a variety of individuals that he has many positive attributes, but that he had not, at the time of this assessment, really integrated these attributes into more healthy or developed ego functioning. It was more as if he knew of these strengths that he should possess, but that he hadn't really put them into action at this point in his life.

Ben's lack of specificity in response to the "What's good about you?" questions is not terribly unusual for a ten-year-old boy. But the pervasiveness of his vagueness is significant. For example, each response requires some follow-up to obtain specific information, such as: "What about your personality is good?" or "What about your lifestyle is good?"

From a psychoanalytic perspective, it is especially significant that Ben mentioned food in his tenth and last response to "What's good about you?" As noted by psychoanalytic researchers, when words representing food appear in a projective assessment process, it signals a possibility of problems in what Freud originally identified as the oral stage of psychosexual development (Fisher & Greenberg, 1985). While it was obviously premature to make much of a single food-related response to this assessment activity, the point is that it can be useful for the counselor to be alerted to the possible significance for Ben of food, nurturance, support, and of having dependable and trustworthy objects (or caretakers) in his life. Additionally, it is interesting that after doing this activity for over seven years with dozens of youth, none have ever mentioned food in response to the question, "What's good about you?"

In session three, I had a rare opportunity to directly view Ben's impulsive anger. I was meeting jointly with Ben and his aunt. They were sitting side by side on a small love seat in my office. They were both positive and upbeat, responding calmly to my questions and to each other. We were discussing Ben's tendency to avoid responsibility for his behavior, when his aunt began laughing at how he recently made excuses for why he could not complete some yard work. Suddenly, Ben took a magnificently violent swing and struck his aunt across her upper chest and shoulder. She and I were both shocked by the sudden, violent nature of Ben's behavior. I stared at Aunt Peggy as tears welled up in her eyes. Her mouth was in the shape of a large O and her breath was shaky. Then I looked at Ben, whose eyes were also filled with tears, but rather than tears of shock, his were tears of hurt and rage. I motioned for him to move away from his aunt, and he did. She indicated that she was physically fine, but emotionally shaken.

After nearly thirty seconds of mostly silence, I turned to Ben and said, "We need to talk about what happened and what made you hit your aunt, but first, you need to know that you can never hit anyone in here again, no matter how you're feeling."

Ben quickly nodded his head and agreed to my terms, but I felt compelled to repeat the limit-setting, this time even more emphatically and with an added dose of authority. "I really need you to understand this Ben. No one is allowed to hit anyone else in here. No one! If you ever hit or kick someone in here again, no matter what the reason, I will call the police and have you ticketed for assault."

Ben's eyes widened and head nodded. He began to explain himself, "She laughed at me . . ." but I found myself cutting him off, "Just a minute. I need to check in with your aunt."

"Peggy, are you okay?"

"Yeah."

"Do you need any help?"

"No. I'm okay?"

"I want you to let me know when you're ready to talk about what just happened. Ben is ready to tell me about what he was feeling just before he hit you. But I want to wait until you're ready to talk about this too."

"That's okay. I'm okay now. We can talk."

"Good. Let's go over the rules again. Ben, you know now that there's no hitting. I also want both of you to know that as we talk about this, our goal is to figure out what happened, so it doesn't happen again. I don't want to call the police, but I will if someone hits someone else again. Also, when we discuss this, I want you to listen to each other and if things are getting too heated, then you both need to promise to stop talking and listen to me. Are these rules okay?"

Both Ben and Aunt Peggy agreed. My hope was that by re-setting rules and limits very clearly and by invoking a higher authority (the police or superego), I could support the ego-functions of control or restraint and understanding or insight. In addition, by telling them I would be in charge if things got too heated, I was trying to lend some ego-functions in case their emotions and impulses escalated. From the psychoanalytic perspective, this intervention might be conceptualized as me serving as Ben's superego (conscience and ego ideal) by telling him that it is not acceptable behavior to physically assault another person. At the same time, I was imposing a potential external negative consequence to guide his ego in future behavior moderations.

Despite the fact that I often work with delinquent youth and impulsive boys, it is extremely rare that I actually view—in-vivo—aggressive physical behavior inside my office. Perhaps this is because of the natural inhibiting factors of counseling and perhaps because I usually take steps to prohibit such behavior. But in Ben's case, the aggressive behavior erupted suddenly and there was little chance to stop it. In fact, Ben had been talking openly about his challenges at home and was earnest and upbeat immediately before striking his aunt. Fortunately, Ben was only ten years old, and so his aunt was stunned but unhurt. Nevertheless, two positive developments emerged from this aggressive incident. First, it was an opportunity to set clear and unequivocal limits with Ben, the sort of limits that he had been unable to set for himself and that his aunt had been yelling about at home, but had been unable to enforce. Second, the precipitating stimulus for Ben's violence was clear. In the instant before he struck, his aunt had disparagingly laughed at something Ben had said.

At the time, I conceptualized Ben's sudden anger as a response to what he experienced as a sudden abandonment of emotional support (his aunt's laughter). It was as if they were emotionally together and then suddenly she left him completely bereft of support and so he struck out in vengeance. Another word that seemed to capture this dynamic was betrayal. Based on his behavior and explanation, Ben viewed his aunt's laughter as a deep interpersonal betrayal. Put into a traditional psychoanalytic metaphor, this was a situation where for Ben, the good, nurturing, and supportive milk he had been drinking up had suddenly turned sour (and so he bit his caretaker). In fact, Ben's relationship with his biological mother and aunt seemed to involve parallel processes: Initially his mother was with him and then abandoned him, and now his aunt, who had been a former "chum" was growing increasingly critical of him and, at some level, he seemed to fear that she would abandon him as well.

## Case Formulation

Ben, his aunt, and I formulated three main goals for Ben's counseling. These were: (1) anger/aggression control or management (strengthening of ego functioning and internalization of superego-based inhibitions); (2) increased positive or prosocial behaviors in the home and at school; this goal was based on Ben's general negativity toward authority figures, his picking on his brother, and his strained, physically aggressive peer relations (more strengthening of ego functioning and internalization of a trustworthy and dependable authority figure self-object); and (3) improving Ben's compliance with his aunt's directives at home (this also included helping his aunt become more competent at stating and enforcing limits and in complimenting Ben for positive behaviors in an effort to help him strengthen his ego functions and internalize a more consistently supportive self-object).

The initial plan was for Ben to see me on a weekly basis. (His sessions were paid for by Medicaid.) The strategies and techniques I planned to employ with Ben included: (1) continuing to develop a positive therapeutic alliance with him through intermittent playful activities, discussions of topics of interest to him, as well as by modeling a serious work ethic regarding "dealing with his anger, aggression, and social problems," (2) using a variety of techniques (including cognitive-behavioral strategies designed to strengthen his ego functioning) to help him understand and control his aggressive impulses, (3) becoming a reliable and supportive male figure in his life (with all the appropriate limits to my role as dictated by professional and ethical guidelines), and (4) coaching his aunt in ways that allowed her to be less critical, more supportive, and more able to set reasonable limits and follow through with them if they were violated.

My biggest fear in Ben's case was his impulsive anger combined with his aunt's fragility as a caretaker. I worried that he would continue his pattern of misbehavior and that she would give up her caretaker role.

This scenario would provide Ben with another abandonment experience and deepen his internalization of an untrustworthy authority figure. I also worried that Ben felt such self-loathing that he would act in ways to fulfill his negative self-prophecy (Willock, 1987).

## The Middle Sessions

After our first sessions, Ben and I (and his aunt, who occasionally met with us adjunctively) set to work on his anger, impulsiveness, and emotional management skills. We often worked on developing his ego functions using contemporary cognitive-behavioral anger management and emotional education strategies; when working with youth, these educational approaches are not inconsistent with psychoanalytically informed counseling.

Ben was a reluctant, but willing participant in counseling. After about six sessions, his aunt told me (while Ben took a bathroom break) that he liked me and liked coming to see me. This was partly due to the fact that we played checkers, chess, cards, ate snacks, and talked incessantly about how it felt to win and lose and what strategies he used for playing games. But I also felt that his quick attachment to me was a function of his father hunger, something that his previous female therapist probably could not satisfy.

To Ben's credit (and his aunt's as well), they took a number of steps that helped diffuse Ben's potential for having a full-blown father transference toward me. These steps included having Ben get a Big Brother, having Ben spend time with his maternal grandfather, and obtaining assistance from other social service agencies. Additionally, Ben was almost always cautious and sometimes ambivalent in his approach to me. During some stretches of counseling he forgot our meetings nearly as often as he remembered them, and although this was a scheduling inconvenience, I made sure that Ben was always greeted with positive anticipation and never punished for missing sessions. I took this stance principally because I believed that his forgetting sessions were more a function of his fear of closeness and rejection than behavioral acting out. In addition, I did not interpret this behavior because it would have been far too threatening to expect Ben to face his simultaneous longing for a father figure and fear of rejection. Moreover, at the age of ten and even later in our counseling together, Ben might not have been able to grasp the interpretation. As a consequence, I saw my role as a supportive figure who did not judge or reprimand, but who was reliable, trustworthy, fun, safe, and able to help him discern appropriate from inappropriate behavior. Our time together was designed to make up for the absence of a reliable, trustworthy, fun, safe, and discerning male figure in his life so that he could begin to internalize these qualities.

Ben and I had the luxury of working together intermittently for over seven years. I say intermittently because Ben often missed many sessions and, at one point (when Ben was fourteen), I took a five-month sabbatical. Several months prior to my departure I discussed my upcoming absence with Ben and his aunt, and we arranged for him to meet with another male counselor. Unfortunately, this arrangement lasted only about three sessions partly because Ben missed two appointments and partly because he didn't think that his substitute counselor "really cared" about whether he showed up or not. When I returned from my trip, Ben returned to counseling with me and displayed perfect attendance for six consecutive weeks.

Toward the end of our work together, Ben began drinking alcohol and smoking marijuana recreationally. At one point, he was caught in possession of marijuana and sentenced to probation. Like most youth, Ben initially minimized the significance of his substance use. Later, after gently reviewing his use intermittently for several sessions, he admitted that he liked how marijuana made him feel. In particular, he claimed it helped him relax, helped him not care so much about things, and helped him cope with anxiety and nervousness. Three issues and opportunities came to the surface during this time that warrant further discussion.

First, Ben did not describe his marijuana use as helping him deal more effectively with his anger. In fact, at this point in counseling, Ben was managing his anger rather well (especially for a sixteen-year-old male). The pot seemed to help him deal with other less pleasant emotions, such as disappointment and fear. Overall, his descriptions of why he used marijuana helped me begin to conceptualize Ben's emotional issues as having evolved beyond the oral aggression he had exhibited so frequently early in counseling. Disappointment and fear, although challenging emotions, were based less in early primitive betrayals (oral stage) and more in later performance-based anxieties (phallic stage). Again, we want to emphasize that Freud's stages are certainly not state-of-the-science developmental theory, but that they can help (along with newer developmental models) with understanding issues and developmental progress.

Second, Ben's drug-related legal problems stimulated the counseling process. This happened in several ways. As he explained his substance use and experiences with me, he could do so without reprimand, without lecturing, and without fear of abandonment or betrayal. During this time, all I had to do was listen, explore, question, discuss, and express empathy for his legal situation, the dysphoric emotions he was trying to manage, and the sheer panic that his drug-related legal problems elicited from his aunt. From a broad psychoanalytic perspective, these discussions provided an opportunity for a corrective emotional experience (Alexander & French, 1946). From a more specific psychoanalytic perspective (object relations), Ben had the opportunity to internalize a calmer and more sympathetic adult authority figure.

Third, as a part of his probation, Ben had to make several appearances in court. These appearances provided me with an opportunity to discuss Ben's anxiety over the loss of control he was experiencing. It also was an opportunity for me to support him in ways that he may have never previously experienced. Ben's aunt was so emotionally distraught over his drug use that she refused to accompany him to his court hearings. Consequently, I was left with several choices. First, I could help him manage the situation alone partly by expressing empathy for his anxiety and partly by expressing confidence in his ability to handle the situation independently. Second, I could encourage him to find another comforting person to be with him in the courtroom. Third, I could offer to meet him at the courtroom and provide the emotional support directly.

In the end, I asked Ben if he wanted me to come to the court hearings and sit next to him as he waited for the judge to hear his case. This decision easily could be seen as my acting on a countertransference impulse to be Ben's hero or father figure. To be honest, I have to admit this explanation remains a possibility.

My rationale (or rationalization) for offering to accompany Ben to court was that I felt I was in the best position to provide him with direct emotional comfort and support. This comfort and support would hopefully be in direct contrast to the emotional abandonment he generally experienced during times of stress or crisis. My further hope was that my presence might give him a better chance to begin using internal skills (rather than drugs) for coping with anxiety.

I let Ben know that I was not always 100% available to be with him at the courthouse because of my practice schedule, but that with planning, I could probably attend. Ben expressed a desire for me to attend, and I was able to be there for two of his three hearings. Again, this may be a rationalization, but I believe my presence with him during these hearings, from any theoretical orientation, may have been the best therapeutic activity he and I ever experienced together. In particular, I have a vivid memory of showing up at the courthouse and the look of relief on Ben's face. But even more importantly, to sit next to him on a bench in the courtroom for thirty minutes, listening to him breath, noticing him battling his anxiety, whispering supportive (and sometimes irreverent) comments into his ear was, at least for me, the pinnacle of supportive counseling. He was also deeply appreciative of these shared moments.

During about the same time as his legal troubles, I began feeling a need to talk with Ben about sex and sexuality. Beginning when he was around thirteen, I had begun routinely inquiring about whether he had any romance in his life and he occasionally gave me a few hints that he had some brief girlfriends, but that he had not engaged in any serious sexual activities and that, in many ways, he was quite frightened of girls. At one point I recall being aware that Ben and I had sometimes come close to talking directly about sex, but that generally we had danced around the subject (although, when he was fifteen years old we had discussed homosexuality, and I explored whether he felt any homosexual urges, which he, rather gently for a teenager, brushed aside noting that he was interested in girls, but had nothing against gays or lesbians).

The idea of talking directly about sex with Ben, much in the same way a parent would talk with his/her child about the birds and the bees, kept returning to my mind. For several weeks I pondered this possibility, trying to make sure that my motive for talking was not too laden with unresolved issues about my own parents' inability to discuss the issue directly with me. Eventually, I decided that because in some ways I was serving as Ben's surrogate father, it was my responsibility to talk with him about sex and that this talk should include at least some personal disclosure. Conceptually, this was an example of the more contemporary intersubjectivity or two-person model of psychoanalytic therapy where the counselor reveals more of him- or herself in an effort to deepen the understanding of the client's issues. Overall, it seemed necessary, appropriate, and potentially healing for me to talk about my impulse to discuss sex with him, my motives for such a talk, and to share minor personal revelations while exploring his thoughts and feelings about sex.

At the next session I began with a quick check-in, and when as usual, Ben indicated that he had little he really wanted to talk about, I said, "I've been thinking we should have a serious talk about sex."

Ben's eyes widened, but rather than let him resist, I rambled on into a monologue that I had wanted to get out before he could object.

> I'm sure you know a lot about sex from talking with friends and from the movies and magazines. But I've been wondering if anyone has ever sat down with you and had a serious talk about the birds and the bees. I know it's sort of old-fashioned, but I decided we should have that kind of talk, just because I don't know if any

other adults in your life, especially men, will ever sit down and talk with you about this.

To his credit, Ben responded the way he often did when faced with a serious issue. He said, "Okay. That's fine with me." He then expanded on his initial compliance by saying, "Well, of course we covered that in school. In sex ed. But nope, no adult has ever really brought this up. Well, I guess my aunt left a book in my room once, but that's about it."

And so we proceeded. I told him my parents had never had the sex talk with me either. I asked him to tell me some of what he knew and he complied, albeit without much detail. I brought up pornography, and we agreed that looking at too much porn was generally a bad idea. We talked about respecting women as sexual partners, about accepting it when women didn't want to have sex, about the myth of blue balls, and about Viagra, premature ejaculation, and birth control. Ben confessed that he was still a virgin, and I shared back that I was a virgin "for a long time, too." Throughout our conversation, Ben was his usual cautious self and provided me with limited disclosures. Finally, at the end of our session, I thanked him for tolerating my need to talk with him about sex. He appeared relieved and returned the thanks with what appeared to be sincerity, but without any particular enthusiasm (sort of a "Hmm, that's interesting" response).

## Termination Phase

When I initially started learning about psychoanalytic theory and therapy, I thought, somewhat rigidly and perhaps idealistically, that counseling had a clear beginning, middle, and ending. In particular, I thought there was a clear ending, time when counseling ended and contact between counselor and client stopped forever.

I also recall a time when working with a young female medical student toward whom I held at least a bit of positive countertransference, being unable during our final meeting to utter the clear and concise "good-bye" that I knew was most appropriate. Instead I heard the words "See you later" slip out of my mouth. Around the same time, I noticed that my own well-respected and experienced psychoanalytic therapist seemed to struggle with the same issue. When I said to him at our final meeting, "Well, I guess we won't see each other again," he responded with, "There are always conferences."

In my work with teenage clients I have discovered that termination is not always clean and simple. There *are* always conferences, and supermarkets, video stores, basketball games, public lectures, and college. And so counseling ended, as usual, sort of.

In our final session, Ben and I reminisced over milkshakes at a local restaurant. Something about it felt very unprofessional and another part felt just right and very psychoanalytic. I bought him a burger and fries and occasionally snuck a few fries off his plate. Of course, I said, "I'll probably see you around town." And we talked about saying "Hi" to each other when we ran into each other (just as we had been doing for the past seven years).

It was about four months later when I ran into Ben at a local video store. We said "Hi" just like we'd planned. I told him it was "Very nice to see him" and that he "Looked great," both of which felt true from my perspective. It wasn't much later when I heard from Ben. I received a graduation announcement. I responded by sending him money (a reasonable amount that I tell myself and my young clients that I am always willing to provide on an annual basis for significant events, such as graduation or fundraising requests). I also enclosed a note where I expressed my pride in him for having such persistence and success in school. A month or so later, I heard back from Ben. His note was simple and direct, the kind of communication I had grown to expect from him. It read:

> Dear John:
>     Thank you for all your support over the years. You were a great influence, even when I didn't want to be influenced. I owe a lot to ya, and it seems very miniscule in comparison to all you have given me, but thank you.
>     Ben N.

I haven't seen Ben for several years. But I am fairly certain that he learned and grew from his counseling with me, not in the sort of leaps and bounds expected by managed care companies and short-term counseling models, but slowly and surely, with two steps forward and one step back. I also think he benefited from counseling because when I look back and reminisce about the experience, I can easily recognize how much I learned from him.

## Summary

A working knowledge of psychoanalytic theory can be very helpful for school and mental health counselors. Although brief counseling approaches, including cognitive, behavioral, and solution-focused, are growing in popularity, there is still a strong rationale for thinking like a psychoanalyst—at least sometimes.

The advantages of thinking psychoanalytically range from the self-scrutiny of countertransference to the importance of considering the counseling relationship as a potential healing relationship. No other theoretical approach appreciates and attends to the richness of the individual's internal mental life as the psychoanalytic approach. In essence, the requirement from psychoanalytic theory is that we pay great attention to what the client or students feels, what she or he thinks, and how she or he behaves; we are also challenged to do the same regarding our feelings, thoughts, and behaviors while counseling. Learning to respect and understand the individual's complete experience is one of the great benefits of thinking psychoanalytically.

The counseling case presented above was designed to illustrate an eclectic psychoanalytic approach to counseling with a teen and preteen. No doubt many traditional psychoanalysts would argue about whether the case accurately represents psychoanalytic theory in action. For example, many theorists might take issue with our position that it is altogether possible to apply cognitive behavioral strategies to enhance client self-control within the context of a psychoanalytic model. Nonetheless, we believe that in many ways, as long as the counselor is considering psychoanalytic concepts, she or he is practicing psychoanalytically informed counseling.

Ben, in the case example, showed his poor ego development through impulsive aggression and poor peer relations. His ambivalence and mistrust of adults ran deep and was probably rooted in a fixation or developmental arrest at the oral stage of Freud's psychosexual development (or Erikson's crisis of trust versus mistrust). To address this issue, the counselor not only used cognitive behavioral educational approaches, but also became a calm, consistent, reliable, and fun adult presence with whom Ben could identify. Ben's response to this counseling opportunity was consistent with his ambivalence and mistrust of adults, but in the end, it appears that he was able to use the counseling to further develop his ego strength and potential for success in life.

Learning about and applying psychoanalytic principles to counseling are challenging for counseling professionals. We must admit that it is often easier to think like a solution-focused or behavioral counselor. However, if you want to deepen and enrich your understanding of counseling process and of your clients and students, we strongly recommend that you try thinking like a psychoanalytic theorist from time to time. You just might discover you like it.

# Annotated Bibliography

Cohen, C. (2000). Object-relations theory: Cultural and social implications for psychotherapy with individuals who are deaf. *Smith College Studies in Social Work, 70,* 35–49.
Through a case study, the author provides practical applications for working from a psychoanalytic framework with diverse individuals. The author integrates psychological, sociocultural, and linguistics components to the therapeutic process. Furthermore, there is an informative discussion of deafness as a culture, rather than a disability as often perceived by the dominant culture.

Freud, S. (1966). *Introductory lessons on psychoanalysis.* Norton.
This great introduction to psychoanalysis resulted from Freud's lectures during his only visit to the United States. It addresses the foundations of his theory, such as the meaning parapraxis, dream analysis, and a basic theory on neurosis.

Gay, P. (1998). *Freud: A life for our time.* New York: Norton.
The author, who is also a psychoanalyst, provides a detailed biography of Freud's life. The author discusses Freud in many different roles, such as father, friend, and psychologist, through previously published and unpublished literature, as well as letters written by Freud.

Greenberg, J. R., and Mitchell, S. A. (1983). *Object relations in psychoanalytic theory.* Cambridge, MA, Harvard University Press.
This book is one of the seminal texts in object-relations theory. It is clear, comprehensive, and provides in-depth coverage of this fascinating and challenging topic.

Hamer, F. M. (2002). Guards at the gate: Race, resistance, and psychic reality. *Journal of the American Psychoanalytic Association, 50,* 1219–1237.
This enlightening article is written by an African American psychoanalyst who discusses how racial differences and similarities impact the therapeutic process, the relationship between race and resistance, and the fluidity of race in the context of therapy. It is worth reading regardless of theoretical orientation.

Hergenhahn, B. R. (1994). *An introduction to theories of personality* (4th ed.). Englewood Cliffs, NJ: Prentice Hall.
This textbook provides a meaningful introduction to important psychoanalytic theorists. The author introduces not only Freud but also Carl Jung, Adler Alfred, and Karen Horney. Although an introductory text, the discussions are in sufficient depth to provide a basic framework.

Javier, R. A. (1996). Psychodynamic treatment with the urban poor. In R. Perez-Foster, *Reaching across boundaries of culture and class.* New York: Aronson.
This is a key article encouraging clinicians to utilize a psychoanalytic framework with diverse individuals. It also provides useful practical applications.

The author discusses how he has adopted theoretical constructs to success-fully treat poor people through an insight-oriented therapeutic process.

Lotto, D. (2001). Freud's struggle with misogyny: Homosexuality and guilt in the dream of Irma's injection. *Journal of the American Psychoanalytic Association, 49,* 1289–1313.

This is a valuable article for those interested in Freud's struggle with negative projections toward women. The author provides an interpretation for Freud's famous dream, connecting it to his childhood experiences, intense relation-ships with males, and desire to "overcome" his own homosexual tendencies.

Masson, J. M. (1984). *The assault on truth: Freud's suppression of the seduction theory.* New York: Farrar, Straus and Giroux.

As former director of Freud's archives, Jeffrey Masson has insight and inside information regarding virtually every aspect of Freud's history and theo-ries. In this historical account, Masson criticizes Freud for abandoning his seduction theory. This book is much more than a simple critique of Freud, it is a glimpse into the struggles that led him to contend that most sexual abuse of psychiatric patients is a fantasy constructed by the patient.

Okimoto, J. T. (2001). The appeal cycle in three cultures: An exploratory com-parison of child development. *Journal of the American Psychoanalytic Associ-ation, 49,* 187–210.

This is a research article comparing mother–child relationships in three different cultures. The findings suggest empirical differences in child development across Caucasian Americans, overseas Japanese, and Chinese-Vietnamese immigrants living in the United States.

Ringstrom, P. A. (2001). Cultivating the improvisational in psychoanalytic treatment. *Psychoanalytic Dialogues, 11,* 727–754.

When we think about psychoanalysis and psychoanalysts, the image of a distant, analytical figure probably comes to mind for most of us. In con-trast, Ringstrom's work emphasizes the importance of spontaneity and gen-uineness in the counselor–client encounter.

St. Clair, M., and Wigren, J. (2004). *Object relations and self psychology: An intro-duction.* Belmont, CA, Brooks/Cole.

This basic text provides an excellent introduction to object-relations the-ory and the self psychology of Heinz Kohut.

Wheeler, S., & Izzard, S. (1997). Psychodynamic counsellor training—integrating difference. *Psychodynamic Counselling, 3,* 401–417.

This is a noteworthy article that discusses how to prepare counselors-in-training to become culturally and racially aware. It presents a model that integrates psychodynamic concepts while embracing sociopolitical concepts in preparing counselors to work more competently within a contemporary, diverse society.

Wilson, M. (2003). The analyst's desire and the problem of narcissistic resistances. *Journal of the American Psychoanalytic Association, 51,* 72–99.

In this interesting article, the author discusses how important it is for therapists to "remove" themselves (i.e., their desires and wishes) from the therapeutic relationship. If therapists remain flexible, resistance on their part diminishes, and patients can more freely give meaning to their own experiences.

# References

Adler, A. (1956). *The individual psychology of Alfred Adler.* New York: Basic Books.

Ainsworth, M. D., Blehar, M. C., Waters, E., & Wall, S. (1978). *Patterns of attachment.* Hillsdale, NJ: Erlbaum.

Alexander, F., & French, T. M. (1946). *Psychoanalytic psychotherapy.* New York: Ronald.

American Psychological Association. (2006). Evidence-based practice in psychology. *American Psychologist, 61,* 271–285.

Bankart, C. P. (1997). *Talking cures: A history of Western and Eastern psychotherapies.* Pacific Grove, CA: Brooks/Cole.

Bowlby, J. (1969). *Attachment and loss, Vol. 1.* Attachment. New York: Basic Books.

Cernoch, J. M., & Potter, R. H. (1985). Recognition of maternal axillary odors by infants. *Child Development, 56,* 1593–1598.

Chambless, D. L., Baker, M. J., Baucom, D. H., Beutler, L. E., Calhoun, K. S., Crits-Christoph, P., et al. (1998). Update on empirically validated therapies, II. *The Clinical Psychologist, 51,* 3–16.

Cohen, C. (2000). Object relations theory: Cultural and social implications for psychotherapy with individuals who are deaf. *Smith College Studies in Social Work, 70,* 35–49.

Cooper, G., Hoffman, K., Powell, B., & Marvin, R. (2005). The circle of security intervention: Differential diagnosis and differential treatment. In L. J. Berlin, Y. Ziv, L. Amaya-Jackson, & M. T. Greenberg (Eds.), *Enhancing early attachments: Theory, research, intervention, and policy* (pp. 127–151). New York: Guilford Press.

Corey, G. (2005). *Theory and practice of counseling and psychotherapy* (7th ed.). Belmont, CA: Brooks/Cole.

Dass-Brailsford, P. (2003). A golden opportunity in supervision: Talking about countertransference. *Journal of Psychological Practice, 8*(1), 56–64.

Erikson, E. H. (1963). *Childhood & society* (2nd ed.). New York: Norton.

Eysenck, H. J. (1952). The effects of psychotherapy: An evaluation. *Journal of Consulting Psychology, 16,* 319–324.

Fairbairn, W. R. D. (1952). *Psychoanalytic studies of the personality.* London: Tavistock Publications and Kegan Paul, Trench, & Trubner.

Fenichel, O. (1945). *The psychoanalytic theory of neurosis.* New York: Norton.

Fisher, S., & Greenberg, R. P. (1985). *The scientific credibility of Freud's theories and therapy.* New York: Columbia University Press.

Fonagy, P., Kachele, H., Krause, R., Jones, E., Perron, R., & Lopez, L. (1999). *An open door review of outcome studies in psychoanalysis.* London: International Psychoanalytic Association.

Freud, A. (1966). *The ego and the mechanisms of defense* (Vol. 2). New York: International Universities Press.

Freud, S. (1949). *An outline of psychoanalysis.* New York: Norton.

Freud, S. (1965). *The origin and development of psychoanalysis.* Washington, DC: Regnery Gateway.

Freud, S. (1966). *Introductory Lessons on Psychoanalysis.* New York: Norton.

Gallagher-Thompson, D., & Steffen, A. M. (1994). Comparative effects of cognitive-behavioral and brief dynamic therapy for depressed family caregivers. *Journal of Consulting & Clinical Psychology, 62,* 543–549.

Goldfried, M. R., & Davison, G. C. (1994). *Clinical behavior therapy* (2nd ed.). Oxford, U.K.: Wiley.

Hamburg, P. (2004). The supervisory alliance. *American Journal of Psychotherapy, 58*(2), 259–261.

Hamer, F. M. (2002). Guards at the gate: Race, resistance, and psychic reality. *Journal of the American Psychoanalytic Association, 50,* 1219–1237.

Hergenhahn, B. R. (1994). *An introduction to theories of personality* (4th ed.). Englewood Cliffs, NJ: Prentice Hall.

Javier, R. A. (1996). Psychodynamic treatment with the urban poor. In R. Perez-Foster, *Reaching across boundaries of culture and class.* New York: Aronson.

Kivlighan, D. M. J. (2002). Transference, interpretation, and insight: A research-practice model. In G. S. Tryon (Ed.), *Counseling based on process research: Applying what we know.* (pp. 166–196). Boston: Allyn & Bacon.

Kohut, H. (1984). *How does analysis cure?* Chicago: University of Chicago Press.

Lotto, D. (2001). Freud's struggle with misogyny: Homosexuality and guilt in the dream of Irma's injection. *Journal of the American Psychoanalytic Association, 49,* 1289–1313.

Luborsky, L. (1984). *Principles of psychoanalytic psychotherapy: A manual for supportive-expressive treatment.* New York: Basic Books.

Mahler, M. S. (1968). *On human symbiosis or the vicissitudes of individuation.* New York: International Universities Press.

Masson, J. M. (1984). *The assault on truth: Freud's suppression of the seduction theory.* New York: Farrar, Straus and Giroux.

Miller, P. (2002). *Theories of developmental psychology* (4th ed.). New York: Worth.

Miller, W. R., & Rollnick, S. (2002). *Motivational interviewing: Preparing people for change* (2nd ed.). New York: Guilford Press.

Mohr, J. J., Gelso, C. J., & Hill, C. E. (2005). Client and counselor trainee attachment as predictors of session evaluation and countertransference behavior in first counseling sessions. *Journal of Counseling Psychology, 52,* 298–309.

Moss, D. (2003). On hating in the first person plural: Thinking psychoanalytically about racism, homophobia, and misogyny. *Journal of the American Psychoanalytic Association, 49,* 1315–1334.

Norcross, J. C. (Ed.). (2002). *Psychotherapy relationships that work.* New York: Oxford University Press.

Okimoto, J. T. (2001). The appeal cycle in three cultures: An exploratory comparison of child development. *Journal of the American Psychoanalytic Association, 49,* 187–213.

Renik, O. (1993). Analytic interaction: Conceptualizing technique in light of the analyst's irreducible subjectivity. *Psychoanalytic Quarterly, 62,* 553–571.

Ringstrom, P. A. (2001). Cultivating the improvisational in psychoanalytic treatment. *Psychoanalytic Dialogues, 11,* 727–754.

Rosenberger, E. W., & Hayes, J. A. (2002). Therapist as subject: A review of the empirical countertransference literature. *Journal of Counseling and Development, 80,* 264–270.

Russell, M. J., Mendelson, T., & Peeke, H. V. S. (1983). Mothers' identification of their infants' odors. *Ethology and Sociobiology, 4,* 29–31.

Snyder, D. K., Wills, R. M., & Grady-Fletcher, A. (1991). Long-term effectiveness of behavioral versus insight-oriented marital therapy: A 4-year follow-up study. *Journal of Consulting & Clinical Psychology, 59,* 138–141.

Sommers-Flanagan, J., & Sommers-Flanagan, R. (2004). *Counseling and psychotherapy theories in context and practice: Skills, strategies, and techniques.* Hoboken, NJ: Wiley.

Sommers-Flanagan, J., & Sommers-Flanagan, R. (2007). *Tough kids, cool counseling: User-friendly approaches with challenging youth* (2nd ed.). Alexandria, VA: American Counseling Association.

Strupp, H. H., & Binder, J. L. (1984). *Psychotherapy in a new key.* New York: Basic Books.

Sue, D. W., & Sue, D. (2003). Counseling the culturally diverse: Theory and practice (3rd ed.). Hoboken, NJ: Wiley.

Wallerstein, R. S. (2002). The growth and transformation of the American ego psychology. *Journal of the American Psychoanalytic Association, 50,* 135–169.

Weisz, J. R., Weiss, B., Han, S. S., Granger, D. A., & Morton, T. (1995). Effects of psychotherapy with children and adolescents revisited: A meta-analysis of treatment outcome studies. *Psychological Bulletin, 117,* 450–468.

Wheeler, S., & Izzard, S. (1997). Psychodynamic counsellor training—integrating difference. *Psychodynamic Counselling, 3,* 401–417.

Willock, B. (1987). The devalued (unloved, repugnant) self: A second facet of narcissistic vulnerability in the aggressive, conduct-disordered child. *Psychoanalytic Psychology, 4*(3), 219–240.

Wilson, M. (2003). The analyst's desire and the problem of narcissistic resistances. *Journal of the American Psychoanalytic Association, 51,* 72–99.

Woody, S. R., Luborsky, L., McLellan, A. T., & O'Brien, C. P. (1990). Corrections and revised analyses for psychotherapy in methadone maintenance patients. *Archives of General Psychiatry, 47,* 788–789.

# CHAPTER SEVEN

# Erik and Joan Eriksons' Approach to Human Development in Counseling

## Michael J. Karcher and Kristine Benne

Joan and Erik Erikson developed a theory of human development that charts stage-wise progression in the social, emotional, and cognitive skills that individuals use in their relationships with significant others across the lifespan. Initially, this theory was referred to as a bio-psycho-social theory of human development, but over time and across their careers of writing about human growth, the Eriksons placed more emphasis on charting how individuals manage interpersonal tasks and demands than on the biology of Freud's drive psychology that served as the initial impetus for the model. In fact, the biological dimension of the theory, drawn in part from Freud's model and from the ways in which physiological maturation affects the demands and tasks placed upon individuals, has been the least referenced component of the theory. Instead, the psychological and social constructs have come to signify the theory and most directly reveal its use in counseling.

Best known are the key constructs of industry, identity, and generativity. Yet these constructs, at least as descriptions of individuals' behaviors and beliefs, belie that this is a theory about social as much as psychological development. The theory addresses the psychosocial demands placed upon us and our development in response to changing interpersonal situations from birth to death, all of which are embedded in relationships with significant others. Therefore this theory, when

## ABOUT THE CHAPTER AUTHORS

### Michael Karcher

In 1994 I was living in Boston, working as a school counselor trainee at Curley Middle School in Roxbury, and reading developmental theory with a passion. My friend, Dennis Barr, was able to spend time with the Eriksons at one of their famed sing-alongs in their house in Cambridge. I hoped to meet the Eriksons. I possessed all of their books (and had read almost half of them) and felt a connection with them partly as a function of the time I, too, lived in Vienna. I remember where I was, in the basement counseling center of the school, when I heard on the radio that Erik Erikson had passed away. I like to think I was very close to meeting them.

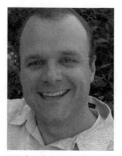

**Michael J. Karcher**

*Michael J. Karcher*, Ed.D., Ph.D., is an associate professor of education and human development at the University of Texas at San Antonio. He received a doctorate in human development and psychology from Harvard University and a doctorate in counseling psychology from the University of Texas at Austin. He conducts research on school-based and cross-age peer mentoring as well as on adolescent connectedness and pair counseling. He currently conducts the Study of Mentoring in the Learning Environment (SMILE) funded by the William T. Grant Foundation (www.utsasmile.org). He lives in his hometown of San Antonio with his wife Sara and their son Reed.

### Kristine Benne

In 2003 I had the privilege of taking a counseling theories class taught by my co-author on this chapter, Dr. Michael Karcher. Through his teaching and obvious passion for developmental theory, my interest was sparked. Since then I have sought out readings and research by Erik and Joan Erikson. My excitement for developmental theory was solidified by Joan Erikson's *The Woven Life Cycle*. I would encourage anyone who enjoys our chapter to read this selection.

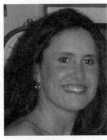

*Kristine Benne* graduated from the University of Texas at San Antonio (UTSA) with a Master of Arts in counseling. While at UTSA, Dr. Michael Karcher gave her the opportunity to work on and eventually manage a three-year grant-funded project called the Study of Mentoring in the Learning Environment (SMILE). The SMILE project focused specifically on the effectiveness of school-based mentoring. Kristine currently is working on the steps to become a licensed professional counselor (LPC) and has recently accepted a position providing case management and psychosocial support services for children and families. Kristine resides in San Antonio with her husband Michael and their two dogs Sophie and Ellie.

**Kristine Benne**

viewed more deeply, is about the tension of human growth in relationships and the resulting balance between needs for intimacy and connectedness, as well as for individuation. Viewed from this perspective, the Eriksons' theory provides a unique lens to the work of counselors, from those in community settings working with adults to those counselors in schools who try to bridge the lives of children and adults through child-focused interventions.

## The Eriksons' Biopsychosocial Model of Human Development: An Overview

All introductions to the work of Erik Erikson present his psychosocial stages of development. These are well known. Nevertheless, we review them here as well. We do this partly to reveal how most of what has been written about the Eriksons' approach may be considered andro(male)- and ethno(white)-centric if not considered within the larger scope of what Joan and Erik wrote during their professional careers. Namely, most of the stages in his model—certainly the stages most often referenced and studied by researchers who wrote about Erik Erikson—are the stages describing how the individual develops through individuation, through separation and increasing distinctiveness. These, as we are slowly learning through research in the fields of psychology, counseling, and other social studies, may not be the best terms for describing the essential characteristics of healthy developmental processes for women and people from ethnic minority groups. Therefore, something is missing, at least in the usual descriptions of this theory.

We feel, however, that when the work of Joan and Erik Erikson are considered together, in their totality, a different picture emerges. We will lay out this picture visually and descriptively in the sections that follow. In the second half of the chapter, we apply this wider picture to a case study involving a school counselor supervising an adult mentor working with a younger mentee in a school setting.

There is no doubt that Erik Erikson, in most of his seminal works, addressed the issues of culture, race, and marginality as well as perhaps any theorist of his era. In *Childhood and Society* (1950), Erikson prominently places descriptions of psychosocial development among Native Americans. As fodder for this work, both of the Eriksons lived in these indigenous communities, which allowed them to write about culture as a participator rather than from the distanced perspective of an academic writer. In *Identity: Youth in Crisis,* Erik Erikson applied the concept of identity across gender and culture. Identity is a construct we take for granted, but it was not until Erikson identified, named, defined, and illustrated identity as a life stage that it became part of common parlance. Before him, the construct was virtually not discussed in psychology.

Nevertheless, the Eriksons' works have not been beyond reproach from cultural and feminist critiques. In *Identity: Youth in Crisis,* Erikson himself introduced two chapters that highlight the limitations of his theory. Descriptions of the core characteristics of development among White males are not sufficient to fully capture the experiences of women and ethnic minorities. Therefore, generalizability of his theory may be called into question. Yet in two chapters in *Identity,* "Womanhood and the inner space" and "Race and the wider identity," he set the stage for the wider applied developmental perspective that we introduce here.

## Eriksonian Theory and the Marriage of Two Minds: Joan and Erik

Erik was clear that in most of his writings Joan played a central role. *A Way of Looking at Things* (Schlein, S., 1987), an edited compilation of Erikson's works, opens with a quote from Erik: "[I]n this whole collection there does not seem to be one bit of good writing that was not shared by [Joan] in thought as well as in formulation" (p. ix). The ways in which Joan may have widened Erik's theoretical perspective may be best illustrated in the content of *Wisdom and the Senses* (Erikson, J., 1988), which she alone penned. What Joan's perspective brought to the corpus of Erik's (and her) work is attention to the central role of relationships in psychosocial development. Yet this emerged most prominently in an essay in 1968 that revealed the connection between psychosocial development and what E. Erikson referred to as the "radius of significant relations."

Consistent with models of ethnic identity development and gender development, such as those of Jean Phinney and Carol Gilligan respectively, E. Erikson directly embeds each psychosocial crisis in the group of individuals with whom the developing person has the most significant relations at that point in development. Erikson's theory is commonly viewed as characterizing development in terms of the increasingly abstract and wider perspectives that individuals bring to their self and personal development over time. Less often does one find this sequence of individual development fully embedded within those groups constituting one's radius or sphere of influence, which also become more differentiated over time with each developmental advance. At each stage of development, the individual moves into a new relational context, such as into the neighborhood or school, as well as a new psychosocial role, such as by becoming a romantic partner or a parent. As we review the well-known psychosocial stages of development below and cover more directly their relations to the work of counselors, we highlight what appear to be the healthy and unhealthy reactions to each developmental crisis. We reveal how the Eriksons viewed each of these crises as embedded in interpersonal relationships.

We also wish to highlight a point of view not always prominent in chapters on Erik Erikson's theory, namely, the construct of virtues or basic strengths. Erikson believed these basic strengths (i.e., hope, will, purpose) emerge from the healthy movement through each developmental crisis requiring that the individual experiences both intense connection as well as differentiation, balancing two opposing but interrelated developmental reactions. These reactions—intense experiences of intimacy and autonomy—take place, of course, with and against those individuals within the radius of one's significant relationships. Therefore, we argue, understanding how development occurs within relationships and against a backdrop of prior development in relationships reveals the ways in which counselors can assist clients through a tandem focus on connectedness and distinctiveness as interrelated propellers of growth.

## ABOUT ERIK & JOAN ERIKSON

### Erik H. Erikson

Erik H. Erikson was born on June 15, 1902, near Frankfurt, Germany. His parents were both of Danish descent but separated before Erik was born. His mother, Karla, relocated their family from Denmark in order to be near friends and eventually settled in Karlsruhe, Germany. At the age of three Erik became ill and was treated by a local pediatrician, Dr. Homburger. Karla married the Jewish doctor, creating a new family for Erik, but signaling a difficult phase in his life. Tall, blonde, and blue eyed, he was picked on by his Jewish neighbors. In response, he attempted to fit in at school by becoming a "German Superpatriot" but found that his Jewish heritage was not appreciated by his peers, and their anti-Semitism was offensive to him. Feeling as though he did not fit in with either culture, Erikson became sensitive to the adolescent's struggle to establish an identity through a series of societal affiliation choices.

Growing up, Erik was an avid reader and loved the arts. He was extraordinarily interested in human relationships, specifically the relationship between parent and child. However, he was not interested in academics and did not do well in school. Instead of going off to a university, Erik became a wondering artist. He traveled across Europe learning about art and the human existence. He would call this time of his life his moratorium. He had difficulty establishing a self-identity and, despite their differences, Erik was always grateful to his stepfather for funding his search.

At the age of twenty-five, Erik found himself back in his hometown preparing to study and teach art when he received a life-changing letter from his old friend Peter Blos. Peter asked Erik to come to Vienna to teach at the Hietzing School. He not only taught at Peter's school but also studied Montessori education. These six productive years in Vienna would profoundly change his professional and personal paths in life. During his time in Vienna, Erik met the Freud family and began training in child psychoanalysis under Anna Freud. He focused on becoming a psychoanalyst, eventually graduating from the Vienna Psychoanalytic

Institute. During this time, Erik met his future wife, Joan, and his story became theirs together (and is detailed in her biography below).

## Joan Erikson

Joan Serson was born in the small town of Gananoque, Ontario. Her Canadian father, John, was the local Episcopal pastor. Her American mother, Mary, came from a wealthy New York railroad family. Often hospitalized for depression, Mary contributed little stability to the family. John seemed to favor Joan's youngest sibling and acted indifferently toward Joan. He died when Joan was only eight, and for the remainder of her youth, Joan lived on and off with her grandmother, Nama. Childhood left Joan angry at her parents but appreciative of Nama for providing her only source of nurturing support.

Her childhood difficulties motivated Joan to leave home as soon as possible. College presented just that opportunity. She received more formal academic training than Erik, including a B.A. in education from Columbia and a Masters degree in sociology from the University of Pennsylvania. She was interested in completing a Ph.D. and traveled to Germany to work on her dissertation. There Joan was analyzed by one of Freud's first disciples, Ludwig Jekels. In 1929 she traveled to Vienna and interviewed for a teaching position at the Hietzing School, where she first noticed Erik. In that same year, Erik attended a Mardi Gras masked ball and was formally introduced to his future life partner.

Within months of their introduction at the ball, Joan and Erik became involved in a serious relationship. In the spring of 1930, Joan discovered she was pregnant and wanted to marry Erik. Surprisingly, Erik entered into marriage reluctantly and had to be persuaded by friends. He was concerned that his family would be disappointed that he was marrying a non-Jew. Ultimately, it was their reminding him of his mother's plight as a young single mom and of the absence of his own biological father that convinced him he should act responsibly for his new family. Erik and Joan married soon after and moved to a rural cottage outside of Vienna. Their emotional union solidified the professional relationship that Erik Erikson credited for all of his work. Although Erik was given most of the professional accolades, by his own admission Joan provided significant contributions at every step of the process. Together they not only pioneered a theory but also produced three children, Kai, Jon, and Sue. In 1933, when Hitler took power in Germany, the Erikson family migrated to the United States, and Erik became the first child analyst in Boston.

Leaving Vienna marked a geographical separation from Freud that allowed the Eriksons more autonomy to expand the psychoanalytic theory beyond its focus on biological drives. Studying different cultures helped to facilitate a shift of focus from strict biology to a biopsychosocial framework. This shift began when Erik Erikson traveled to the Sioux Indian reservation of South Dakota to observe children. Unable to balance the beliefs of their own culture with the demands of American society, the Sioux children were left in a state of confusion and apathy. The Eriksons documented firsthand how society has a significant effect on the personality development of a child and believed that understanding the social context was key to understanding a child's personality development. Armed with this fundamental idea, Erik Erikson went on to head a longitudinal study at Berkeley, which followed "normal" American children for an entire generation. Through his work on this project and his study of diverse cultures, the theory of the eight stages of psychosocial development was born. The Eriksons can be credited with expanding the psychoanalytic theory to include environmental factors, specifically the cultural and social context of the individual.

Erik and Joan Erikson went on to write twelve books, including the acclaimed *Childhood and Society* (1950), and continued to teach, consult, and provide therapy throughout their careers. Erik Erikson worked for many prestigious institutions, including Harvard Medical School and Yale. He died in Harwich, Massachusetts, in 1994. Joan died in 1997.

## Trust Versus Mistrust

Erikson's theory of psychosocial development begins in infancy with the developmental crisis of trust versus mistrust. This is the hallmark experience of connection and intimacy against which other experiences will be judged. By striking a balance between trust and mistrust within one's first significant relationship—that is, with the [maternal] caregiver—the virtue of hope emerges.

Trust can be fostered in the infant through familial love and support. When an infant cries and the primary caregiver responds in a positive way, the issue that has upset the child is remedied (e.g., hunger or isolation). At that point in time, trust begins to take hold in that relationship. As the primary caregiver continues to respond to the infant's needs in a consistent manner, the experience of a safe, predictable world is created for the infant. By contrast, when an infant's needs are satisfied rarely and inconsistently, feelings of mistrust develop, and trust becomes harder to achieve both in the present and most likely in later relationships.

Mistrust, however, is not development's enemy. Mistrust can be a critical, adaptive reaction, which can help to ensure survival in some contexts and relationships (J. Erikson, 1988). Rather, it is the balance between trust and mistrust that endows the individual with a healthy character. Consider the child who knows to run away from the stranger who offers the child a ride home from school. However, the virtue of hope emerges among those individuals who develop an enduring belief that, although life will continue to fluctuate through moments of succor as well as of fear, safety can be experienced within the radius of one's significant relations. Attachment research confirms that these beliefs, established early in this primary relationship, tend to be lasting and color the lenses through which one views later relationships.

## Autonomy Versus Shame and Doubt

Autonomy, while not central to our case study other than through its role supporting the development of subsequent virtues, provides perhaps the best example of the kind of differentiation that we feel has been highlighted too much in prior work on Erikson's theory. Similar in nature to the concepts of individuation and individualistic, autonomy and autonomous suggest the person stands alone, on no one's shoulders. Yet this notion of the self-made man is exactly the sort of ethnocentric and androcentric representation of development that need not be ascribed to Erikson's work.

This stage highlights a second key assumption held by the Eriksons but often omitted when discussing their model, namely, that the healthiest resolution of a developmental crisis is to achieve a balance between the two crisis reactions characteristic of each developmental stage (e.g., between complete autonomy and complete shame and doubt). Albeit momentary from a lifespan point of view (as it is likely to be revisited countless times in later developmental crises), this balance creates a healthy tension through which development occurs best.

During the second stage of psychosocial development, toddlers begin to exercise their autonomy through evolving motor and verbalization skills (Schlein, 1987). The toddler begins to investigate the world around him or her, testing the limits at every turn. The crisis constitutes the child's need to find a balance between feelings of confidence resulting from newfound autonomy and feelings of shame and doubt at unsuccessful efforts to separate and stand alone. The toddler faces the double demand to demonstrate self-direction and to attain the approval and affection of primary caregivers (E. Erikson, 1964) through which the virtue of will or willpower is developed. Yet sustainable, genuine willpower—the type that can be drawn upon during subsequent developmental crises—can only be developed through the experience of both autonomy successes and failures.

The way this developmental crisis occurs and gets resolved is somewhat at odds with feminist critiques of the role of connectedness in girls' development (Brown & Gilligan, 1992; Chodorow, 1978; Gilligan, 1980) and crosscultural differences in parental rewards for autonomous behavior. Girls' efforts to express autonomy are not rewarded the same way as with boys', and this can complicate this developmental crisis for them. When examined from a sociocultural and historical perspective, girls (and children of both sexes in many societies) are kept close to the family (literally) and rewarded for conforming (figuratively). Joan Erikson also observed that even in Western societies, overanxious parents inadvertently inhibit their toddlers' autonomy by evoking shame and doubt by inconsistently reprimanding the toddler for curious, exploratory behavior (J. Erikson, 1988). This suggests that although there appears to be a positive valance applied to "autonomy" strivings and a negative valance applied to feelings of "shame and doubt," healthy development requires that both be experienced, in tandem, for a resilient experience of willpower to develop.

## Initiative Versus Guilt

The third stage of psychosocial development presents the crisis between initiative and guilt, which represents another in this series of stages that seems to favor the differentiation and individuation processes. Notice, however, that the emergence of this crisis occurs as a result of the child actively engaging with playmates in a new, nonfamily environment (J. Erikson, 1988). The crisis occurs when the child initiates contact with the surrounding world through social exploration and through manipulation of objects. This personal enterprise invites the development of perspective taking, such as the sense of guilt that results from an awareness that a child experiences when she or he has disregarded other people's boundaries through an age-appropriate initiative. Indeed, not experiencing guilt when one's own needs affect others adversely is consistent with definitions of conduct disorders among children and narcissistic personality disorders during adulthood.

During this stage, goal setting emerges and actions become purpose driven; purpose is the virtue that develops through a balanced reaction to this crisis. Children also begin to purposefully manipulate objects such as toys by taking them apart, not out of destructiveness, but out of a genuine curiosity. However, if children encounter consistently severe punishment or reprimand for these actions, initiative may decrease and children may become paralyzed with guilt (Muuss, 1996).

A skill that is awakened during this stage and that is used in an increasingly elaborate and abstract fashion throughout the teen and adult years is role taking. It also can provide a powerful clinical tool, such as in Gestalt therapy's "empty chair" technique, or even in the cognitive-behavioral approaches to imagining successful resolutions to a difficult circumstance. It also provides the foundation for the role-taking or perspective-taking skills that are required in late adolescence to experience mutuality and intimacy in relationships (Selman, 1980). From a counseling perspective, role playing allows children to act out negative feelings, which can evoke manageable feelings of inner guilt as the child destroys something loved and needed (J. Erikson, 1988). Winnicott's (1965) *transitional object* phenomenon is an early, developmentally critical example of this need to engage in fantasy to symbolically act out feelings of anger that result from the guilt a child experiences when her or his behavior has threatened the radius of significant relations.

## Industry Versus Inferiority

Children across societies receive the instruction and preparation they need to enter and navigate their social and future worlds (E. Erikson, 1959). The child learns that by producing things, he or she is recognized in a positive manner (E. Erikson, 1968). The developmental crisis occurs when the child tries to tolerate both the joy of working hard toward a job well done and the feelings of inadequacy that result from the inevitable failures that precede the mastery of any skill. An important factor in the outcome of this stage is the ability of significant adults to recognize and emphasize with the positive achievements that the child produces (E. Erikson, 1968).

This technique is central to fostering hope in the counseling relationship. Clients are like children in that when a sense of industry is effectively nurtured, the person will strive for recognition of successfully completed assignments or tasks and will seek out more work, culminating in a feeling of workmanship or competence in her or his abilities (Muuss, 1996). However, the child must internalize feelings of competence in her or his abilities through the attention and accolades of others (for children, of significant adults); but if satisfaction becomes dependent solely on the external feedback of others, feelings of uselessness and inadequacy can overpower feelings of industry. Through this stage, as a result of securing a balance between industry and inferiority, and through the mastery of some but not all available tasks, the virtue of competence emerges ( J. Erikson, 1988).

Erik Erikson was one of the first "culturalists," those psychodynamically oriented theorists who embedded development within a wider culture of intergroup relations. (Two other culturalists are Karen Horney, who described the impact of gender socialization on psychodynamics and development, and Sullivan, who described the way in which anxiety is borne out of close relationships with significant others.) Erik Erikson described most directly how culture informs self-awareness and psychological crisis resolution. For example, when considering the experience of youth of color during this developmental crisis, he suggests that often it is at this point the child "finds out immediately that the color of his skin or the background of his parents rather than his wish and will to learn are the factors that decide his worth as a pupil or apprentice" (1968, p. 125). In this case, the powerful influences of media, social stratification across cultural lines (e.g., seeing no one who looks like you in high prestige jobs), and the often unconscious responses from passersby who convey one's difference simply by shifting their eyes or clutching their possessions, all threaten to trump the influences of those in one's radius of significant relations. Both become internalized. Feelings of inferiority are bred not out of the actual trial-and-error performances made toward skill mastery but also by those ascriptions of worth that are unrelated to one's effort but reflect a caste or lot in life as a function of one's race, sex, or economic status. Again, Erik Erikson was clear that the experience of each developmental crisis was not just unique to the individual but also differentiated along the lines of group membership. Counselors must keep this second layer of influence in mind at all times to best and deeply understand their clients.

Erik Erikson also provided examples wherein an overemphasis on industriousness can undermine one's faith and joy in work. Erik Erikson argued that if the child identifies too heavily with his or her industrious side, play and imagination may be sacrificed too early, leading the individual to believe that the only thing that makes him or her worthwhile are others' perceptions of her or his effectiveness in the world of work (E. Erikson, 1968). This proposition foreshadows the concept of a false self that subsequently emerged in several objection relations theories of psychopathology, such as in the work of Sullivan, Kohut, and Winnicott. If one's experience of industry precludes appreciation of it as a process rather than a goal—that is, if productivity remains external and is not internalized as meaningful to the individual—she or he may become beholden to the wishes of others. Surely the Eriksons would have had something to say about the way in which high-stakes testing might adversely affect the development of youth, particularly those in underachieving schools.

## Identity Versus Role Confusion

Identity development is the last of the stages that are commonly described almost entirely as if its achievement did not depend upon the youth *signifying* a radius of important others. Of course, the challenges one faces in pursuit of personal identity require sustained effort by the individual to select out her or his uniqueness from the confusion of the many possible values, beliefs, goals, and behavior traits. A reluctance to work actively toward personal identity can result in role diffusion, and such an inability to define oneself can result in a subsequent estrangement and seclusion from others.

There is a temporality, or time-centeredness, involved in this stage that has been absent in the stages up to this point. Youth will explore and reflect upon past, present, and future selves in their attempts to find continuity (Muuss, 1996). Foremost, however, the formation of one's identity requires that youths rely on their peers for guidance and support in their exploration of new values and ideologies (E. Erikson, 1963). That is, while the stage of identity development heralds unprecedented use of emerging skills in abstract thinking (and perspective taking practiced earlier), it is even more so a social process involving others. This is why a sense of fidelity or loyalty becomes the virtue that is developed at this point—not just a certainty, focus, or commitment to ideas alone but also loyalty to others through one's identification with them. It is partly for this reason that some have argued that intimacy precedes identity and perhaps especially so among girls. The virtue of fidelity becomes ever harder to maintain over time, surprisingly, because of the advances in one's, ability to entertain possible and various ideological perspectives. Fidelity reflects the ability to maintain allegiance despite the contradiction of value systems that emerge over time (E. Erikson, 1964). This is the stage at which decisions must be made about who one is and who one is going to be; but perhaps more difficult, this is a time of choosing with whom one will form an allegiance and from whom one must turn away in order to maintain ideological consistency.

## Intimacy Versus Isolation

A reading of many developmental psychology text books might lead one to think Erik Erikson did not see others playing a central role in development after trust is formed and before intimacy is brought to the table. At this point in the young adult's life, finding another person with whom to develop an intimate sexual relationship becomes the goal. Love is the virtue to be developed. An intimate relationship involves sacrifice, compromise, and an ethical strength to commit oneself to a relationship (E. Erikson, 1963). However, in order for one to give her or his complete self to the relationship, there has to be a self to give, just as for one to identify with others in the formation of an identity, there must have developed some interpersonal connections that have been given priority. In other words, the development of identity is crucial in order to successfully navigate this stage of psychosocial development, but identity also was dependent on an earlier form of connectedness. Yet truly intimate relationships involve sharing of one's life, work, goals, and ideologies (J. Erikson, 1988), which require more complex cognitive and identity development than have been present prior to adolescence. For intimacy to occur, cognitive developments such as mature perspective-taking abilities are necessary but not sufficient (Selman, 1980). If identity has not begun to be established, mature love cannot grow because individuals will bring little to the relationship in terms of a unique self. In this case fear of engulfment can occur and the individual may retreat into isolation as has been well described by Kohut (1971) and Winnicott (1965). Clearly, this is not the first stage in which love has surfaced; however if love was lacking in one's earlier stages, if connectedness at prior stages was weak and insincere, the young adult at this point is likely to disengage from this normative pursuit of connection, choosing solitude instead of intimacy (J. Erikson, 1988).

## Generativity Versus Stagnation

The seventh stage of psychosocial development finds a mature adult dealing with the challenge of generativity versus stagnation. The virtue to be developed is care through a broadening concern for what one has created (E. Erikson, 1964). Generativity is the need to selflessly guide the next generation (McAdams & de St. Aubin, 1992; Schlein, 1987). This can be accomplished through either applying this drive to the individual's own offspring or by feeling responsible for the larger society (J. Erikson, 1988). The mature adult wants to be useful and effective, contributing to the world. Adults feel a need to impart their own knowledge and teach younger generations (E. Erikson, 1964). The counterpull of stagnation can occur when the adult focuses internally, ceasing further psychosocial development. The adult falls into a repetitive routine within the social and work worlds, with the only concern and focus being on oneself.

## Integrity Versus Despair

The eighth stage of psychosocial development finds an aging adult entering twilight of his or her life. The developmental crisis of this stage is to find a balance between integrity and despair. The virtue to be developed is wisdom based on accumulated knowledge and mature judgment through life (E. Erikson, 1964). As adults reflect upon their lives, one challenge is to appreciate and integrate previous life experiences while minimizing feelings of despair or resentment. However if the adult feels as though her or his life has been wasted, feelings of discontentment can become overwhelming. Despair can not only contaminate the self but also drive away significant others, further strengthening the associations between despair, isolation, and feelings of failure. As an individual reviews her or his life story, the developmentally ideal result is a sense of acceptance and overall integrity for a life well lived. (See Table 7.1 for a summary of the Erikson's developmental sequence.)

TABLE 7.1    A Developmental Sequence in Virtue Development as the
Product of the Weaving Tension of Developmental Growth

| | Developmental Crises and Resulting Self-Developments | Basic Strengths or Virtues | Radius of Connectedness in Significant Relations |
|---|---|---|---|
| I. | Trust vs. Mistrust | HOPE | Maternal Persons |
| II. | Autonomy vs. Shame, Doubt | WILL | Parental Persons |
| III. | Initiative vs. Guilt | PURPOSE | Basic Family |
| IV. | Industry vs. Inferiority | COMPETENCE | Neighborhood, School |
| V. | Identity vs. Role Confusion | FIDELITY | Peer Groups and Outgroups; Models of Leadership |
| VI. | Intimacy vs. Isolation | LOVE | Partners in Friendship, Sex, Competition, Cooperation |
| VII. | Generativity vs. Stagnation | CARE | Divided and Shared Household |
| VIII. | Integrity vs. Despair | WISDOM | "Mankind" "My Kind" |

*Note.* Adapted from *The Human Life Cycle* (E. Erikson, 1971). Copyright 2005 by Michael Karcher.

# Underlying Assumptions of the Theory

Erik Erikson's eight stages of psychosocial development include several core assumptions that set the foundation for the larger theory. The first assumption is that although the stages are linear and generally occur at certain ages, rates of progression through the eight stages will vary depending on individuals' internal (i.e., biological) and external (i.e., social and cultural context) circumstances and prior experiences. People continue to develop, in part, because biological changes propel them into new tasks imposed by new contexts and accompanying interpersonal demands. Thus, the stages and their corresponding age ranges are not meant to be restrictive or finite but rather represent the central developmental crises that individuals most commonly deal with at particular points in the life cycle.

A second element of this first assumption about the diversity of developmental pathways is that the residual experiences of past crises reactions as well as the seeds of subsequent developmental crises are present in every stage: Prior crisis resolutions provide the foundation upon which current developmental crises are played out; each crisis reaction and resolution, then, sets the stage for future crises. For example, although individuals in their late twenties and early thirties tend to face head on the developmental crisis of intimacy versus isolation, the residue of trust versus mistrust struggles from earlier stages and the identifications that emerged from the crisis of identity versus role confusion inform how intimacy is approached (e.g., how much trust is bestowed on others) and with whom (typically people consistent with the identifications chosen earlier).

All of which brings us to a second important assumption. Each stage should not be looked at as a success or failure but as a process, the results of which are the strengths and virtues we carry with us (and continue to cultivate) throughout life. It is true that each stage represents a crisis, but it is the individual's ability to strike a balance between the two poles that facilitates growth and development. An individual should and will experience struggles at each stage of her or his psychosocial development. Why? Because like the effect of fire on metal, challenges and strong reactions to each crisis make the resultant resolution and virtues stronger.

The fourth assumption is that life demands constant rebalancing. No crisis resolution is finite and immutable. That the individual finds a balance between the two poles during the initial crisis resolution does not mean that the issues just overcome will not arise again later. New life stages provide multiple opportunities to rework prior crisis resolutions.

The fifth and final assumption that we highlight is not one that stands out in most discussions of the Eriksons' model of psychosocial development, namely, that life is about a weaving back and forth between developmental priorities. Each priority reflects a greater or lesser emphasis on connectedness and individuation, but at no point can the developmental crises that reveal these priorities be seen in isolation from each other. Just as each crisis has a positive and negative reaction, each crisis also reflects the need to establish a balance that leans either more toward connectedness or more toward individuation. Notably, as Selman's model of interpersonal negotiation strategies reveals, as individuals mature, the width of the gap between connection and individuation narrows. Selman and Schultz (1990) suggest that based on how individuals respond to conflict—viz. in terms of

which participant changes or transforms her or his own needs and wants—
the person can be characterized as acting in more self-transforming or
other-transforming ways. As people mature from their use of egocen-
trism toward the use of cooperation as interpersonal conflict resolution approaches, these two styles (self- and other-transforming) become
less extreme or distinct. Like the Eriksons' stages, which are viewed
for the most part as occurring in a predictable sequence, Selman (1980)
also presents a series of states in which social cognition, namely
perspective-taking abilities, unfold in a predictable fashion across the
lifespan. In Selman's final stage of social cognitive maturity, collaborative interpersonal negotiation strategies emerge wherein the self- and
other-transforming styles become indistinguishable because collaboration reflects accommodation and assertiveness simultaneously. Similarly, as individuals approach the stages or developmental priorities of
generativity and integrity, it becomes hard to determine whether these
stages reflect expressions of connection or separation because these priorities reflect both. That is, both models illustrate that as the individual matures, there is a developmental movement toward unity
where previously in development there were clearly competing poles
and clearly evidenced tension between them.

An assumption we add to those above, all of which can be found
easily in the voluminous writings of the Eriksons—an assumption that
we think has been less commonly reflected in prior writings on the
Eriksons' theory—is the importance of connectedness as a propeller of
the better known self-developments: industry, initiative, and identity.
Yet when one takes seriously the role of the "radius of significant relations" that accompanies each of these developmental priorities for individuation, it becomes clear that connectedness and individuation or
self-developments go hand-in-hand. For this reason, much as Kegan
(1982) has described in *The Evolving Self*, we have arranged the Eriksons' stages figuratively.

In Figure 7.1 the stages are arranged two dimensionally rather than
in their usual linear fashion. In this figure, the second dimension is that
of the continuum between connectedness and self-developments reflecting the developmental priorities of individuation. The width of the spiral illustrates the distinctiveness of connectedness and individuation at
these points in development, with the smallest gap being at the start
and end of life. In other words, in this life cycle the individual is most
"at odds" with herself or him toward the early middle of life when the
tension between self and connectedness developments are most in conflict.
This time in the life cycle also may be when the internal experience of

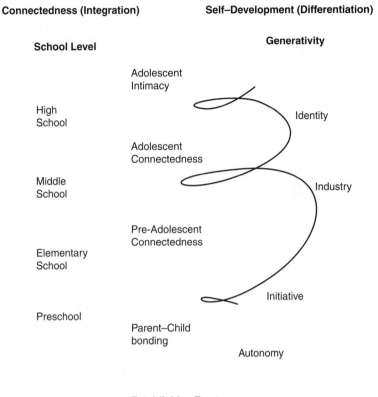

**Connectedness (Integration)**          **Self–Development (Differentiation)**

**School Level**                              **Generativity**

Adolescent
Intimacy

High
School                                          Identity

Adolescent
Connectedness

Middle
School                                          Industry

Pre-Adolescent
Connectedness

Elementary
School

Initiative

Preschool

Parent–Child
bonding

Autonomy

**Establishing Trust**

***"Weaving tension of developmental growth"* (Joan Erikson)**

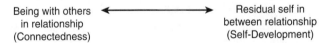

Being with others   ⟷   Residual self in
in relationship            between relationship
(Connectedness)           (Self-Development)

FIGURE 7.1   A Figural Representation of the "Weaving Tension of Developmental Growth" Copyright 2005 by Michael Karcher

tension and developmental imbalance are most different between men and women. In the Eriksons' work, it seems that the male experience has been given priority and has been held out as the main example, which has sometimes been viewed as either the only or the most important way in which the self and connectedness developmental tension is experienced. This is unfortunate, because their framework clearly affords an application to how both men and women deal with the different social and biological forces that bear on this developmental crisis. It is perhaps for this reason that Eriksons' framework of developmental tension between self and connectedness is elaborated on by Kegan and has also been used by Belenky, Clinchy, Goldberger, and Tarule to give voice to the unique expression of this tension for women in *Women's Ways of Knowing* (1986). Works of others at the Stone Center and that of Carol Gilligan also explore this tension.

## The Role of the Eriksons' Theory of Human Development in Counseling and Supervision

Erik Erikson's theory has been used at times as a lens for examining the developing individual's life in relative isolation in terms of individual achievements—for example, to say what stage the *individual* is at or that *she or he* successfully resolved a developmental crisis. We believe, however, that he did not intend for it to be used in that way. Only by embedding one's understanding of another person within the "radius of their significant relations" (as the Erikson's called it in *Insight and Responsibility*) and then placing the totality of these relations within their sociocultural, gendered, and historical context can a full understanding be approximated.

For these reasons, no intervention, counseling, consulting, or other help is likely to take hold unless it directly or indirectly affects that web of connections within the client's radius of significant relations. Joan Erikson (1988) suggests "if any intervention can break the *dullness of the graying pattern,* it will be the experience of an intimate relationship. Only by means of such a genuine mutuality can empathy slowly retrieve some of the lost vitality of the insecure basic strengths" (p. 99).

What form of intimate relationship develops between the counselor and client, or in what manner a counselor is able to help facilitate meaningful and intimate relationships for the client outside the therapeutic relationship, varies according to intervention structure and goals. The intimate relationship may be the client-counselor relationship. It may be the relationship that forms within a counseling group or the family relationships that are made more meaningful through family counseling. But from an ecological perspective, the counselor also can work in a consulting or supervisory role with people whose role it is to establish strong, meaningful, and intimate relationships with others, such as the teacher with a student, a boss with her staff, or a mentor with her mentee.

# Kerry, Sam's Mentor

Sharon is a school counselor at an urban middle school in a large metropolitan area. She has been at the same school for five years and has been a school counselor for eight years, after four years as an elementary school teacher. In her graduate studies in school counseling, she became interested in the lifespan model written by the Eriksons and wrote her thesis on its use in school counseling. Although her thesis focused on how teachers' developmental crises may interact with their students' crises and how she could use the Eriksons' model to help facilitate teacher–student relationships, currently she is experiencing a supervision challenge she did not anticipate.

In the fall, Sharon set up a school-based mentoring program at her school in which she invites adults working in local businesses, retirees, and both college and graduate students to work one hour a week with her middle school students. Sharon enlisted all of the known mentoring best practices and created a strong program. For example, she spends two hours with potential mentors training them, provides them a one-hour school orientation, and makes available ongoing training. She, of course, has the school run background checks on potential mentors, but she also uses innovative procedures to match mentors with mentees, makes available a variety of academic and recreational activities for the mentors and their mentees to engage in, and maintains regular contact with the mentors and mentees to monitor the development of their relationship. It is in this last capacity, as a supervisor of mentors, that Sharon has found the Eriksons' model particularly useful.

Kerry is a mentor working at Sharon's school once a week with Sam. Sam is a Latino youth who has average grades at school, is social and well accepted by peers, but who is at risk for involvement in local gangs. While Sam has fairly good relationships with teachers at school, he has more contact, time-wise, with older teens in his neighborhood who discourage his afterschool involvement in homework or extracurricular sports. Having an older brother who is a member of a gang, and to whom Sam looks up, creates a considerable challenge to dissuading Sam from spending time with kids in his neighborhood who are involved in gang activities.

This problem has risen to the foreground in Kerry's mentoring relationship with Sam. While Kerry spends much of her effort trying to engage Sam in instrumental or goal-oriented mentoring activities and conversations, such as about the value of a high school diploma, the benefits of participating in school-sponsored sports, and the benefits of being successful in school, Kerry feels the constant pull on Sam's attention from the world he encounters after school each day.

Sam is from a large family. His mother works two jobs and Sam does not know his father. Sam does not participate in any youth clubs or religious organization, and does not have any particularly strong connections with teachers at school. Given this absence of other adult role models in Sam's life, Kerry feels particularly responsible for providing guidance to Sam that will help redirect his attention away from gang activities and potential membership. Using the Hemingway Measure of Adolescent Connectedness (Karcher, 2003; Karcher, Holcomb, & Zambrano, in press) as a screening tool to assess the degrees of connectedness Sam reports across his radius of significant relations, Sharon has found that Sam has high levels of connectedness to peers and far less connectedness to teachers, which is a sign that Sam is more engaged outside school than to school and relies more on peer relationships to shape his inchoate, developing identity. His connectedness to school, however, is high, suggesting that strengthened relations with adults at school may be what could benefit him most.

Although Sam reports a healthy sense of competence both in his neighborhood and at school, Sam grapples with the burden of choosing a path: join a gang or become more involved with school activities. His loyalties are constantly being questioned and tested by peer and adult influences. Sam struggles to choose one world to which he can assign his loyalty and experience the virtue of fidelity resulting in identity development. Sam sees Kerry as a positive influence in his life but is uncomfortable with the pace and depth of their relationship. Thus at this point, Kerry may actually be jeopardizing Sam's commitment to a better life.

Through their weekly discussions, Sharon has discovered that Kerry has become emotionally overinvolved, attempting to serve a savior role in Sam's life. It is spring. The school year is winding down. With summer looming and threatening to further expose Sam to unsupervised time with friends and "associates" in his neighborhood, Kerry has become anxious and almost obsessed with protecting and caring for Sam. This has become most problematic in that Kerry has talked about wanting to meet with Sam regularly over the summer. She even discussed taking Sam to the beach for a few weeks in the summer to help get him out of his neighborhood. But Kerry has not discussed any of this with Sam's mother, and summer contact outside of the school is not condoned or sanctioned by the parameters of Sharon's school-based mentoring program. Sharon is faced with the task of enforcing the rules of the mentoring program without offending Kerry and jeopardizing the supportive presence of Kerry in Sam's life. What Sharon has noticed through her discussions with Kerry is that there is a dearth of other significant, important relationships in Kerry's life, such that Sam seems to be the most significant person in her life at this time. Kerry seems to focus on Sam's life and struggles to such an extent that she neglects her own social life and interpersonal relationships.

Kerry works at a local television station as a news anchor. She is known by virtually everyone in the community, but she has virtually no friendships and has never mentioned involvement in a romantic relationship. Although Kerry is a very interesting person with lots of interests and a clear sense of who she is professionally, interpersonally Kerry is hard to profile. Her connectedness with others seems only surface deep, not superficial, but simply not given enough time to allow her relationships with others to mature and provide meaning in her life.

One final element of this situation is that Sharon knows that if this mentoring relationship works out, Kerry is likely to encourage others at the station to mentor youth, and there is the possibility that the station might even run a service announcement that could bring even more mentors to Sharon's school. So Sharon has many reasons to want to make this match work out well.

As Sharon begins to think seriously about how best to reach out to Kerry, she turns to the materials in Kerry's mentor application. Because Sharon once read that high scores on generativity measurements may contribute to longer-lasting, more meaningful mentoring relationships, Sharon has each mentor who applies complete the Loyola Generativity Scale (McAdams & de St. Aubin, 1992) and the Measures of Psychosocial Development (MPD; Garbarino, Gaa, Swank, McPherson, & Gratch, 1995), which provide an assessment of dimensions of generativity and levels of successful crisis resolution for each stage (rather than providing a "level" of development). In Kerry's case, it appears that she has a solid foundation in her developmental history relating to the tasks of industry and identity development, but her strength of the virtues of love and care seem to have been hampered by her prior avoidance of challenge and exploration in romantic relationships. This underdeveloped experience of intimacy now seems to be undermining her ability to develop the virtue of caring, that is, of exploiting her desire for generativity. Kerry's efforts to master a form of caring that is not rooted in her own intimacy needs seem to be inhibiting her ability to step back from her mentoring relationship and see how her own history and developmental needs may be contributing to her assessment of what she must do to be "a good mentor."

Thus far in Sharon's supervision of Kerry, she has found Kerry most receptive to the Eriksons' theoretical constructs, but these have all been understood by Kerry in terms of how the constructs explain Sam's situation and developmental needs, not her own. Kerry seems to really understand and appreciate that Sam is struggling with his own inchoate movements toward the establishment of a consistent identity. Sam has developed both academic and social skills through a successful period in which industry strivings led him to explore all of his options for skill development. Kerry also sees that, while Sam's mother is not currently available, when Sam was younger he had strong, consistent, positive experiences within his early maternal and family relationships. Thus it is easy for Kerry to see present in Sam the virtues of hope, will, purpose, and competence. Kerry understood well when Sharon used the Eriksons' model to explain the elements of Sam's success efforts to develop a balance between identity and role confusion. Kerry could see how Sam was wrestling to view himself consistently across his worlds and how, feeling the developmental imperative to experience fidelity in his relationships across contexts, Sam has come to feel the need to become either a good student or a connected member of the "associations" in his neighborhood.

Kerry is not devoid of insight into her own processes, but she struggles to see how her own need to experience love through successfully balancing intimacy and isolation experiences is playing into her mentoring relationship. For example, when Sharon was explaining the striving for identity versus role confusion that Sharon thought Sam might be experiencing, Kerry could connect this to her own career choices and see how making those decisions helped firm up her own sense of self. But Kerry was less able to see how her identity crisis resolution occurred, in part, through her identification with others and specifically the peer groups that defined her identity. Kerry, not experiencing much closeness or affiliation with others at work, saw her identity as a news anchor defined by a set of tasks, skills, and duties. She downplayed the meaning of her affiliation with others in the field of broadcasting, and she did not see how her choice of career also led her to experience isolation from people in other arenas in her life. She did not connect how her career left her little time to spend with family, nor did she link it to her severed relationships with her teammates in college when she abandoned her goal of becoming a professional athlete for broadcasting.

Most striking was Kerry's inability to see how a lack of intimacy in her current life might be contributing to her deeply felt urgency in terms of "saving" Sam. Kerry understood Sam's relationship with his mom might help serve to buffer him from deepening involvement with his older brother's associates, but she did not see how such relationships contributed to her own mental health and psychosocial development.

Sharon asked Kerry if she could try to provide Kerry some more personal insights into the mentoring relationship by discussing the assessments Kerry had completed as part of her application. Kerry agreed, and Sharon began a discussion of the nature of their supervision by assuring confidentiality regarding what was discussed. Following this, Sharon began to ask Kerry about her experiences related to identity and intimacy in the past and more recently. Over the course of two meetings, Kerry shared that she had grown up in a tough neighborhood in Philadelphia where her first love was Lucas, a boy who was actively involved in gangs. He remained involved with gang activity in Philadelphia after Sharon left for college. Through later communications with mutual friends, Sharon learned that Lucas may have been shot and killed during gang activities. Sharon never sought confirmation of Lucas' death, but she related a series of other hostile, aggressive interpersonal relationships she had in high school and later in college; Kerry commented that she lost trust in people as a result of those experiences. She especially lost trust in men through some unpleasant experiences in college and explained that since then she has just focused on her work. Through discussions with Kerry about the lack of intimate relationships in her life, Sharon helped Kerry see her self-imposed isolation and deep desire for intimacy.

As Sharon helped Kerry apply the tenets of Erik and Joan Eriksons' theory to her life and relationship with Sam, Kerry became clearer about how she was trying to meet multiple developmental needs of her own in her work with Sam. She could see how her own intimacy needs were affecting her own resolutions of identity and generativity strivings. Feeling incomplete interpersonally, Kerry experienced intimacy vicariously by seeing herself as Sam's savior, even as a secondary maternal figure for him. Kerry could see how her own failing to experience love resulted in a lack of intimate relationships throughout her adult life, inhibiting her ability to genuinely give that love back to society through caring for others like Sam. She was not able to achieve a sense of herself as generative because she worried that if she could not save Sam then she was a failure. All this underscored that above all Kerry was getting her intimacy needs met through her intense, personal, and involved dialogues and interactions with Sam. In that light, Kerry could see both how taking Sam on a trip over the summer met her needs more than his and could be seen as inappropriate.

## Summary: How the Eriksons' Theory Helps Counselors Mentor the Mentor

Joan and Erik Eriksons' theory of human development charts a stagewise progression in human development in relationships across the lifespan. The Eriksons placed primary emphasis on charting how individuals manage developmental tasks and relational demands in context. Best known are the self-developments of industry, identity, and generativity that Erik Erikson described. Yet these constructs do not fully capture the true role of social and cultural processes in the theory of psychological development that the Eriksons pioneered. Their theory addresses the psychosocial demands placed upon us and our development from birth to death in response to changing interpersonal situations, all of which are embedded within a radius of relationships with significant others. Therefore, we have described their theory as best characterized by the weaving tension of human growth in relationships and the resulting tension between needs for connectedness and for individuation that Joan articulated in her book *Wisdom and the Senses* (1988).

Viewed from this perspective, the Eriksons' theory provides a unique lens for the work of counselors, from those in community settings working with adults to those counselors in schools who try to bridge the lives of children and adults through child-focused interventions. In the case study, a school counselor helped mentor a school-based mentor using the core principles of the Eriksons' theory. The counselor helped the mentor, Kerry, understand her own inability to achieve a satisfactory balance between intimacy and isolation in her own life. This allowed Kerry to comprehend her own intense feelings about Sam. She gained a greater ability to stand back and observe her relationship with Sam as but one of several positive adult influences in his life. She was better able to see that regardless of *his* choices, she was not a failure if Sam did not succeed in school or go to college. On a more positive note, a full examination of Kerry's own developmental achievements, crisis resolutions, and experiences from the vantage of the Eriksons' sequence of virtues helped her reflect back on the important role her own family and adult mentors had in facilitating her own hope, will, purpose, competence, and identity. Through an introduction and application of the Eriksons' theory by the counselor, Kerry better understood that she would need to achieve a greater sense of intimacy with others if she was to fully exploit her own trust and initiative in mature, interpersonal relationships with others. This development in relationships, and more specifically relationships embedded within a given culture at a given time in history, is the legacy of the Eriksons that may prove to be the most lasting.

# Annotated Bibliography

## On Theory Validation

Belenky, M. F., Clinchy, B. M., Goldberger, N. R., & Tarule, J. M. (1986). *Women's ways of knowing.* New York: Basic Books.
This book details the Eriksons' theory as it applies uniquely to the lives of women, in part by extending the model presented by Kegan (1982) wherein the processes of separation, individuation, and connection across the lifespan are considered key developmental catalysts. This book also builds on the work of Gilligan (1988), who has highlighted the primacy of relationship and connection in the psychosocial development of women.

Kegan, R. (1982). *The evolving self: Problem and process in human development.* Cambridge, MA: Harvard University Press.
Robert Kegan's work extends the Eriksons' work and integrates it with several other developmental theories to illustrate the processes of separation and individuation throughout the life cycle, but it is unique in its inclusion of connection and intimacy as key developmental processes as well. The "wind tunnel" diagram we present in Figure 7.1 elaborates on Kegan's model. This diagram illustrates how the Eriksons' work typically has been used to detail the processes of individuation. However, Kegan does a wonderful job of showing how these developmental priorities of intimacy and autonomy, which vary systematically and predictably across the lifespan, manifest in people's self-understanding, career choice, and interpersonal challenges. Kegan has gone on to write about the application of this theory to groups, to the workplace, and to adult development more specifically. These works provide a nice illustration of the influence the Eriksons' work has had on later theorizing.

Ochse, R., & Plug, C. (1986). Cross-cultural investigation of the validity of Erikson's theory of personality development. *Journal of Personality & Social Psychology, 50,* 1240–1252.
These authors created a self-report measure of Erik Erikson's model of personality development. The focus of the article, beyond reporting on measurement development, is to suggest that individuals' sex and race may play a role in the timing of identity resolution. For example, in this study of South Africans, White women resolved their identity crisis earliest, and Black men the latest. They also found evidence of greater experiences of

intimacy among women than among men, which is an assumption made in our chapter as well.

Sorell, G. T., & Montgomery, M. J. (2001). Feminist perspectives on Erikson's theory: Their relevance for contemporary identity development research. *Identity, 1,* 97–128.

The authors of this article, as well as the three experts who subsequently comment on this essay in their own commentaries (found in the same journal, volume 2), do a nice job of placing the Eriksons' work within its sociopolitical context. They critique the emphasis of biology in the biopsychosocial model, but recognize it reflects to some extent Erik Erikson's debt to Freud. More importantly, perhaps, is their effort to highlight androcentrism in the Eriksons' work. The Eriksons' work provides, at times, an overly male-centered perspective on human development. It is this autonomous, separation-focused aspect of the Eriksons' theory that we have tried hard to counter in our chapter by merging the work of both Eriksons.

## On Eriksonian Measurements for Use in Counseling

Kowaz, A. M., & Marcia, J. E. (1991). Development and validation of a measure of Eriksonian industry. *Journal of Personality & Social Psychology, 60,* 390–397.

Marcia is a key researcher of identity theory, and this work focuses squarely on the stage of identity. Although the measure that was developed for this study has not been used much subsequent to this publication, the article does a nice job of both illustrating the essential elements of measurement validation and of teasing apart the underlying construct of industry in the Eriksons' model.

McAdams, D. P., & de St. Aubin, E. (1992). A theory of generativity and its assessment through self-report, behavioral acts, and narrative themes in autobiography. *Journal of Personality & Social Psychology, 62,* 1003–1015.

This article is useful in that it provides both a theoretical extension of Erik Erikson's generativity construct and a measure. The psychometric properties of the Loyola Generativity Scale are reported, and interesting findings are presented (e.g., that fathers reported greater generativity than men who had not fathered children). The article is important in that it provides a definition of generativity with greater specificity than had existed previously. Namely, the authors suggest it includes a cultural demand, an inner desire, generative concern, belief in the species, commitment, generative action, and personal narration, each of which is detailed in the article.

Phinney, J. S. (1992). The multigroup ethnic identity measure: A new scale for use with diverse groups. *Journal of Adolescent Research, 7,* 156–176.

Jean Phinney changed the landscape of ethnic and intergroup understanding by taking Erik Erikson's identity development processes and using them as a lens through which to view ethnic identity. This scale has been used frequently in studies that attempt to examine how a youth's stage of ethnic identity exploration may relate to psychological phenomenon, such as depression and self-esteem, and behavioral correlates of ethnic identity, including academic achievement and affiliation with their own and different ethnic groups. The stages of identity exploration, moratorium, and achievement can be better understood by learning how Phinney applies these Eriksonian terms to the processes of ethnic identity.

# References

Belenky, M. F., Clinchy, B. M., Goldberger, N. R., & Tarule, J. M. (1986). *Women's ways of knowing*. New York: Basic Books.

Brown, L. M., & Gilligan, C. (1992) *Meeting at the crossroads*. Cambridge: Harvard University Press.

Chodorow, N. (1978). *The reproduction of mothering : Psychoanalysis and the sociology of gender*. Berkeley: University of California Press.

Erikson, E. H. (1950). *Childhood and society*. New York: Norton.

Erikson, E. H. (1959). *Identity and the life cycle*. New York: Norton.

Erikson, E. H. (1964). *Insight and responsibility*. New York: Norton.

Erikson, E. H. (1968). *Identity: Youth and crisis*. New York: Norton.

Erikson, J. M. (1988). *Wisdom and the senses*. New York: Norton.

Garbarino, J., Gaa, J. P., Swank, P., McPherson, R., & Gratch, L. V. (1995). The relation of individuation and psychosocial development, *Journal of Family Psychology, 3*, 311–318.

Gilligan, C. (1988). Remapping the moral domain: New images of self in relationship. In C. Gilligan, J. V. Ward, & J. M. Taylor (Eds.), *Mapping the moral domain* (pp. 3–19). Cambridge, MA: Harvard University Press.

Karcher, M. J. (2003). The Hemingway: Measure of Adolescent Connectedness: Validation studies. *ERIC* no. ED477969; *ERIC/CASS* no. CG032433. Retrieved February, 20, 2002, from www.adolescentconnectedness.com.

Karcher, M. J., Holcomb, M., & Zambrano, E. (in press). Measuring adolescent connectedness: A guide for school-based assessment and program evaluation. In H. L. K. Coleman & C. Yeh (Eds.), *Handbook of School Counseling*. Mahwah: Erlbaum.

Kegan, R. (1982). *The evolving self: Problem and process in human development*. Cambridge, MA: Harvard University Press.

Kohut, H. (1971) *Restoration of the self*. Madison, CT: International Universities Press.

McAdams, D. P., & de St. Aubin, E. (1992). A theory of generativity and its assessment through self-report, behavioral acts, and narrative themes in autobiography. *Journal of Personality & Social Psychology, 62*, 1003–1015.

Muuss, R. E. (1996). *Theories of adolescence* (6th ed.). New York: McGraw-Hill.

Schlein, S. (1987). *Erik H. Erikson: A way of looking at things*. New York: Norton.

Selman, R. (1980). *The growth of interpersonal understanding: Developmental and clinical analyses.* New York: Academic Press.

Selman, R. L., & Schultz, L. H. (1990). *Making a friend in youth: Developmental theory and pair therapy.* Chicago: University of Chicago Press.

Stern, L. (1990). Conceptions of separation and connection in female adolescents. In C. Gilligan, N. P. Lyons, & T. J. Hanmer (Eds.), *Making connections: The relational worlds of adolescent girls at Emma Willard School* (pp. 73–87). Cambridge, MA: Harvard University Press.

Winnicott, D. W. (1965). *Maturational processes and the facilitating environment. Studies in the theory of emotional development.* Madison, CT: International Universities Press.

# CHAPTER EIGHT

# Lifespan Developmental Issues for Women

## Rita Sommers-Flanagan and Monica Carlson Roscoe

Because of the gains made by first and second wave feminist activists, women in the United States have access to education, health care, and life options that were undreamed of by their grandmothers. On the surface, this might lead students and practicing counselors to assume that the developmental challenges and trajectories of females are much more similar to males now. And to some degree, they would be correct. However, such an assumption glosses over a vast array of subtle and not-so-subtle differences between male and female developmental paths. In addition, cultural norms and expectations for women's roles and development vary greatly among the clients we might work with in the United States.

This chapter is designed to help readers recognize basic feminist tenets relevant to the many aspects of human development that are affected by gender. Did it matter to your parents if you were a girl or a boy? Can you remember feeling confusion or shame about your attempts to fit in as a boy or a girl? Did you ever feel limited, angry, or constrained because of being born male or female? How would your own life be different if you'd been born the other sex?

Normal developmental milestones are inextricably influenced by sex and gender. This chapter uses nine factors, shown in Table 8.1 (p. 234), to help counselors glimpse the developmental implications of sex and gender in the lives of women.

## ABOUT THE CHAPTER AUTHORS

### Rita Sommers-Flanagan

Writing this chapter on lifespan developmental issues for women was both rewarding and frustrating. As we were putting the finishing touches in place, an e-mail arrived from Maggie, a brilliant young woman working on her Ph.D. at a prestigious university. She was furious that her advisor had just informed her that childbearing was not a realistic option for women academics who wished to be tenured in top-tiered institutions. Thus while the lifespan developmental challenges for women have changed over the centuries, they have not abated. Both male and female helping professionals need to be aware of the particular issues faced by women in many cultures. I hope this chapter helps you envision ways to be of help to Maggie, and all the other wonderful women developing their potential over their entire lifespan.

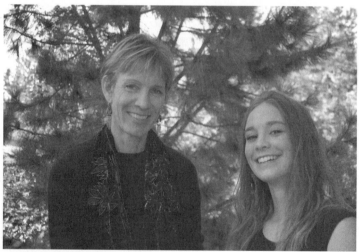

**Rita Sommers-Flanagan and her daughter**

*Rita Sommers-Flanagan* is a tenured professor of counselor education who somehow managed to bear two wonderful daughters. Professional interests include ethics, professional development, and the efficacy of human helping interventions. Besides teaching at the University of Montana, Rita is a consultant for the Missoula

Vet Center and shares, with her husband John Sommers-Flanagan, a part-time consulting position at Trapper Creek Job Corps.

## Monica Carlson Roscoe

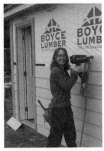

*Monica Carlson Roscoe*, M.A., works as a school counselor at Hellgate High School, while pursuing a counselor education program Ed.S. at the University of Montana. Her professional interests include both school counseling and mental health counseling. She has held professional internships or had work experiences in a variety of settings in Missoula, including Early Head Start; elementary, middle, and high schools; and a university student affairs program. She and her husband live in Missoula, Montana, where she enjoys good friends, hiking, singing, and building.

**Monica Carlson Roscoe**

Readers do not have to identify themselves as feminists to make use of this chapter. The fact that humans are born with features that cause most to be identified as either male or female is uncontested. Most would agree that this differentiation has cultural and psychological implications that are primary and profound, and which are often a source of pain, conflict, and/or confusion as we grow and develop across the lifespan. Furthermore, women do not need to see themselves as feminists to benefit from understanding some of their developmental challenges through feminist scholarship and through a feminist therapeutic lens. The developmental challenges don't change, although the desired outcomes will vary with each individual.

The authors of this chapter are both female and feminists. One is Lutheran, one Catholic. One is twenty-something, one is fifty-something. One has parents who wished she were a boy. One has parents who wish she'd have more children than she wants. Both have careers, husbands, gardens, advanced degrees, and body insecurities. Both have faced struggles around when/if to bear children. We have lived and will continue to live the developmental challenges faced by women that are discussed in this chapter. We hope the discussion serves as both a source of information and an invitation to reflection for practicing and developing mental health professionals. Our intention is to help increase both awareness *and* sensitivity to the unique developmental challenges faced by women across the lifespan.

## Feminist Theoretical Overview

This chapter explores dimensions of female identity development through a feminist theoretical lens. As you know, the theories presented in this book are each situated in a particular context. By context, we mean such influential factors as the time and place in which the theory first came into being, and the background, training, and politics of the theorists. Patricia H. Miller (2002) points out:

> When a person develops or adopts a particular theory, she takes on a whole set of beliefs concerning what questions about development are worth asking, what methods for studying these questions are legitimate, and what the nature of development is. . . . There are unwritten rules of the game that are very much a part of the theory as it is practiced. (p. 5)

By definition, human development theories make claims about what it means to be human and what dimensions of being human are worthy of note. Since the early 1960s, feminists in many academic fields, including counseling, theology, philosophy, medicine, and psychology have maintained a steady stream of research and analysis pointing to the constriction of theory resulting from a nearly exclusive male, White, Western European version of normative human development. The costs of this constriction can hardly be overestimated. Women and people from other racial or cultural backgrounds have been pathologized, ignored, exploited, urged back into destructive relationships, shamed, lied to, and sometimes, abandoned in their confusion and need simply because their developmental trajectory did not match the dictates of the normative model. Feminist theory has much in common with multicultural theory, but feminists tend to examine the role of power more directly, and feminist inquiry always attempts to understand and include the often-forgotten worldview and experiences of women within any given culture.

Feminist *theory* is more aptly referred to as feminist *theories*. Feminism is by no means a monolithic philosophy, nor a single political stance (Murray, 2001; Sommers-Flanagan & Sommers-Flanagan, 2004).

Different theoretical perspectives undergird the kinds of inquiry feminists undertake, and thus the kinds of data found. Wilkinson (2001) discusses three key theoretical perspectives (feminist positivist empiricism, feminist experiential research, and feminist social construction) and helps the reader understand how both the research perspective *and* the feminist dimension help inform the acquisition of knowledge and the formation of theory.

Obviously, feminist theories as they relate to male and female human development vary according to the method of inquiry and the assumptions in question. For the purposes of this chapter, however, it is comforting to acknowledge that while there is great variation in feminist theory, there is also common ground. Below, we offer four basic tenets of feminism with which we believe virtually all feminists would agree:

1. Feminists believe that all humans are of equal value, deserving of fair and equitable life opportunities throughout the lifespan, regardless of sex, race, culture, socioeconomic status, and/or sexual orientation (Funkerburk & Fukuyama, 2001).
2. Whereas most humans are born with unambiguous anatomical features that cause them to be designated as male or female, this designation is not biologically deterministic for most other human behaviors, skills, abilities, inclinations, or desires (Fausto-Sterling, 2000; Zucker, 2001).
3. Human cultures have developed rules and guidelines for defining gendered (masculine or feminine) behaviors. These rules are fluid and vary from culture to culture, sometimes contradicting each other (Athanasiadou, 1997; Sparks & Park, 2002; Tuana, 1992).
4. Throughout both recorded histories and within current lived experiences in human cultures, the human male has been favored as normative, dominant, and often, the sex preferred by expecting parents (McMullin & Cairney, 2004; Sommers-Flanagan & Sommers-Flanagan, 2004).

Each of these tenets alone has profound implications for human development, but taken together, they provide a compelling case for including a feminist critique of each of the dominant theories of human development, which unfortunately, is not the mission of this chapter! However, also taken together, they provide you with an understanding of the foundational assumptions underlying this chapter.

TABLE 8.1   An Overview of Lifespan Developmental
Issues Affecting Women

| Factors | Feminist Issue | Potential Developmental Implications for Women |
|---|---|---|
| **Sex at birth** | Males are preferred; parents are disappointed if they bear a female child | Conscious and unconscious energy  devoted to parental disappointment<br>Difficulty accepting and enjoying being female |
| **Attachment patterns with caretakers** | Mother is the primary caretaker for young children | Mothers deemed as the source of pathology; absence of father or social structures are ignored<br>Women cope with the devaluation of the feminine due to the need for a male to differentiate from the mother and in essence, oppose all things female |
| **Gender-role acquisition** | Children learn rigid gender roles at an early age | Women are discouraged from expressing "masculine" behaviors and identity<br>Women are encouraged to express "feminine" behaviors and identity |
| **Choices about achievement** | Educational and professional achievement and competition associated with masculinity | Discomfort with competition, managerial styles, and achievement-related attitudes and behaviors<br>Earlier generations of women discouraged from seeking education<br>Downplay intelligence/strengths to preserve femininity |
| **Spiritual or religious identity** | God is referred to as male in many religions, carrying gendered messages for behavior and status of women | Women cope with substandard place given religiously/ spiritually<br>Encouraged to stay in destructive relationships or bear unwanted children due to rigid doctrinal stances |

| | | |
|---|---|---|
| **The arrival of menstruation, breasts, and thighs** | Media norms are tall, thin, prepubescent-looking women, with the exception of large breasts | Thinness becomes an obsession<br>Women experience depression and eating disorders more than men<br>Women associate negative meanings and receive stifled education surrounding menarche |
| **Romantic and social relationships** | Beautiful, preened women favored<br><br>Men's violence against women widespread | Women endure competition with other women based on desirability<br>Mental, emotional, and physical harm to women |
| **Career, reproduction, and family roles** | Rigid societal roles rooted in a patriarchal system | Unresolved issues surrounding personal choices<br>Experience discrimination for unpopular choices |
| **Midlife and aging** | Societal preference for young women | Devaluation of aging mental and physical self |

## Clinically Relevant Aspects of Feminist Theory

In order to address women's development across the lifespan, it is essential that we identify some of the major attributes and milestones that are particularly salient to and influenced by one's gender. Therefore, we offer a nonexhaustive list—the same used in Table 8.1—to help guide our consideration of gender-influenced aspects of the development of a woman's identity:

- Sex at birth
- Attachment patterns with caretakers
- Gender-role acquisition
- Choices about achievement
- Spiritual or religious identity
- The arrival of menstruation, breasts, and thighs
- Romantic and social relationships
- Career, reproduction, and family roles
- Midlife and aging

No woman reading this chapter will be without significant life experiences in each of the categories named above. We would like to encourage readers to take time to think about their own struggles and triumphs in these domains, or their fears about those yet to come. Perhaps more than other theoretical orientations, feminists believe our own subjective experiences are welcome and important as we strive to understand the developmental challenges and needs of our clients. As counselors, we are not the objective expert, but rather a guide, chosen by the client, to help enable the client to heal, gain insight, or achieve her/his goals.

These nine aspects are listed in roughly the chronological order in which they might first appear in a woman's life in our current culture. Of interest clinically is the fact that once these aspects have appeared and begin to exert developmental influence, they never conclude or completely go away. What woman among us not only remembers the mixed emotions associated with breast development and pubic hair, but also occasionally revisits some form of those emotions? For a compelling first-person account, read the chapter "Fighting Fire" in Judy Blunt's (2002) powerful memoir, *Breaking Clean*. What follows are brief descriptions of how both sex and gender enters into these developmental dimensions from a feminist perspective.

## Sex at Birth

> A female embryo, then, is the result of a lack or an incapacity, a deviation from the proper form.
>
>                    — (Artistotle as quoted in Tuana, 1992, p. 25)

The vast majority of women are born identifiably female and chose to stay that way throughout their lives. However, we would be remiss if we didn't note that there are a significant number of humans born with unusual and less defined physical, genetic, and hormonal features, some of whom adopt a gender identity of female, and some of whom do not (Berenbaum, 1999; Zucker, 2001). In addition, there are women who choose to become female using surgical and/or hormonal interventions. The psychological impact of being born or developing in a way that violates the "rules" for being male or female can hardly be overstated. The Pulitzer Prize winning novel, *Middlesex*, by Jeffery Eugenides, explores these themes in great depth.

Even for those who are born unambiguously female, there might still be a psychological price. For both social and economic reasons, the majority of first-time parents in our culture (Markle & Nam, 1982) and in many others, prefer to have a boy (Mazurana & McKay, 2001). In some cultures, this preference is so pronounced that female fetuses are aborted because they are female. In fact, social scientists in some countries are becoming alarmed at the skewed population demographics resulting from this practice, and one can hardly imagine a more telling enactment of male as normative and preferred (United Nations, 1996). In the United States, data are not available regarding sex-based selective abortions, but the impact of male baby preference is psychologically costly. If you happen to be born a female under those conditions, you may spend significant conscious or unconscious energy compensating for this parental disappointment, and fully accepting and enjoying the sex you were born may be a lifelong task.

## Attachment Patterns with Caretakers

> Understand: I am my mother's
> novel daughter: I
> have my duty to perform.
> — (Piercy, 1980, p. 43)

Many psychoanalytically oriented feminists have explored the ramifications of mothers being the primary or only caretaker for infants and young children (Chodorow, 1989). As an aside, we should note that mothers have long been accused of being the source of their children's pathologies or developmental struggles, while the absence of fathers and necessary social support continues to be largely ignored. We will cover more on this when we address reproduction, parenting, and family roles. Theorists believe females attach differently to their mothers (the usual primary caretaker) than do males. Put simply, toddler girls come to realize that they are the same sex as mommy, and began to identify as such (Chodorow, 1989). They have a same-sex role model close at hand. As the quote beginning this section, daughters see their future "duties" enacted by their mothers from birth on. Boy toddlers come to realize they are different than mommy, and thus their gendered developmental task is to be different than mommy. If they have no immediate same-sex role models, this leads to a shallow identification with males in the media, literature, or video games, and a developmental strategy that opposes all things "female."

Of course, attachment is far more multifactoral and complex than this (Mackay, 2003; Turnbull, 1997). However, it seems clear that the sex of our caretakers and close family members and the quality of our relationships with them play a role in the ways we develop our own gender and sexual identities.

## Gender-Role Acquisition

> Sugar and spice, and everything nice
> That's what little girls are made of.
> — (Traditional)

Theorists suggest that after birth, humans gradually realize they are no longer attached to their mother's umbilical cord, and are therefore separate beings (Mahler & Pine, 1975). Further, researchers and theorists suggest that the second identity-shaping realization that humans have is that of their biological sex. As early as eighteen months, toddlers can indicate if they are a boy or a girl. Soon after, they begin to attend to what their cultures tell them is "right behavior" for persons of their sex. Authenticity is a concept very relevant in women's development. In our experience, the origin of not being able to find one's own voice begins with "right behavior" or behavior intended to please and pacify others rather than behavior coming from a desire to grow and to express one's authentic self and gifts. One developmental implication for women that is common in the literature is the idea of finding one's own true voice. This challenge originates from stifling the direct and genuine expression of one's ideas and feelings in order to please others and keep the peace.

Most of you can think of examples of these cultural messages. Not long ago, I (RSF) was standing in line at an ice cream shop. In front of me was a little girl, not more than three years old, in a taffeta gown, perhaps acquired by being someone's flower girl. She was drawing a great deal of admiration for her fancy dress, pretty hair, and engaging giggle. Ahead of her, a boy about her age was dragging his baseball bat along, in full uniform. The comments he received had to do with performance and play. "Hey, slugger. Hit any home runs?" No one mentioned his pretty eyes, complimented him on his calm demeanor, nor asked him where he'd shopped for his uniform.

Of all the nurture/nature debates, gender is probably the most profound and most complex. How much of being "feminine" or "masculine" is genetically and hormonally determined, and how much is shaped by the environment? In our opinion, these are outdated questions. Both biology and environment make significant and interactive contributions to human potential and behavior. The more relevant question is not "how much?" but rather, as Anastasi (1958) urged so many years ago, "How?" And when we ask "How does our culture shape gendered identities and behaviors?" it's difficult to even begin to count the ways. From the ways our parents handled us as infants, to family expectations, to school, to television, movies, and magazines, to peer pressures—the messages drum a steady, stereotypic beat into our heads, directly and profoundly affecting our gendered behaviors and identity.

## Choices About Achievement

> My own sex, I hope, will excuse me, if I treat them like rational
> creatures, instead of flattering their *fascinating* graces, and view-
> ing them as if they were in a state of perpetual childhood,
> unable to stand alone.
> — (Mary Wollstonecraft as quoted in Mahowald, 1994)

From preschool on, gender plays a role in our choices about achievement. Researchers have shown that boys tend to seek out hierarchically organized group interactions, whereas girls tend to prefer reciprocal, one-on-one interactions (Beneson, 1996). Much later in life, this finding is reflected in comfort with competition, managerial styles (Pines, Dahan-Kaley, & Ronen, 2001), and many other achievement-related attitudes and behaviors.

While still terribly disproportionate globally, educational opportunities are available to both girls and boys in our culture. Though some of your midlife clients may have been told "the only reason young women should go to college is to get their Mrs. degree," most girls today are *not* overtly given this message, but are encouraged to pursue their educations and excel in areas of interest. This does not mean that achievement has become gender neutral. Many of our teenaged female clients complain that "boys don't like smart girls." And they seek to find ways to hide or downplay their achievements in order to preserve their "femininity."

## Spiritual or Religious Identity

> Dear God,
> Are boys better than girls? I know you are one, but try to be fair.
> — (Quoted in Tucker, 1992, p. 97)

In the vast majority of instances, across time, culture, and faith systems, God is referred to as male. In some religions, the maleness of God is literal and unquestioned. In others, it is symbolic, with occasional God metaphors being female. In both dominant religions and many mythologies, women have been saddled with "original sin," and the mistreatment of women and misogynistic practices of all sorts have thus been justified. Many feminist religious scholars have convincingly disputed such rigid stances and interpretations (Meyers, 1988; Ramshaw, 1994; Trible, 1973), but the fact remains that religious beliefs, for girls and women, carry many gendered messages that at least on occasion may contradict their lived experiences.

Clinically, counselors will often find women struggling with religious doctrinal messages interpreted to dictate constricted options or outright psychological or physical harm. These might include staying in abusive relationships or being forced to carry an unwanted pregnancy to term because the doctrine asserts that such is God's will. Feminists from within all major religions object to these narrow, misogynistic interpretations of divine will. For instance, visit the website www.qantara.de for views of Islamic feminists. Regardless of your personal stance, it is likely that many adult female clients will be facing life development issues in these areas. Counselors should not shy away from helping clients explore their faith messages and spiritual beliefs as they evolve in the counseling relationship.

## The Arrival of Menstruation, Breasts, and Thighs

> Girls must go through a physiological process of developing a woman's body, which ushers in their objectification.
> — (Tolman & Brown, 2001, p. 143)

The bodily changes that accompany puberty have long been a source of conflict and shame for females in many dominant cultures. Breast size and shape is a fixation of Western European culture, especially in that large breasts are valued, but the normally corresponding rounded belly and larger thighs and hips are greatly devalued. Menarche is an event that carries many layers of meaning for girls. Unfortunately, research suggests most of these meanings are still negative and constrictive (Ver Halen, 2004).

Besides the symbolic and social meanings associated with menstruation and breast development, pregnancy becomes a possible reality for adolescent girls. Pregnancies generally require the actions of both a male and a female, but as has been true for most of recorded history, it is the female who bears the brunt of an unwanted pregnancy. Besides the obvious physical concerns, there are enormous psychological, social, and practical considerations that have life-changing developmental ramifications (Tolman & Brown, 2001). To further complicate these matters, providing adolescents with accurate sex education remains an ongoing political struggle in our culture.

Body image concerns are becoming a feminist developmental issue at earlier and earlier ages. Prepubertal girls are sexualized in advertising, and thinness can become an obsession for girls as early as fourth grade (Kilbourne, 1999). According to many researchers and the DSM IV, eating disorders are vastly more common in girls and young women than in boys and men (American Psychiatric Association, 2000). Around this same time, for complex reasons still under investigation, depression becomes much more commonly diagnosed in females than in males (Kutcher et al., 2004).

## Romantic and Social Relationships

> Within the hidden culture of aggression, girls fight with body language and relationship instead of fists and knives. In this world, friendship is a weapon, and the sting of a shout pales in comparison to a day of someone's silence.
>
> — (Simmons, 2002, p. 3)

Feminists have pointed out that while men in our culture are driven to acquire material success in order to attract a mate, women are urged to preen themselves, using beauty and "sexiness" to compete with each other for male attention. This sets women up for complicated social relationships. They don't know what they want, so much as they know they want to be wanted (Young-Eisendrath, 1993). Further, women who find they are not attracted to men, but are instead lesbian or perhaps bisexual, have many developmental challenges from childhood on because of the continued heterosexual bias in the culture and widespread homophobia.

In their chapter on gender and relationships, Dion and Dion (2001) cite numerous studies exploring relationship satisfaction. Both men and women indicate a desire for a least some egalitarian qualities in intimate relationships, but young women and same-sex couples tend to endorse this value more strongly. Further, while a majority of couples endorse this value, only a small minority claim that their current relationship is egalitarian. There are likely to be many reasons for this gap, and exploring it could provide fertile ground for counselors working with women who want, but do not have, egalitarian relationships.

While relationship struggles of all sorts and magnitudes will be a dominant clinical theme for women, perhaps the most difficult for counselors to work are those with partner violence. United States Department of Justice reports indicate that on average 1.5 million women are raped or physically assaulted by an intimate partner and over a thousand lose their lives every year (Rennison, 2003). Research shows the many complex and damaging clinical concerns in this area, from crippling self-blame (Fine & Carney, 2001) to denial of personal disadvantage (Crosby, Pulfall, Snyder, O'Connell, & Whalen, 1989). Counselors who work with women who've experienced intimate violence know the road to recovery is long and difficult, requiring significant counseling skill and great patience.

## Career, Reproduction and Family Roles

> Choosing motherhood or refusing it has proven to be much more complicated than the seventies feminism had imagined.
>
> — (Burman, 1995, p. 9)

> Today we have much more extensive data on people like the Aka and the Efe, where infants from birth are passed among multiple caregivers with whom they become very familiar and are quite at ease. Far from growing up less secure, such infants are if anything more so.
>
> — (Hrdy, 1999, p. 495)

Both science and religion regard mating, reproduction, and the rearing of offspring as central to life, and as such, these areas present profound lifespan developmental challenges for human females. The male wish for control over female reproductive choices has a long, long history, the account of which would fill volumes of scholarly books. Feminists believe that women should have the final say over whether and/or when they use their bodies to produce offspring.

Further, as humans bearing the vulnerable and care-intensive next generation, women need appropriate levels of assistance from the "tribe" or collective society. This support could come in many forms:

- an economy that allows them to care directly for the infant full time,
- a society that provides such possibilities to fathers,
- employment conditions that enable both parents to provide quality direct care, or
- high-quality group or individual caretakers that allow parents to pursue vocational interests without causing the infant any developmental delays or losses.

The world of work itself is fraught with concerns for feminists, from lower wages for women doing the same work to denied advancement based on overt or hidden gender-based criteria. Complicating these difficulties are assumptions about infant needs, attachment, and parenting roles. While there is no evidence that men are unsuited to care for infants (Silverstein, 1996), many attachment theorists, researchers, and writers seem to take a biased, guilt-inducing stance that mothers must be the primary, or stay-at-home, parent to ensure a psychologically healthy child.

Needless to say, midlife women clients will have many concerns, and possibly unresolved issues, surrounding choices they've made about education, employment, and having and raising children. Feminist theorists locate the source of the damage and struggle in the patriarchal and misogynistic messages in our culture, rather than "pathology" in the women.

## Midlife and Aging

> The old gray mare, she ain't what she used to be, many long
> years ago.
> — lines from an old country-western ditty

Consistent with society's emphasis on females as sexual objects and baby-machines, aging can be especially hard on women (Chrisler, 2001). Menopause is the conclusion of child-bearing potential, and can carry many messages of outlived usefulness for women. Very few *Playboy*-type magazines focus on the sexiness of gray hair, wrinkles, sagging breasts and buttocks, or creaky joints. However, feminists reject these narrow definitions of female identity and value, and like Joan Erikson (wife, and co-theorist with Erik Erikson) identify great meaning and value in the final stages of life, whether male or female (Erickson & Davidson, 1995).

# Clinical Cases

Here we provide two cases from the clinical work of the first author. These cases illustrate the importance of lifespan considerations in working with women from a feminist theoretical perspective. We hasten to add that male clients could easily benefit from a feminist orientation as well. The first case example details a year-long women's therapy group. The second is an account of working with a young victim of abduction and rape.

## A Women's Therapy Group

For over a year, I (RSF) had the privilege of leading a women's therapy group. The five members ranged in age from forty-two to fifty-six, and all were struggling with midlife identity, relationships, career choices and changes, and aging. The backgrounds of the members varied a great deal, but the work they accomplished was remarkable. The following descriptions have been altered to protect the identities of the women, but their concerns and life stories are highly representative of midlife women's developmental issues.

Georgia was a forty-two-year-old English instructor at a community college. Her husband, Gil, had recently been killed in a motorcycle accident, leaving Georgia with two preteens, many debts, and a deep, bitter grief.

Millie, a forty-eight-year-old half-Kootenai, half-Irish woman was a stay-at-home mom. She had married at age eighteen, and was a very active member in her Mormon church. Her husband and she fought constantly, and she was questioning how long she could stay in the marriage, even though her religion and values were strongly against divorce. The couple only had one child, much to their disappointment.

Candace was a fifty-six-year-old woman whose second husband, Ben, had left her abruptly for a woman twenty-three years younger than he. She was reeling from this loss, drinking "more than I should be," and torturing herself with questions of why he did this.

Linda was a fifty-year-old Latina woman with a grown daughter and a teen-aged daughter, divorced for seven years. The girls' father had moved away, and did not send child support for the daughter still at home. Linda struggled with finances and with her relationship with her daughter.

Sarah was a fifty-two-year-old school nurse. She had originally come to therapy because she had been caught stealing things from a local grocery store. After working for three months in individual therapy, she decided she wanted to continue her work in group. She was strug-gling with depression and had mild suicidal ideation. Her estranged husband had been diagnosed with cancer, which limited the time he could spend with their two teen-aged children.

The group met weekly for two hours. As part of the treatment model, I kept notes in essay form that I mailed to the women during the middle of each week, thus highlighting the issues, and providing an exten-sion of the sense of community. From these notes, all fifty-five of them, I offer the following quotes and synopses of themes that emerged and reemerged in our work together. You will see a direct connection between the concerns and challenges facing these women, and the top-ics of feminist theoretical concern listed in the first part of this chapter. In fact, it might be interesting for you to take the list of milestones (repeated for your convenience) and check off how many times you encounter each topic in the group members' accounts below.

- Sex at birth
- Attachment patterns with caretakers
- Gender-role acquisition
- Choices about achievement
- Spiritual or religious identity
- The arrival of menstruation, breasts, and thighs
- Romantic and social relationships
- Career, reproduction, and family roles
- Midlife and aging

Early in our meetings, the topic of our own worth in the world came up. From feminist theory, we know that women have been devalued, objectified, and had their worth narrowly defined in relationship to pleasing or serving men. Here's the essence of an exchange addressing this deep, human concern:

*Millie:* "I don't trust anyone who says they love me. What are they wanting from me? I'm pretty sure I never quite measure up. He makes it pretty clear that I'm not as important as his friends, but he wants me around, to cook, and of course, for sex. But he seems to like men better for what I'd call a real relationship. Same with my dad. He related to my brothers like humans, but to me, like I was some kind of burden or something."

*Linda:* "When I was with Bill, I never knew if he knew who I was. Sometimes, he even made jokes that I was a life-support system for a nice pussy."

*Georgia:* "Wow. That's ugly. I can't remember it being that bad with Gil, really. But the kids don't seem to think of me as human. I'm just the go-fer, chauffer, bottle washer, cook, and laundry queen. And I can't keep up, and I find myself wishing I had a mom who could take care of *me* instead of me being everything to everyone."

The group members nodded knowingly, and the room was filled with a kind of sad silence. Glances around the room gradually led to eye-contact among members, which led to one member quietly saying, "Maybe we can sort of be each other's moms in here." The warmth only increased when Millie quipped, "Yeah, well that might be okay, but my church doesn't believe in that rebirthing stuff."

A summary paragraphs from one of these early groups said:

> We meditated on the ways we have been treating ourselves with regard to this concept of love. We cannot know if others are loving us in healthy ways if we are not loving ourselves first. If, in fact, we love ourselves, why do we tolerate others treating us unlovingly? Is it loving to tolerate being treated badly? To ourselves? To others? Do we even believe we are worthy of love, from ourselves or others?
>
> We observed the pain involved in having our own goodness used against us, used to control us or put us down. This is the opposite of love. Our chance to grow is retarded or reversed. We remembered the Beetles' song "I used to be cruel to my woman. I kept her from the things she loved." Love is a basic trust. It is not a nonrenewable resource.

The group continued to work on the notions of love and relationship, fighting to overcome what some feminist call the harsh and narrow beauty standards for women, with shared and take-home readings from various feminist poets and commentators.

*Candace:* "One time before he left, Ted looked at me and said, 'God, Candace. You bend over like an old lady.' I'm fifty-six. What's he expect? She's thirty-two and got a nice, tight ass. What can I do, have cosmetic surgery back there?" (Laughter, and then tears)

*Sarah:* "He's afraid. Afraid of aging himself, and dying. And it gets put on you—but only when they're basically healthy themselves.

When Glen was diagnosed with cancer, he did this amazing reversal. When it gets real, the young chicks don't look so good. Now he's looking for a full-time nurse, and I'm not going there. Or at least, I wish I wasn't. God, I feel so damn guilty. The kids need so much, Glen needs so much, the kids at school need so much, and I can't keep it up. I want a normal, adult relationship with a nice, normal man."

*Candace:* "I thought Ted was normal. Or as normal as men get. And look at him. I don't get it. How did I pick him? He's as shallow as, as, as I don't know. Shallow as a mirror."

*Georgia:* "I wonder if we train them to be. Shallow, I mean. Like always worrying about how everyone looks, and talking bad about our own bodies and stuff."

The group members shifted uncomfortably in their chairs, aware of their judgments about themselves and each other on all the shallow domains humans worry about.

Here's an entry from about this time in group:

> We talked about old habits of picking "defective" people to be intimate with. It is easier to try and be a hero (the perfect lover, or mother, or whatever) and love someone into maturity, than to try and be with someone who is basically healthy, and therefore might see OUR faults and imperfections. Intimacy is not safe or easy. Perhaps we have picked intimate others who are in fact not capable of true intimacy because we can blame them for the lack, rather than explore our part in it all. If an adult relationship is healthy, nurturing has to be a two-way street. Regression, play, exchange of control, holding, caring, crying, needing, listening, being tough, developing—all essential, and in relationship, they need to be roughly equal.

Taking up space is a figurative and literal feminist issue for women in our culture. This issue came up as one woman came to group stating she'd been worried all week about how much time she had taken up the week before.

*Sarah:* "I have to check in on this. I felt horrible all week because I think I talked too much last week. I'm sorry." (She is near tears.)

*Georgia:* "Sarah, you needed that time. We were worried about you." (Others nod.)

*Sarah:* "No, I didn't need that much time. I open my big fat mouth, which matches my big fat thighs, and I just don't have control. So I try not to talk at all. What's with me? Why can't a little be enough?"

The group worked hard to both reassure Sarah and to explore what it meant to share the time in group in ways that felt fair. I noted that this was a very exciting sign of group maturity—the women were daring to ask questions about their impact on each other in the here-and-now, which takes a lot of trust and courage. Mutuality in relationships is a central feminist value. We talked about the give and take necessary in relationships.

*Linda:* "I don't regret the giving I have done. I regret not getting anything back, and not seeing how much that hurt me. This group is something different for me. I feel like I can listen, and give like that, and I can talk, and give ideas, and get ideas. And feel like there's some kind of balance."

The group talked about our responsibility to care for ourselves and how confusing, exhausting, and disappointing that can be. We covered the practical things like getting the right therapy, the right attorney, and budgeting, and the deeper, more painful things.

*Linda:* "When I shouted 'Why don't you love me?' and he didn't even answer, how come I stayed on anyway?"

*Sarah:* "I know I stayed too long out of fear of being along, but now that I'm basically alone, I am afraid of trying again."

The decisions surrounding whether to stay in a less-than-healthy relationship are always complex, but in midlife, the added dimensions of aging and limited chances for anything better come into play. Counseling can often help women explore societal messages about what to expect in a relationship and what it means to be alone. Trying again certainly has its risks, as Candace went on to point out.

*Candace:* "Yeah, and you should be. I tried again with Ted, and look where it got me. My first husband left me for a woman who could have babies. Did I tell you all he wrote me and said he's got three grandkids? What a jerk. Like I want to know that right now."

*Millie:* "Candace, did you not want kids, or what?"

*Candace:* "Oh, no. I wanted them. But not right away, and then those first years went by, and we tried. I'd had an abortion in high school. Had to drive to another state to get it. I still blame myself. I still wonder if that's what made me unable to get pregnant. We didn't do any fancy fertility stuff, but I think maybe that's because he'd started having affairs anyway."

Two or three of the women nodded knowingly and we observed how easy it is to blame ourselves when we've been betrayed. "In here," one woman said, "I can see things through all your eyes. It makes me see myself in your eyes, too, and I feel worth something to you, and worth something to myself."

The challenges of raising children were often discussed in group.

*Georgia:* "Gillian is driving me crazy. She'll be twelve in a month, and she wants a midnight curfew, and brand name clothes, and she can push my buttons so fast . . . I wonder if it's guilt. She reminds me of myself at her age, except my dad wasn't dead. I think I could handle it better if I, well, if she wasn't so pushy."

*Millie:* "I wish Jimmy would be a little pushier. He's a fat, unmoving blob in front of the television, and I can't get his father to do a thing about it. Jimmy puts a pillow on each ear when Mark starts yelling, and just shuts down. He has no friends, and hates church. He, well. I hate to admit this, but he embarrasses me. Being fat myself is one thing, but a fat kid . . . that makes it worse."

We talked about how children provide mirrors for us, and how the child within us can do the same. Children will not trade material security for false, tense, destructive relationships. Children seek love and security. They ask, over and over again, "Do you love me?" and "Can I trust you?" They are not fooled by half-answers, and they are not comforted by empty promises. However, they, unlike adults, cannot often remove themselves when the answers are wrong. Is our frozen state related to that somehow? Are we afraid to be adults? And how do we help our kids come out differently? We talked about our wish to be a stay-ahead-of-the-storm kind of parent, and the impossibility of that sometimes. We talked of needing to help our kids learn to be assertive, not aggressive. We all learned to be submissive, and to hold back, even to the point of self-destruction. Now, we are learning self-care and assertiveness as a second language. Many of our kids seem

to be learning the opposite—we noted the quote from Salvador
Minuchin, "It is a sad and dangerous society that promotes individualism, greed, and isolation while modeling violence and aggression
for its youth."

As group continued, and the sense of community deepened, I wrote
the following paragraph as part of the summary for week thirteen.

> Why do we struggle with intimacy, authenticity, and vulnerabil-
> ity? Because it is the very center of human development. As S. said,
> "If being a mature, balanced woman were easy, there'd be a whole
> bunch of fantastic people walking around out there." We talked
> about the group's purpose for each of us. For some, it is to move
> beyond words into the experience of self. For some, it is to dare to
> put real words on what has been too frightening to speak. For all
> of us, it is a place to struggle to become more integrated, evolved,
> and whole. As C. said, "This group is a place where, if I decide I
> want to, I can let people know about me." It is also a place where
> we can peer inside, and let ourselves know what's in there. The only
> expectation is this: that we come to offer and receive deep encour-
> agement on our journey, to listen for and honor the wise voices
> within ourselves and each other. The group is like the clichéd onion.
> We go deeper as the layers are removed, and sometimes, we cry.

Of all the emotions the group experienced and discussed, predictably,
anger was the hardest.

*Linda:* "Civilized women don't know how to get angry. They don't
speak it. They hold it together, no matter what. People say, 'Oh,
that Linda, she holds it together.' No matter what kind of shit is
coming down. I hold myself together, tight, but sometimes, I think
I'm going to blow the lid right off. There's a volcano in there,
somewhere."

*Sarah:* "What about in group? Could you let it blow in here? I asked
myself that last week, when Millie was saying how she went to talk
to that elder at church."

*Linda:* "Yeah. No. I don't know. I feel like we let things rip in here,
but only at other people, not each other."

*Millie:* "So, Sarah, you were angry at me? For what?"

*Sarah:* "For listening to those f— fools. It's like you're a trapped bird,
or something. And I want you to be free. I'm sorry, but I just don't

believe God isn't some kind of big Daddy with some kind of cosmic silent wife and spirit babies. I think we are all like God, if there is a God. Doesn't it say that somewhere, about male and female both being in God's image?"

The group surrounded Sarah and Millie, caring, but open to exploring how it felt to have someone angry, and to notice where the anger came from, and how it hit us all. The women realized, again, how much the group had come to mean, and how hard intimate relationships of any kind are.

The group met for a total of fifty-five sessions before collectively deciding it was time to "graduate." We covered wide-ranging topics, including addictions, forgiveness, sexual concerns, caring for older parents, caring for grandchildren, body image, grief, rejection because we were aging, and fear associated with such losses. It was a very gratifying experience as a therapist. My own life concerns and fears were often mirrored in the themes we addressed, and I was often challenged to grow and develop right along side these courageous women. While there is no way to report even a fraction of the amazing insights these women had and connections they made to each other, we hope the excerpts provide you with insights about how these themes play out in women's midlife development.

As feminist theory would predict, midlife enlightenment, or consciousness-raising, has a profound developmental effect for women who have the chance to glimpse the role culture has played in their identities. These women no longer apologized for being born female, for having "imperfect" bodies, for being unable to meet everyone's needs, for smelling like, walking like, throwing like, laughing like, or being a "girl." They had resolved to face being alone, or being in relationships, in ways that kept their core identity intact. They had come to care about each other very deeply, and experienced healing from the scars inflicted by culturally endorsed female-to-female jealousy, cruelty, and suspicion.

## A Young Teenage Victim of Rape

One day, many years ago, a call came into my (RSF) small, part-time private practice, from a teacher at one of our local high schools. She asked if I would see a fourteen-year-old rape victim who was having a terrible time in school. There was a small crime victim's fund that would pay a modest fee, but the family had no health insurance and very limited resources. Although I didn't need any more clients, and I already had a number of low-to-no fee clients, I sighed and agreed. As anyone whose professional development has included becoming a feminist counselor knows, the referring community quickly becomes aware of how to get a feminist to accept a client. Because this is not a text on professional development, we won't go into a lengthy explanation. Suffice it to say, suffering rape victims are difficult for feminist counselors to turn away.

Tabitha swung her long blond hair over her shoulders, keeping one strand to chew on as she filled out intake forms and went over my informed consent form with me.

**Tabitha:** "So, if I told you I feel like killing myself or tracking down those bastards and shooting them, you'd tell the cops?" *(Tabitha was reading the section listing reasons mental health professionals might need to break confidentiality. Of course, this is especially clinically relevant to someone who has been violated by rape—and it needs careful, caring discussion. Tabitha's normal adolescent need for privacy and self-determination had been mangled by being raped. She needed to feel safe above all. Only in a very safe environment will she be able to talk about the rage, helplessness, violent urges, flash-backs, and other rape sequelia.)*

**Rita:** "Nope. Sounds like we've got plenty to talk about, though. What that statement means is that counselors like me need to listen really, really carefully. We need to help people stay safe and alive. It seems pretty normal that you might feel like killing yourself or killing those creeps sometimes. And it's just fine to talk about that as much as you want. I don't need to tell anyone. BUT if I decide that you're telling me in a way that makes me worried that you might actually do it, then I would work with you on a plan to stay safe and to keep out of trouble. And that could involve other people if I thought that was what was needed. The whole idea is to keep you safe. Does that make sense?"

**T:** "Yeah. But who would you tell?"

**R:** "Tabitha, the first person I would tell is you. If I'm worried to the point of needing to break our confidentiality, I'll tell you first. Deal?"

**T:** "Okay. What about my mom?"

**R:** "What about her?" *(In counseling with young women, I often find a need to involve their mothers or older sisters. Remember, feminist developmental theory posits that the culture pits women against each other, isolating and doing great damage in the process. Female family members are no exception. Sometimes, mature feminist development is enhanced by forgiving and/or making peace with other women in the family.)*

**T:** "Like, are you going to tell her everything?"

*R:* "Nope, again. In a few minutes, we'll have her come in and I'll explain this to both of you, but basically, most parents are fine with not being told everything. On the other hand, sometimes, it's nice to have your mom know a few things about how it's going. You and I can decide together about that, if it's okay with your mom, and if that's okay with you."

The abduction, which included multiple sexual assaults, had taken place a month before Tabitha came to see me. She had been walking home after school when a car pulled along side and asked if she wanted a ride. In the car were two nice-looking men in their early twenties. She accepted the ride, and the beer they offered. Eighteen hours later, she was allowed to jump out of the moving car onto a lawn near her home. Both men, who we'll call Frank and Jake, had raped and molested Tabitha many times throughout the ordeal.

Adolescent development from any theoretical perspective takes into account the impact of hormones, body changes, and the rapid development of sexual personhood. Feminist developmental theorists are especially aware of the impact of cultural mixed messages to the female adolescent. She is given many messages about her worth being directly connected to stereotypic sexually desirable features, such as large, shapely breasts, and a long, thin body. Any adolescent female in our culture will struggle with her body image. A raped adolescent will have this struggle intensified enormously. About three months into our work together, Tabitha told me the following:

*Tabitha:* "I hate my body. It isn't fair that I got Granny's shape. You've seen Mom's boobs. They're big. I'm totally flat."

*Rita:* "Yeah, bodies are hard to love sometimes. I'm wondering what made you think of that. I mean, we were just talking about how drunk Frank and Jake were."

*T:* "I know, but that's the thing. They were making fun of me. He had me on the bed and was saying to Jake how he couldn't find my boobs cuz they were so little."

*R:* (feeling a need to kill these guys myself) "Yeah, that's pretty awful. Seems like they wanted to hurt you about every way they could. Too bad their meanness seeped in, and now you have to learn how to like your body again in about a million ways."

*T:* "Yeah. I guess. I've got short legs, too. Do you think my boyfriend could come in with me sometime? He thinks it's cool that I have a shrink."

*R:* "I think we could talk about that. Tell me how that came to mind."

*T:* "Well, it's the body thing. Maybe you could talk to him about it."

*R:* "Pretty hard to be dating, and have feelings for someone, and have your body image be kind of shook up, huh?"

*T:* "Yeah, but he's helping in a way. He says nice things."

*R:* "What are you saying to yourself? I mean, it's nice to have a guy say nice things, but you never know what they're saying it for, really. I wonder if you could find some nice things to say to yourself? Let's get out this mirror, and see what nice things you could say to yourself?"

*T:* (laughing) "What, you want me to make some lezzy talk? Like, 'Oh, Tabitha, what nice blue eyes you have. Oh, Tabitha, what cute short legs you have. Will you go to bed with me?'"

*R:* "That's sort of what I meant, but isn't it weird how our body, and body comments like that are kind of related to sex? Like, what if we just focused on all the cool stuff about your body, but without relating it to sex?"

My work with Tabitha extended over seven years. Of course, it wasn't seven years of weekly contact. At first, we had frequent sessions— sometimes even twice a week. As time went on, the need for contact varied with legal proceedings, life developmental stages, family crises, and so on. As a feminist therapist, I sat with her in the incredible pain of being raped, forced to testify, and ultimately, deal with the fact that neither man was convicted. I also worked (gently and over time) to help her see the various cultural forces and patterns that stood in the way of her healing and development.

Feminist developmental theory asserts that adolescent females are capable of developing intellectual, social, and physical self-sufficiency. However, many aspects of our violent, hyper-sexualized culture, driven by incessant media images, work against the attainment of this independence. In addition, sexual harassment, predatory male attention, and humiliation by teachers, coaches, and parents for "female" behaviors, bodies, or struggles add to the damage. Feminist therapists working with adolescent females must work patiently, accepting the length and challenges of the road to true feminist individuation.

## Summary

Feminist theory of women's development begins with the foundational assumption that female developmental needs share vast common ground

## IMPORTANT FOREMOTHERS

### About Jean Baker Miller

Jean Baker Miller, M.D. is a major contributor to the body of knowledge aimed toward deepening an understanding of women's development among the general public. Her most notable work is *Toward a New Psychology of Women* (1976). Miller's book became a bestseller by succinctly suggesting the psychological consequences of male dominance for women and by positing new ways of envisioning the future for women. She begins by saying, "Humanity has been held to a limited and distorted view of itself—from its interpretation of the most intimate of personal emotions to its grandest vision of human possibilities—precisely by virtue of its subordination of women" (p. 1). To Miller, "dependency" of women, often perceived pathologically, is replaced with "relational ability." Dr. Miller expands a definition of women's development by writing, "women stay with, build on and develop in a context of connections with others" (p. 83). She recognizes the unrecognized strengths of women in making connections and empowering the development of others in a relational context. Dr. Miller also suggests the tasks upon which a model for women can be built: by maintaining ties with one another, becoming oneself, claiming the economic and political power to enhance unbalanced societal institutions, and reclaiming conflict. Further, Jean Baker Miller posits that daughters often fail to recognize the positive attributes of mothers by assuming the dominant culture's judgment of women. Dr. Miller's continues to broaden an understanding of women's development by emphasizing a relational model of women's development, by giving the world a rational view of women, and by creating places to support women's development such as the Jean Baker Miller Training Institute.

### About Carol Gilligan

Carol Gilligan, Ph.D., also jumpstarted a revolution among the general public when she wrote the book *In a Different Voice* (1977). While many feminists insist that there are no differences between males and females, Gilligan asserted that women have differing moral and psychological tendencies than men that should be valued equally by Western society. Carol Gilligan taught along-side Erik Erikson and became a research assistant for Lawrence Kohlberg. Gilligan went on to challenge Kohlberg's work on moral development, emphasizing a feminine ethic of care in contrast to a masculine ethic of justice.

> As we have listened for centuries to the voices of men and the theories of development that their experience informs, so we have come more recently to notice not only the silence of women but the difficulty in hearing what they say when they speak. Yet in the different voice of women lies the truth of an ethic of care, the tie between relationship and responsibility, and the origins of aggression in the failure of connection. (1977, p. 173)

Gilligan also speaks to differing senses of self among women and men. When asked, "How would you describe yourself?" women often fuse their identity with intimacy, referencing themselves as daughter, mother, lover, or friend. In contrast, men will more often reference themselves as "I" or separation. This difference is supported by fairy tales as well. Successful men go off to foreign lands alone to slay dragons while successful women find the perfect mate. The result is an adult population of men who see themselves as separate and of women who see themselves as connected. Gilligan is known for challenging theories of development that were developed by and based on men. She, like Jean Baker Miller, emphasizes a relational orientation in women's development.

with male developmental needs. However, in most if not all cultures, females are devalued, limited, and narrowly defined in relationship to male prerogative and need. This less-than-male status has serious psychological implications for the developing female human, beginning at birth and continuing through old age. In addition, throughout life, women face the physical perils of possible sexual assault, unwanted pregnancies, and partner violence.

Practicing professional counselors who work with women will find their caseloads filled with women grappling with the many demanding dimensions of being female in our culture. Adolescents will be struggling with issues of attractiveness, body image, relationship confusion, conflicting messages about achievement, and the pain of being taught to compete with each other for male attention. Young adult women will struggle with choices related to relationships, careers, childbearing, and the messages of the culture about having it all, being it all, and pleasing men in the meantime. Midlife women will be reflecting back on the outcomes of the decisions just mentioned, juggling family demands, partner demands, aging parental demands, and body and hormone changes, and wondering if they should save money for plastic surgery.

Perhaps we can hope that in times to come, elderly women will have a sense of completion and generativity as they move through the golden years with wisdom and grace. At present, it is more likely that those seeking counseling will be doing so out of a sense of loneliness or frustration with the demands of an aging spouse and adult children who still seek to have their mother meet their needs. Counselors should remember: it's never too late for consciousness raising. It's never too late to encourage women to see themselves as whole human beings, deserving of equal opportunities for work and pleasure, and deserving of respect from themselves, family members, and society at large.

## Annotated Bibliography

Rhonda K. Unger (Ed.). 2001. *The handbook of the psychology of women and gender*. New York: Wiley.
    Forty-seven distinguished contributors wrote the twenty-seven chapters in this handbook. The book provides historical perspectives, details developmental issues, and addresses social roles and systems that impact the physical and mental health of women. It is especially helpful in delineating gender as a powerful culturally determined concept.

## References

American Psychiatric Association. (2000). *Diagnostic and statistical manual of mental disorders* (IV-TR ed.). Washington, DC: Author.

Anastasi, A. (1958). Heredity, environment, and the question "How?" *Psychological Review, 65,* 197–208.

Athanasiadou, C. (1997). Postgraduate women talk about family and career: The discursive reproduction of gender difference. *Feminism & Psychology, 7*(3), 321–327.

Beneson, J. F. (1996). Gender differences in the development of relationships. In Gil Noam & K. W. Fischer (Eds.), *Development and vulnerability in close relationships* (pp. 263–286). Hillsdale, NJ: Erlbaum.

Berenbaum, S. A. (1999). Effects of early androgens on sex-typed activities and interests in adolescents with congenital adrenal hyperplasia. *Hormones and Behavior, 35*, 102–110.

Blunt, J. (2002). *Breaking clean.* New York: Knopf.

Burman, E. (1995). The abnormal distribution of development: Policies for Southern women and children. *Gender, Place and Culture, 2*, 21–36.

Chodorow, N. J. (1989). *Feminism and psychoanalytic theory.* New Haven: Yale University Press.

Chrisler, J. (2001). Gendered bodies and physical health. In R. K. Under (Ed.), *Handbook of the psychology of women and gender* (pp. 289–302). New York: Wiley.

Crosby, F. J., Pulfall, A., Snyder, R. C., O'Connell, M., & Whalen, P. (1989). The denial of personal disadvantage among you, me, and all the other ostriches. In M. Crawford & M. Gentry (Eds.), *Gender and thought* (pp. 79–99). New York: Springer-Verlag.

Dion, K., & Dion, K. (2001). Gender and relationship. In R. K. Unger (Ed.), *Handbook of the psychology of women and gender* (pp. 256–271). New York: Wiley.

Erikson, J. M., & Davidson, J. (1995). *A conversation with Joan Erikson at 92.* Davis, CA: Davidson Films.

Fausto-Sterling, A. (2000). *Sexing the body: Gender politics and the construction of sexuality.* New York: Basic Books.

Fine, M., & Carney, S. (2001). Women, gender and the law: Toward a feminist rethinking of responsibility. In R. K. Unger (Ed.), *Handbook of the psychology of women and gender* (pp. 388–409). New York: Wiley.

Funkerburk, J. R., & Fukuyama, M. A. (2001). Feminism, multiculturalism, and spirituality: Convergent and divergent forces in psychotherapy. *Women & Therapy, 24*(3/4), 1–18.

Gilligan, C. (1977). *In a different voice.* Cambridge, MA: Harvard University Press.

Hrdy, S. B. (1999). *Mother nature.* New York: Pantheon Books.

Kilbourne, J. (1999). *Can't buy my love.* New York: Simon and Schuster.

Kutcher, S., Kusumaker, V., LeBlanc, J., Sabatino, S. A., Lagace, D., & Morehouse, R. (2004). The characteristics of asymptomatic female adolescents at high risk for depression: The baseline assessment from a prospective 8-year study. *Journal of Affective Disorders, 79*(1–3), 177–185.

Mackay, D. E. (2003). The relationship of gender and parental attachment to spiritual maturity. *Dissertation Abstracts International: Section B: The Sciences & Engineering, 64*(4-B), 1908.

Mahler, M. S., Pine, F., &.Bergman, A. (1975). *The psychological birth of the human infant: Symbiosis and individuation.* New York: Basic Books.

Mahowald, M. B. (1994). *Philosophy of woman: An anthology of classic to current concepts.* Indianapolis: Hackett.

Markle, G. E. & Nam, C. B. (1982). Sex predetermination: Its impact on fertility. *Social Biology, 29*(1–2), 168–179.

Mazurana, D. E., & McKay, S. A. (2001). Women, girls, and structural violence: A global analysis. In D. J. Christie, R. V. Wagner, & D. D. Winter (Eds.), *Peace, conflict, and violence* (pp. 130–138). Upper Saddle River, NJ: Prentice-Hall.

McMullin, J. A., & Cairney, J. (2004). Self-esteem and the intersection of age, class, and gender. *Journal of Aging Studies Special Issue: New Directions in Feminist Gerontology, 18*(1), 75–90.

Meyers, C. (1988). *Discovering Eve: Ancient Israelite women in context.* New York: Oxford University Press.

Miller, J. B. (1976). *Toward a new psychology of women.* Boston: Beacon Press.

Miller, P. (2002). *Theories of developmental psychology* (4th ed.). New York: Worth.

Murray, R. T. (2001). *Recent theories of human development.* Thousand Oaks, CA: Sage.

Piercy, M. (1980). *The moon is always female.* New York: Knopf.

Pines, A. M., Dahan-Kaley, H., & Ronen, S. (2001). The influence of feminist self-definition on the democratic attitudes of managers. *Social Behavior & Personality, 29.*

Ramshaw, G. (1994). *God beyond gender: Feminist Christian God-language.* Minneapolis: Fortress.

Rennison, C. M. (2003). Intimate Partner Violence 1993–2001. Retrieved November 11, 2004, from www.ojp.usdoj.gov/bjs

Silverstein, L. B. (1996). Fathering is a feminist issue. *Psychology of Women Quarterly, 20,* 39–54.

Simmons, R. (2002). *Odd girl out.* New York: Harcourt.

Sommers-Flanagan, J., & Sommers-Flanagan, R. (2004). *Counseling and psychotherapy theories in context and practice: Skills, strategies, and techniques.* New York: Wiley.

Sparks, E. E., & Park, A. H. (Eds.). (2002). *The integration of feminism and multiculturalism: Ethical dilemmas at the border.* Washington, DC: American Psychological Association.

Tolman, D. L., & Brown, L. M. (2001). Adolescent girl's voices: Resonating resistance in body and soul. In R. K. Unger (Ed.), *Handbook of the psychology of women and gender* (pp. 133–155). New York: Wiley.

Trible, P. (1973). Depatriarchalizing in Biblical interpretation. *Journal of the American Academy of Religion, 41,* 30–38.

Tuana, N. (1992). *Woman and the history of philosophy.* St. Paul, MN: Paragon House.

Tucker, R. A. (1992). *Women in the maze: Questions and answers on biblical equality.* Downers Grove, IL: InterVarsity Press.

Turnbull, K. C. (1997). Searching for the Oedipus complex: The parental preferences of preschool children. *Dissertation Abstracts International: Section B: The Sciences & Engineering, 58*(6-B), 0419–4217.

United Nations. (1996). Platform for action and the Beijing declaration. New York: United Nations Publications.

Ver Halen, S. M. (2004). The effects of menarcheal and body image changes on public self-consciousness. *Dissertation Abstracts International: Section B: The Sciences & Engineering, 64*(9-B).

Wilkinson, S. (2001). Theoretical perspectives on women and gender. In R. K. Unger (Ed.), *Handbook of the psychology of women and gender* (pp. 17–28). New York: Wiley.

Young-Eisendrath, P. (1993). *You're not what I expected: Breaking the "he said-she said" cycle.* New York: Touchstone.

Zucker, K. J. (2001). Biological influences on psychosexual differentiation. In R. K. Unger (Ed.), *Handbook of the psychology of women and gender* (pp. 101–115). New York: Wiley.

# CHAPTER NINE

# Lesbian Identity Development

## Connie R. Matthews

Counseling research literature has consistently found that lesbians utilize counseling and therapy at fairly high rates. Two of the largest and most representative studies (Bradford, Ryan, & Rothblum, 1994; Sorensen & Roberts, 1997) found that about three quarters of the lesbian respondents had seen a mental health professional at least once in their lives, with many of them having more than one experience with counseling. Other studies (Cochran, Sullivan, & Mays, 2003; Modricin & Wyers, 1990) have found similar results. With such a rate of participation in counseling, it is very likely that most practitioners will see lesbian clients, whether they realize it or not. Unfortunately, counselors are not always prepared to work effectively with lesbian clients, perhaps due to the long-standing ambivalence that counseling and society has about this population.

From the late nineteenth century until 1973, homosexuality was considered a mental illness (Gonsiorek, 1991). This began to change when homosexuality was removed as a classification in the *Diagnostic and Statistical Manual of Mental Disorders (DSM)*. (See the box on Evelyn Hooker for the history of the fight for acceptance within the mental health profession.) Although the process of change involved much political activity within and outside of the American Psychiatric Association (APA), that activity was facilitated by a growing body of empirical evidence, in methodologically sound studies, indicating that gay men and lesbians were no more likely to exhibit mental illness than their heterosexual counterparts (Gonsiorek). Since the changes to the *DSM*, the American Counseling Association (ACA), the APA, and various other mental health associations have passed numerous resolutions recognizing the biases that continue to exist in society and taking positions of affirmation toward working with gay, lesbian, and bisexual clients. Unfortunately, practitioners and training programs have not always kept pace with their professional associations. Rudolph (1988) suggested that this happens because counselors are influenced not only by their professional associations but also by the larger society in which they live. Thus although many counselors want to follow the affirmative approach laid out by the organizations to which they belong, their attitudes and behavior sometimes reflect those of the culture in which they practice. Furthermore, training programs for counselors and other mental health practitioners often fail to adequately prepare them for working affirmatively with gay, lesbian, and bisexual clients.

Studies examining both counselors and training programs have consistently found counselors reporting a lack of preparation for working with lesbian, gay, and bisexual clients and sometimes outright bias in classes or programs (e.g., Buhrke, 1989; Graham, Rawlings, Halpern, & Hermes, 1984; Phillips & Fischer, 1998; Pilkington & Cantor, 1996). Conversely, there is growing evidence to suggest that when an effort is made to provide affirmative training, counselors do show growth in their attitudes, knowledge, and/or skills (e.g., Dillon et al., 2004; Israel & Hackett, 2004; Pearson, 2003; Sevig & Etzkorn, 2001). This is consistent with the work of Matthews and her colleagues, who have found that one of the most consistent predictors of counselors having affirmative attitudes and behaviors toward this population is working in a nonheterosexist environment (Bieschke & Matthews, 1996; Matthews & Bieschke, 2003; Matthews, Selvidge, & Fisher, 2005).

It is likely that unless you work in a very restrictive counseling environment you will work with lesbian clients. Your professional association probably has a formal position about practicing competently and affirmatively when you do. It is less likely that your training program or work site will adequately prepare you to do this. Hopefully, if you are reading this text as part of a class, you are in a program that is more proactive in this regard. Nonetheless, because society at large does not teach us about developing a lesbian identity as well as it teaches us about developing a heterosexual identity, it is important to begin to acquire such an understanding now. It is particularly important to understand healthy lesbian identity development in order to better assess the degree to which client problems are related to unhealthy development or undue social pressure they face as lesbians, or whether their presenting problems have nothing to do with their being lesbians.

## ABOUT THE CHAPTER AUTHOR

### Connie R. Matthews

I am so excited to be a part of this project. I have taught a development course for several years and have longed for a text that went beyond traditional models to include the variety of developmental concerns that many people experience in addition to those linked to chronological growth. This text promises to bring human development to life in all of its complexity and promise. I look forward to learning from it myself and to using it to help students become engaged in this aspect of counseling.

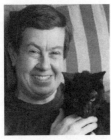

**Connie R. Matthews**

*Connie R. Matthews*, Ph.D., NCC, LPC, is adjunct professor of counseling at Shippensburg University of Pennsylvania. She is actively involved with the Pennsylvania Counseling Association, the American Counseling Association North Atlantic Region, the Society for Counseling Psychology of the American Psychological Association, and the Association for Women in Psychology. Her professional interests include affirmative counseling with lesbian, gay, and bisexual clients, addiction and recovery for women and lesbian, gay, and bisexual clients, and diversity issues in counseling. She lives with her partner Peggy and their cat, RC, who, at nineteen years old and three and a half years into a terminal diagnosis, serves as a model of resiliency.

Furthermore because lesbians themselves may lack such information, they might well expect you to help them in sorting out what can be a stressful but exhilarating process.

# Models of Lesbian Identity Development

## Early Models

The initial work on sexual orientation identity focused on lesbians and gay men. Cass (1979) is generally credited with developing an early model that became a foundation for future work in this area. Her model of homosexual [sic] identity formation included six stages of progression from initial questioning of assumed heterosexuality to full integration of a homosexual identity. It is important to note that Cass and other early theorists tended to use language common at the time, thus referring to gay men and lesbians as "homosexuals." During the gay liberation movement that was emerging at the time, there was a recognition that this term failed to capture an experience that was much more than merely sexual. Counseling scholars and practitioners later moved to referring to gay men and lesbians, as preferred by such individuals themselves, and are currently expanding this language to include terms such as *queer,* which some younger people now prefer as even more encompassing. In this chapter I will attempt to use the language of the theorists and scholars being cited; however, it is critical for counselors to be aware that language and expression are very important, especially for marginalized populations, as they often convey meaning that can either exacerbate or mitigate marginalization. It is vital to understand the nuances that can be conveyed with choice of terminology.

Cass labeled the first stage identity *confusion.* During this stage, an individual begins to question her heterosexuality based on cognitive, affective, and/or behavioral differences between herself and others. During this stage she first wonders whether it might be possible that she is not heterosexual. During the second stage, *identity comparison,* an individual begins to more seriously consider the possibility of being homosexual. This often brings with it considerable turmoil and may be the point at which a person seeks counseling to address the discomfort. The third stage, *identity tolerance,* occurs when someone begins to acknowledge, at least internally, that she is likely lesbian. Such tolerance, however, falls short of being acceptance. Although she can tolerate the idea of being lesbian enough to continue exploring the possibility, she has not yet fully accepted that this is the case and that it might be okay. This is the point at which she will probably make attempts to find others who are considered similar to her emerging lesbian self. *Identity acceptance* is the fourth stage and generally occurs if or when those contacts with others are positive and help the individual to accept the identity of self as lesbian. During this stage, there is generally an effort to reach out more to the gay and lesbian community in an effort to reduce alienation and find an interpersonal place that feels validating. This is further enhanced in stage five, *identity pride,* wherein the individual tends to value homosexuality, while simultaneously devaluing heterosexuality. There is often a preference for associating with others who are gay or lesbian rather than with people who are heterosexual. In the sixth stage, identity *synthesis,* the individual is able to feel comfortable acceptance with a lesbian identity while recognizing that there is considerable diversity among heterosexuals, some of whom are supportive, and some of whom remain threatening.

Within each stage, there are cognitive, affective, and behavioral components that interact to influence the outcome of the stage. Cass (1979) was clear that movement through all six stages is not automatic or assumed once the process has begun. There are developmental tasks to be achieved during each stage and foreclosure is possible at any point if the distress of moving forward seems greater than the tension of subjugating the homosexual aspects of one's identity. Foreclosure is also possible if, especially during the early stages, an individual's exploration leads her to the conclusion that whatever thoughts, feelings, or behaviors led to that exploration, they are not indicative of a lesbian identity. Finally, Cass stresses that there are both private and public aspects to this process. Particularly in the early stages, one might self-identify quite differently from how one presents oneself to others. Cass suggests a coming together of these aspects as one moves through the stages.

Cass (1984) attempted to test this model and found mixed results. Initially she found overlap between the first two stages and last two stages, suggesting a four-stage model might be more appropriate; however, on follow-up she found support for the initial six-stage model. Cass (1996) continues to utilize the six-stage model; however, in her later work she stresses a social constructionist understanding of identity development and emphasizes that hers is clearly a Western model. She does acknowledge the tendency of many clients to be more essentialist in their own understanding and encourages counselor sensitivity in responding to this perspective.

Although Cass (1979, 1984, 1996) argued that her model addressed both lesbians and gay men, several scholars have proposed models of identity development that are specific to lesbians. Gramick (1984) and Chapman and Brannock (1987) offered two of the early models. Brannock and Chapman took more of essentialist approach, arguing that a lesbian sexual orientation exists, even before a woman is aware of it. The lesbian identity development process is largely one of discovery. Gramick described her model as "interactionist" (p. 33), arguing that a woman's interaction with other individuals and social systems influences her perceptions of her experiences and developing awareness of self. Because such social interactions primarily, if not exclusively, portray heterosexuality, it is not surprising that women do not initially recognize early experiences that they might later, in retrospect, identify as lesbian. Such experiences might include crushes on adult women, tender feelings toward particular female friends, or preference for the company of women.

Both models (Chapman & Brannock, 1987; Gramick, 1984) describe an early attraction or connection to other girls or women that predates any conscious awareness of a lesbian identity. Gramick refers to this as "emotional attraction"; Chapman and Brannock call it "same sex orientation." Over time such experiences contribute to a sense of "incongruence" (Chapman & Brannock) or "feeling different" (Gramick), which may not be specifically associated with lesbianism, but which do give her a feeling of being not like other girls or women. This is followed by a period that Chapman and Brannock refer to as "self-questioning/ exploration," which encompasses several experiences that Gramick suggests occur somewhat sequentially. This includes a "cognitive awareness" that lesbians exist in the world and then making a (or several) "lesbian acquaintance." Gramick suggests that such contact is rather limited at this point, although Chapman and Brannock leave the amount of such contact more open-ended. Such contact is often followed by a strong "emotional attraction" to another woman and then having some type of "physical contact" with another woman that an individual can identify as a lesbian experience. Chapman and Brannock suggest that this period might also include some heterosexual involvement as an additional way of sorting out and clarifying feelings and attractions. Gramick's model ends with two stages that include, first, being in a "lesbian relationship" that lasted at least six months and then, eventually "self-acknowledgement" of being lesbian. She argues that being in a relationship, even a bad one, helps to solidify one's identity as lesbian. Chapman and Brannock suggest that self-identification as lesbian precedes involvement in long-term relationships. They describe a stage beyond "self-identification" as lesbian, which they term *choice of lifestyle.* They argue that during this stage a woman actively decides whether or not to pursue women for long-term relationships, although from their essentialist perspective, she maintains a lesbian orientation even if she chooses not to pursue relationships with women.

Both Gramick (1984) and Chapman and Brannock (1987) focused attention on the process leading up to adopting a personal identification as a lesbian. Gramick acknowledged that the process continued beyond that and that the latter process likely included involvement in the lesbian and gay community. Gramick, and to some extent Chapman and Brannock, also pointed out that adoption of a self-acknowledged lesbian identity generated mixed feelings. Although there is some sense of satisfaction, or at least relief, at having figured out the incongruence

## ABOUT EVELYN HOOKER AND OUR FIELD'S STRUGGLE WITH SEXUAL ORIENTATION

In the 1950s Evelyn Hooker mentioned to a colleague that she was interested in studying healthy gay men; the colleague responded that he would like to meet such a person (Hooker, 1996). At the time, homosexuality itself was considered pathological. In other words, a lesbian was considered mentally ill simply because she was lesbian. Furthermore, the prevailing treatment for such a disorder was to attempt conversion to heterosexuality (Gonsiorek, 1991). Thanks to the pioneering work of Hooker who offered the first scientific proof that in masked trials, homosexuals [sic] could not be distinguished from heterosexuals based on tests of mental health and of other researchers who followed her lead, the American Psychiatric Association removed homosexuality from its list of mental disorders in 1973 (Gonsiorek). This was followed by similar action from the American Psychological Association in 1974 (APA, 1975). In both cases such positions became possible through the combined influence of research that discredited the prevailing attitudes of the day, along with savvy political activists within the associations who were bolstered by the gay liberation and gay rights movements occurring in society at large. At present, all major mental health professional associations have adopted positions that reject the notion of homosexuality per se being indicative of mental disorder and/or decry stigma, bias, and discrimination based on sexual orientation (APA, 2000).

The American Counseling Association (ACA) has a history of addressing issues related to sexual orientation proactively. Indeed, the first such action preceded the American Psychiatric Association decision. In 1971, the governing body of what was then the American Personnel and Guidance Association voted to approve adding sexual orientation to antidiscrimination policies and laws (ACA, n.d.). The association reaffirmed its position in 1973, going a step further to encourage its membership to actively work against discrimination based on sexual orientation. Additional related resolutions were passed in 1977, 1979, and 1980. By the mid 1990s, the mental health community was struggling with the question of the ethics of conversion therapy (sometimes called reparative therapy) geared toward converting lesbians and gay men to heterosexuality, or at least celibacy. In 1998, APA passed a resolution that fell short of forbidding its members to practice in such a manner, but nonetheless took a strong stand regarding the role that social bias plays in the distress that lesbians and gay men experience and the lack of scientific support for the efficacy of conversion therapy. A year later ACA Governing Council passed a resolution opposing the use of reparative therapy as a cure for homosexuality (ACA, n.d.).

By the turn of the new century, the mental health professions began moving beyond simply decrying discrimination and maltreatment toward a more proactive, affirmative stance. It is no longer enough to simply not discriminate. With ethical codes based on moral principles that include beneficence as well as nonmaleficence, ACA and APA both developed guidelines for working affirmatively with gay, lesbian, and bisexual clients. The Association for Gay, Lesbian, and Bisexual Issues in Counseling (AGLBIC), a division of ACA, developed "Competencies for Counseling Gay, Lesbian, Bisexual, and Transgendered (GLBT) Clients," which addresses proficiencies that counselors need to have in each of the areas covered by the CACREP curricular standards (AGLBIC, n.d.). These competencies were endorsed by the ACA Governing Council in April, 2004 (ACA Governing Council, 2004). APA likewise has produced "Guidelines for Psychotherapy with Lesbian, Gay, and Bisexual Clients" (2000), which includes sixteen specific guidelines under four broad headings: Attitudes toward Homosexuality and Bisexuality, Relationships and Families, Issues of Diversity, and Education. Both associations have made it clear that counselors and psychologists have a professional responsibility to develop the awareness, knowledge, and skills to work effectively with this population.

one had been experiencing, there is also a realization that a lesbian identity brings with it negative ramifications in a society that prescribes heterosexuality and condemns homosexuality.

Sophie (1986) reviewed six stage theories of lesbian and/or gay identity development and devised what she termed "a generalized model" (p. 41) of lesbian identity development consisting of four stages: first awareness, testing and exploration, identity acceptance, and identity integration.

## Contemporary Model

McCarn and Fassinger (1996) took the lesbian identity literature, literally, to another level when they presented a model that addresses identity development in a manner that incorporates both individual identity
and membership in a group, specifically a stigmatized minority group.
Drawing from the racial identity and gender identity development lit-
eratures as well as the sexual orientation identity development literature, they separate the processes by which an individual identifies herself
individually as a lesbian and as an individual who is part of a minority group. This is an important distinction between McCarn and Fassinger's
model and previous models, which tended to incorporate involvement
in the community into personal identity development. McCarn and
Fassinger more clearly articulate the social realities that might keep one
from more public pronouncements of her sexual orientation despite a
sophisticated level of personal understanding and acceptance. They also
intentionally use the word "phases" rather than "stages" (p. 521) to
describe the components of their model. They suggest that "stages"
suggests a sequential and progressive movement that is not reflective
of the process as it occurs in people's lived experiences. "Phases" allows
for more flexibility in recognizing that there is movement back and
forth as individuals encounter new people and situations. It better
reflects the lifelong process of identity development.

McCarn and Fassinger (1996) describe four phases, which individuals move through at both the individual level and the group level. The
first phase is awareness. At the individual level this generally reflects
a personal feeling of being different. At the group level, this pertains
to a developing awareness that there are a variety of sexual orientations,
not simply heterosexuality. The second phase, exploration, represents
the beginning consideration of one's personal relationship to other lesbians. At the individual level it means attraction to another woman.
At the group level it means examining both one's attitudes toward lesbians and gay men and one's own place, if any, in relation to that group.

The third phase is deepening/commitment, which entails what the
name suggests, a more clearly definable understanding of oneself with
respect to sexuality and intimacy. This includes both one's personal relationships (individual level) and one's sense of oneself as part of a group,
more specifically an oppressed minority group (group level). This phase
also involves greater understanding of the ramifications of such a position, which generally means a combination of pride and fulfillment in
becoming who one was meant to be, but also a measure of anger and

**TABLE 9.1  Models of Lesbian Identity-Development**

| Cass 1979 | Gramick 1984 | Chapman and Brannock 1987 | Sophie 1986 | McCarn and Fassinger 1996 | |
| --- | --- | --- | --- | --- | --- |
| | | | | Individual Level | Group Level |
| Identity Confusion | Feeling Different<br>Cognitive Awareness | Same-Sex Orientation Incongruence | First Awareness | Awareness | Awareness |
| Identity Comparison | Lesbian Acquaintance<br>Emotion Attraction<br>Physical Attraction | Self-Questioning/ Exploration | Testing and Exploration | Exploration | Exploration |
| Identity Tolerance | Physical Contact<br>Lesbian Relationship | | | | |
| Identity Acceptance | Self-Acknowledgement | Self-Identification | Identity Acceptance | | |
| Identity Pride | | Choice of Lifestyle | | Deepening/ Commitment | Deepening/ Commitment |
| Identity Synthesis | | | Identity Integration | Internalization/ Synthesis | Internalization/ Synthesis |

270

despair in realizing the prejudice and discrimination that comes with such an identity. This phase may, but need not, include greater involvement in the lesbian community.

The fourth phase, internalization/synthesis, represents, at the individual level, an integration of one's lesbian identity with the other aspects of one's identity. It denotes an acknowledgement of oneself as lesbian from a broader perspective. At the group level, there is a shift in emphasis from examining oneself in relation to the lesbian/gay/bisexual community to considering oneself a member of that community and examining one's relationships with others both within and outside of the community. No longer the outsider looking in, one becomes the insider looking out. This phase also often brings with it a closer scrutiny of when and in what contexts to disclose one's lesbian identity with others. Although this occurs to some extent during the third phase and to a lesser extent in the second phase, it is during the fourth phase that one more fully negotiates the degree to which being lesbian is part of one's public as well as personal identity. This will become a lifelong process, played out in every new context. McCarn and Fassinger, more than previous models, recognize that there are a great many contextual factors that might influence decisions about how public one can be with respect to being lesbian.

Although McCarn and Fassinger (1996) draw from the racial and ethnic identity development literature as well as the gender identity development literature in developing their model, none of the above models substantially addresses the intersection of lesbian identity development and racial/ethnic identity development. Being both lesbian and a member of an ethnic minority group adds layers to the development process, which counselors must be able to respond to in working with ethnic minority lesbian clients. This is addressed briefly in the next section.

# Using Lesbian Identity Development in Counseling Practice

It is critical that counselors have at least a working knowledge of sexual orientation identity development (Brown, 1996; Pope, 1995; Reynolds, 2003). Pope (citing Elliot, 1990) stresses that the process of identity development for gay men and lesbians is complicated by the fact that, unlike other minority groups, gay men and lesbians usually do not have families who are able to help them through this developmental process. Thus, counselors often play a crucial role in helping lesbian clients address concerns associated with identity development. Bringaze and White (2001) found this to be the case in their study of 262 psychologically adjusted lesbian leaders and role models. Participants were asked to describe some of the things that helped them in the coming-out process; counseling was one of the major factors identified.

As with any type of development, knowing where a client is on a developmental trajectory helps the counselor to better understand how to respond in ways that utilize her current capabilities and help move her forward. Interventions that are highly facilitative in some developmental stages can be counterproductive in others. For example, it might be very facilitative to help a woman in McCarn and Fassinger's (1996) deepening/commitment phase find access to the lesbian community around activities that are consistent with her social, recreational, or spiritual interests. On the other hand, referring someone who is in the earliest stages of awareness of her own same-sex attractions to a lesbian social group might terrify her. It would be much more appropriate in the latter case to encourage exploration, perhaps using cognitive approaches about what being lesbian might mean to that individual (Martell, Safren, & Prince, 2004; Scott & Reyna, 1995). This might be supplemented with psychoeducational activities such as bibliotherapy that is affirmative, yet nonpolitical. Because sexual orientation is such a politically charged issue in the current cultural climate, many activities in the lesbian community involve efforts to change the status quo or to take on the system that oppresses lesbians. Women in the early stages of lesbian identity development are usually not yet ready to take such risks. Nonetheless, they do need exposure to perspectives that affirm them for who they are and who they are becoming. This is where carefully chosen books, videos, and other educational means can be helpful. On the other hand, the woman who is further along in her lesbian identity development might find such seemingly passive approaches frustrating and naïve. Counselors must be familiar enough with educational resources and the local lesbian community to use approaches that are developmentally appropriate (regardless of the woman's chronological age).

Something that separates lesbian identity development from general theories of human development is the reality that developing a lesbian identity also means giving up a heterosexual identity (Reid, 1995). Because we live in a heterosexist culture, all children are assumed to be heterosexual and are raised as such. Heterosexist refers to the cultural notion that heterosexuality is the norm and anything else is aberrant (Herek, 1995). This not only contributes to the sense of marginalization that many lesbians experience, but it also means that everybody is considered heterosexual until determined otherwise. Thus, all women believe themselves to be heterosexual until they begin to become aware of attraction to other females and to experience that sense of "differentness." This can happen at any age and often, although not always, occurs after a short or very long period of heterosexual involvement. Transitioning from a heterosexual to a lesbian identity also means abandoning a majority identity for a minority identity that brings with it prejudice and stigma, as well as loss of privilege (Thompson, 1992).

Kitzinger and Wilkinson (1995) interviewed eighty lesbians who, for at least ten years, had considered themselves heterosexual and were actively engaged in heterosexual behavior, including coitus, but who at the time of the study had established an identity that was "unequivocally lesbian" (p. 97). They took a social constructionist approach in examining the movement from heterosexual to lesbian identity. Through their analysis of the data from the interviews, they identified three sequential themes in this progression, which included the preparatory work of fighting their own heterosexist assumptions and breaking down the barriers to recognition, actually making the transition to a lesbian identity, and then going on with their lives as lesbians. Throughout the process these women were acutely aware of the costs of making such a transition and the consequences of giving up a privileged identity for an oppressed one. Still, a critical factor for counselors to remember is that, of these eighty women, only two or three had any regrets about making this transition. Despite the consequences it might bring, making the transition was worth it. Thus, counselors can play a crucial role in helping women to make the journey from heterosexual to lesbian in ways that affirm a sense of wholeness while helping to reduce the costs of doing so.

Matthews and Bieschke (2001) draw a parallel between lesbians and gay men transitioning to a new identity and immigrants translocating to a new country and culture. They suggest that a number of factors might contribute to both the process and quality of the transition, including such things as the precipitating events, the attitudes of family and friends toward the transition, the client's own internal processes, and early experiences in the new culture. They offer an approach for counselors to use in assessing where a client might be in her development.

In applying models of lesbian identity development, it is also important to consider the context of such development for individual clients. Although the models offer conceptions of a general progression from heterosexual to lesbian identity, the actual experience of this can vary greatly depending on personal circumstances. Age, for instance, can be very important in a woman's experience. This pertains both to the age a woman, or girl, is when she becomes aware of and decides to explore her same-sex orientation and to the historical period in which this occurs. For example, Parks (1999) conducted a phenomenological study of thirty-one lesbians, ranging in age from twenty-three to seventy-nine years. She found that there were distinct generational differences in the experiences of the women as they negotiated the lesbian identity development process, based on the period in which they reached adulthood. She divided the generations into Pre-Stonewall Era, referring to the 1969 riots at the gay Stonewall Inn, generally credited as the beginning of the gay liberation movement; Liberation Era, running from the early seventies to the mid-eighties; and Gay Rights Era, covering the mid-eighties to early nineties. As the contemporary gay liberation and gay rights movements brought attention to lesbian and gay issues, the effect on individuals negotiating a lesbian identity was complicated. Although there was greater visibility of nonheterosexual alternatives, that visibility brought with it a backlash that also made the consequences of such an identity also more evident. It is thus important for counselors to have some familiarity with the changes that occur in society with respect to lesbian and gay issues and the impact they can have on lesbians. Such social forces can influence not only initial identity development but also long-term identity maintenance, which is why contemporary models such as McCarn and Fassinger's (1996) allow for cycling back through phases when new circumstances arise.

Chronological age also has an impact on the identity development process. There is a growing literature on issues facing gay, lesbian, and bisexual adolescents (see, for example, D'Augelli & Patterson, 2001; Savin-Williams, 1990). Adolescence is a period defined by identity-related tasks, yet, rather than being just another piece of the puzzle, negotiating a lesbian identity not only adds another layer but impacts all of the other developmental tasks as well. Presumptive heterosexuality at best marginalizes lesbian teens and can lead to more overt harassment, stigmatization, and even violence (Rivers & D'Augelli, 2001). Furthermore, although heterosexual adolescents often are supported in their developmental trajectories by family and friends, young lesbians lack such support. Even accepting families often lack the knowledge and awareness to be truly helpful with a process they have not experienced—and many families are not accepting. It is not surprising that D'Augelli (2002) found that gay, lesbian, and bisexual youth whose parents were rejecting of their sexual orientation, or who had not told their parents for fear of rejection, experienced more mental health problems than those whose parents were accepting. Large percentages of participants (46% of females; 30% of males) reported fears of losing friends due to their sexual orientation. Youths who did fear losing friends reported more mental health symptoms than those who did not. D'Augelli also found high levels of victimization, with 81% of participants reporting at least one incident of verbal abuse and more than half reporting three or more such incidents; 15% had been physically assaulted, 6% with a weapon. Counselors must be able to help lesbian adolescents respond to such external stressors at the same time that they are dealing with the internal processes related to awareness and exploration of a lesbian identity.

Older lesbians represent another age-group that faces particular concerns with respect to their sexual orientation, although one that has received considerably less attention than adolescents. First, they came into adulthood in a time when being lesbian meant not just minority status, but pathological status (Grossman, D'Augelli, & O'Connell, 2003). Discrimination meant not only lack of privilege but often active penalty, such as loss of children or loss of job. As a result, they might have established patterns of behavior that reflected the realities of the time. This might include compartmentalization of their public and private lives (Reid, 1995; Ritter & Terndrup, 2002) as well as the language they use to describe themselves. Second, as lesbians age, the realities of lack of privilege may become more salient as partners realize that under current law many cannot inherit property from each other even when their property is jointly owned, are not entitled to each other's benefits, and may not even be able to make decisions regarding care for each other.

Encountering such situations might pose very real practical problems as well as the potential for revisiting what it means to be lesbian in a heterosexist culture. It is important to remember, however, that despite these problems, the few studies that have been done have found that older lesbians do not seem to experience inordinate amounts of distress and seem overall to be well-adjusted (Reid, 1995; Ritter & Terndrup, 2002). Counselors should be prepared to expect variability in responses among older lesbians to immense social changes over the course of their lifetimes, any of which might represent healthy adjustment or internal struggle. Counselors should also be knowledgeable enough to help older lesbians negotiate the practical ramifications of aging in a culture that fails to recognize their needs.

Another contextual area where awareness is critical is the intersection of ethnicity and sexual orientation. Lesbians who are also members of ethnic minority groups face multiple levels of development and multiple levels of oppression, yet the professional literature has only recently begun to address this. Morales (1990) has noted that ethnic minority lesbians and gay men live in three separate communities: the gay and lesbian community, the ethnic minority community, and the larger society. Each of these communities fulfills some of the developmental needs of ethnic minority lesbians, but none of them fulfills all of the needs. For example, the lesbian community exists in the context of a larger society that is often racist and ethnic minority communities often reflect the heterosexism of the broader culture (Chan, 1989; Greene, 1998; Liu & Chan, 1996; Loiacano, 1989; Morales, 1990). This leaves little safe haven for lesbians trying to exist in both cultures; in society at large they are oppressed on both fronts.

Ethnic minority families can offer a buffer against the racism of the larger society as well as provide guidance in negotiating racism to achieve healthy development because they have lived, and continue to live, through this experience themselves. In most instances they have little or no frame of reference for helping their children to develop and manage a lesbian identity at any age. Indeed, their own heterosexism may contribute to further shaming of the child. Thus, it is not unusual for ethnic minority lesbians to choose not to disclose their sexual orientation rather than risk losing the support of their families in a racist world (Greene, 1998; Liu & Chan, 1996). Likewise, the strong sense of family among many ethnic minority cultures can lead them to find ways to support their children, even when they condemn their sexual orientation. Often this occurs through an unspoken agreement not to discuss the subject. Although this can work for ethnic minority lesbians, it can also lead to criticism by a lesbian community that stresses the importance of being open, thus sometimes forcing them to choose between being involved in their ethnic communities, including their families, and the lesbian community.

These are just a few of the contextual issues that must be considered when thinking about lesbian identity development. Counselors need to be aware of the ways in which lesbian identity development impacts and is impacted by development of other aspects of one's identity, including other minority identities. To illustrate some of the concepts related to lesbian identity development, let's take a look at Sarah.

# Sarah's Case

## Sarah

Sarah was born in 1950 into a middle-class family. She prefers the term *working class*. Her father was a mason and her mother an elementary school teacher by training who stayed at home while her children were young. The oldest of three children, Sarah has a brother a year and a half younger than she is and a sister a year and a half younger than the brother. Throughout her life she has felt close to her family, although not necessarily intimate. Although she loves and respects her family, she has also always felt different from them. Indeed, she has often joked about looking for her real family since surely she had been sent home with the wrong parents when she was born.

Sarah's family lived in a neighborhood full of families much like her own. There were always children to play with and Sarah got along with most of them. She was an active child who tended to prefer games that involved running, climbing, and movement; however, she was also somewhat reflective and enjoyed opportunities to be creative. She sometimes thought she might like to be a writer. She would develop passions for reading and music in young adulthood, but growing up she liked to be outside and active. She loved sports and played everything her brother played. Indeed, one of the early disappointments in her life was the fact that girls were not allowed to play Little League baseball. Even at a young age she felt an acute sense of unfairness because she was a far better ball player than most of the boys on her brother's team. Her parents made frequent comments about her needing to act more like a "young lady," but because most of the neighborhood activities involved both boys and girls, these comments usually passed rather quickly. Furthermore, Sarah did like cooking and took on most of the housecleaning responsibilities fairly early on, so this seemed to satisfy them that she would someday settle into more feminine pursuits.

One point of frequent contention was clothes. Sarah was not the frilly type; her mother was. As a result, Sarah and her mother would argue often about what Sarah would wear. As a young child this usually meant that Sarah protested the outfits her mother made her wear. As a teenager these arguments usually focused on her mother's complaints about the things Sarah chose for herself. Sarah grew to hate the color pink because this became the symbol of compromise when she was allowed to wear the kind of clothes she wanted (shorts or jeans) as long as they were pink. She knew that this was intended to protect her femininity. As a child, Sarah never could figure out what the fuss was about. As an adult, things began to make more sense.

Throughout her life Sarah has had both boys/men and girls/women for friends. Her closest connections were always to girls, but she enjoyed the freedom of the boys' activities, especially growing up. This was increasingly more of a struggle with her parents the older she got. As a teenager, it became more complicated for her as well. She was aware that her girlfriends were becoming more interested in boys romantically; she felt that she should too but found such attempts to be rather forced. She dated some, but was less than enthusiastic about it. She enjoyed the boys' friendship but couldn't quite get "interested" in them. Indeed, as social restraints made it harder for her to be involved in sports and other active endeavors, she found herself less interested in being with boys. She would much rather go to the movies or socialize with her girlfriends and sometimes felt hurt when they chose to go out with a boy instead of her. She could never really articulate what she was experiencing; she just felt sad.

College changed some of this. Although Sarah's mother had attended a local teacher's college, Sarah was one of the few in her family or her neighborhood to go to college. She probably would not have gone to college herself had it not been for a rather persistent school counselor who saw a lot of potential in Sarah. Although postsecondary education was not in their plans for Sarah, her parents were able to acknowledge that she was smart, "especially for a girl," and were open to sending her to the teacher's college her mother had attended. The school counselor persuaded them that a liberal arts college a few hours away might be a better fit for Sarah and helped them through the process of finding the resources to allow this to happen.

The school was indeed a good fit. The college included in its mission a commitment to social justice, and Sarah attended during the height of the civil rights and peace movements. She became very active in a variety of social justice activities and felt that she had found her niche. As was typical for her, she made many friends among both men and women. She felt that she had finally found some kindred spirits. Because there was a sense of everybody being in the movement together and it was a social period of relaxing sexual mores, there was less emphasis on coupled dating and more of a sense of group interactions. This worked for Sarah. She had casual relationships with a few of the guys and it was fun, but she felt less pressure, at least initially, to be in a serious relationship. This seemed to change as the group got closer to graduation, when everyone started thinking more about settling down.

One of the guys in the group seemed particularly interested in Sarah, and she liked him, too. Although she knew that she did not share his passion, she also knew that she was expected to marry. She expected this of herself. It seemed inevitable that she and Jesse would marry, and they did, right after graduation.

Although Sarah would not describe her marriage as exciting, she was more or less content. Within five years they had two children, a boy, Michael, named for Jesse's grandfather, and a girl, Frannie, named for Sarah's grandmother. Both Sarah and Jesse were high school English teachers. Sarah stayed home with the children for the first few years, but finances dictated that she go back to teaching. She and Jesse had initially worked in the same school, but when Sarah reentered teaching, it was at a different school. Although initially disappointing, Sarah found that she enjoyed being in a place where she could be seen as herself, rather than as Jesse's wife. Indeed, she thrived in the new school. The students, faculty, and administration all loved her. She found her self volunteering, or being volunteered, for committee and extra-curricular work. This posed some scheduling problems in balancing home and school, but Jesse was pleased enough with the new energy he was seeing in Sarah that he tried to be as helpful as he could. As time went on, though, he began feeling that this energy was pulling Sarah away from him rather than toward him. He particularly struggled with the friendships she was making that did not include him, especially friendships with some of her male colleagues.

At the beginning of her third year, a new teacher, Kelly, joined Sarah's team. The two worked well together and immediately became friends. They spent a lot of time together both at work and outside of work. Kelly was single and did not have family locally, so Sarah began inviting Kelly to spend time with her family. The children immediately took a liking to Kelly. Although he resented some of the time she spent with Kelly, Jesse was mostly pleased to see her focused on a woman because it meant that she was spending less time with some of the men. Over time, Sarah found herself growing very fond of Kelly. She had a hard time putting her finger on it, but Kelly was special. She felt alive with Kelly. During the winter, Kelly mentioned that she was going to be starting a master's program at the local university (formerly the teacher's college Sarah's mother had attended). She suggested Sarah consider doing so as well. Sarah thought this was a good idea and was able to convince Jesse that the increase in salary once she got her master's degree would help with family finances. Sarah and Kelly took courses together and Sarah found that she really looked forward to this. She was especially happy that this gave them a chance to be together almost every day over the summer. She also found herself very disappointed and sad when she and Kelly were not able to get together, especially if Kelly had plans that did not include her.

Sarah recognized these feelings as similar to those she had in high school when her girlfriends would make plans with boys instead of her. She also started to wonder what it might be like to kiss Kelly. They were physically close, hugging hello and good-bye, usually accompanied by a kiss on the cheek. These thoughts, however, were different; they both scared and excited Sarah. One night in the fall Jesse had taken the children to a football game. Sarah and Kelly stayed home to work on a project for school. When they finished, they turned on the television and watched a sitcom that happened to have a lesbian theme. This was the 1980s, and such themes found their way into television shows occasionally. Sarah and Kelly both became uncomfortable, giggling and making small talk. Kelly then asked Sarah if she ever had feelings like that for a woman. This led to both of them revealing similar feelings toward each other. Although nothing but conversation happened that night, it would not be long until they moved on to kissing and eventually, a sexual relationship. As with her earlier thoughts about kissing Kelly, Sarah found this both frightening and exciting. She was well aware of the turmoil it would bring to her family if the true nature of their relationship were discovered.

Sarah was not ready to make any major changes in her life. She did, however, begin changing her normal routine, going to bed well before Jesse did so that she would be asleep before he came to bed. He was not usually inclined to wake her up to have sex, and this was something she would rather avoid. Sex with Jesse had never been passionate, but it was okay. This changed when she and Kelly became involved. Sex with Kelly really was making love.

Working together and being in a master's program together gave Sarah and Kelly plenty of time together and plenty of reasons to be together other times. They lived in relatively small town, so there weren't many outlets for two women to socialize together as a couple or to meet other women like themselves. This was a new experience for both of them, and neither was quite sure what to make of it. There were a couple of occasions when they were able to go away together for professional conferences in bigger cities. On one occasion they went to a gay bookstore and on another occasion they went to a gay bar. They found both experiences exciting and frightening. They feared for their jobs even though they were hundreds of miles from home, and Sarah feared the repercussions if Jesse should discover what she was doing. At school they were always very careful to maintain a professional relationship. They had a rule not to talk about anything but school-related issues and never to touch under any circumstances. They even tried to avoid looking directly at each other out of fear that somebody might notice the connection they had with each other.

Eventually Jesse did grow weary of the time Sarah and Kelly spent together. He tried to support Sarah's efforts in graduate school, but it wasn't something that interested him and he frequently made it clear that he wanted his wife back. The children loved Kelly and tended to respond to her as another parent; however, they were clearly unnerved by the increasingly frequent arguing between Sarah and Jesse. Sarah's parents loved Kelly as well because she was very attentive to them but neither of them could understand why Sarah and Kelly wanted to spend so much time in school when the both already had college degrees.

A critical juncture came when Sarah and Kelly were nearing the end of the master's program. Jesse was looking forward to it and to having life return to "normal." Sarah was distraught over the thought of Jesse expecting her to spend more time with him and less time with Kelly. A professor in the master's program had been encouraging Sarah to go on for doctoral work. Jesse "forbade" her even to consider this. Kelly encouraged her to pursue it. Sarah's parents could not imagine why she would even want to do this. She had a good job and a good family; why would she want to disrupt everything so much. The university she was considering was about a hundred miles from home. Sarah and Kelly had been doing some exploration about the lesbian community in the area where the university was located.

At thirty-three years old, Sarah made a bold decision. She applied to the doctoral program without telling Jesse or her parents. She was accepted to begin study in the fall of her thirty-third year. Late in the spring she announced to Jesse that she would be leaving to go to school in the fall. The children would stay with him. She had not intended to tell Jesse about her relationship with Kelly, but he asked. He likely would have found out anyway because Kelly had accepted a teaching position in the town where the university was located. The two of them were planning to live together. Sarah tried to be as honest with Jesse as she could. His initial reaction was quite negative, and Sarah was afraid for awhile that he would prevent her from ever seeing her children. In his initial anger Jesse told Sarah's parents the truth behind her leaving. Jesse told Sarah that they cried when he told them, but they did not raise the issue with Sarah. After that Sarah and Kelly talked with the children. They were shocked, confused, and angry and directed much of this at Kelly. The turmoil created tension between Sarah and Kelly, but they followed through with their plan.

That was twenty-two years ago. When Sarah completed her doctoral program, she took a teaching job at another university where Kelly then began a doctoral program in another field. Eventually the two of them ended up teaching at a university about two hundred miles from their hometown. Teaching at the university level felt safer than the public schools. After a period of activism in the women's and gay rights movements during and shortly after their graduate school years, Sarah and Kelly settled into a quiet life in a university town. Michael and Frannie continued to live with Jesse when they lived at home, but they spent a lot of time with Sarah and Kelly as well, especially in the summers. Michael initially seemed to adjust to Sarah and Kelly's relationship better than Frannie did, but Frannie's acceptance grew over time. Both are now married with children of their own who adore their Grandma Sarah and Nana Kelly. After his initial volatile reaction, Jesse made efforts to accept the situation. This got easier when he became involved with and eventually married another woman who was quite content to focus on being with him. Jesse and Sarah remain cordial if not friendly, seeing each other primarily at events focused on their children.

Sarah and Kelly enjoy their life at the university. Although the surrounding area is somewhat conservative, there is more openness at the university. They don't flaunt their relationship, but they own a home and a couple of cars together and are open with their friends. They socialize with both heterosexual couples and lesbians. Although they try to support the lesbian community at the university, this is not the focus of their lives. Indeed, life has been good for them until the past year.

The ruling in Massachusetts that opened the door for gay marriages (see Human Rights Campaign, n.d., for information on *Goodridge et al. v. Department of Public Health*) also opened a floodgate of backlash from a conservative president up for reelection. Suddenly, gay marriage was at the forefront of people's attention. With it brought increased awareness of the vulnerabilities of lesbian and gay couples. Sarah began thinking more about this issue, both pragmatically and philosophically. She realized that she and Kelly were not too far from retirement. Although they had taken what steps they could to protect themselves and each other, she was acutely aware that there really was not much protection. They were not entitled to each other's benefits and when one of them died the other would have to pay a large sum of money in taxes to keep the house—and that was only if neither of their families tried to intervene. The same was true should one of them become ill or disabled. They had drawn up powers of attorney but still feared that their biological families could interfere. Sarah was becoming more and more aware of the privileges she had when she was married to Jesse that she did not have in her relationship with Kelly.

Sarah has found herself becoming increasingly active in the local gay and lesbian community. Kelly sometimes goes along, but often does not. She sometimes criticizes Sarah for trying to act like a student again. Although initially this situation was little more than annoying, lately things seemed to be deteriorating. Sarah had suggested that the two of them go to Massachusetts to get married. She realized that it would not change things pragmatically, but she thought that symbolically it might help her to feel better about the conservative backlash—and a part of her had always felt sad that she and Kelly could not marry when their relationship was so much stronger that hers and Jesse's. Kelly reacted to the suggestion with annoyance and this hurt Sarah. They have tried talking about the situation but seem to be at a stalemate. Their relationship is not in jeopardy, but they do seem to need some help in moving forward. At Sarah's suggestion, they decided to get counseling. The following dialogue occurred during the intake session as they discussed what brought them in:

*Sarah:* "I was just so hurt when you got annoyed at me for suggesting we go to Massachusetts to get married. It wasn't that I expected you to agree with me, but when you got so irritated that I even brought it up, I was hurt. I know that you love me, but it felt like you were saying that our relationship isn't worth fighting for."

*Kelly:* "It's not a question of fighting for our relationship. We're together aren't we? And we've been together for over 22 years. What difference will a silly piece of paper make at this point? It won't even be recognized here. It won't mean anything. It won't change anything about our lives."

*S:* "It would feel like a statement—that our relationship is important enough to be recognized."

*K:* "Recognized by who? A bunch of bureaucrats? We're out to our family and friends. The people who are important to us do recognize us as a couple. What does it matter what other people think? You married Jesse—did that make it a better relationship?"

*S:* "No! You know my marriage to Jesse was nothing compared to what we have, but that's what upsets me so much. When I married Jesse, who I hardly loved and felt no passion for, it was like the whole world applauded. Had I chosen to stay married I would have been "protected" for life—I would have been eligible for his social security benefits, able to inherit our joint property, able to do joint retirement planning, able to take care of him if something happened. Nobody applauds us. It took years of patience and struggle for some to even accept us. We can't take care of each other financially, or even medically, the way we ought to be able to. Things won't change if people like us don't fight for what's important to us."

*K:* "I have what's important to me. . . ."

## Examining the Case

This case demonstrates a number of things that have been addressed in this chapter. Although not all lesbians are involved with men before settling into a lesbian identity, such a situation is not unusual. Furthermore, even if they are never sexually or romantically involved with men, all women are raised to believe that they will be. Sarah always expected that she would marry and have children. This was the life course she expected to follow and follow it she did. There was nothing particularly unusual about her childhood, although in retrospect she could see that she always struggled with social prescriptions. Some might have considered her a tomboy growing up. Was this related to the fact that she would later recognize and develop her lesbian identity? There is no way to know. It might have had more to do with gender role expectations for women. What she did later recognize as likely related was her lifelong connection to women and her lack of deep attraction to men. Recall that she always enjoyed having men as friends. Contrary to myth, being lesbian is not about hating or being repulsed by men. It is about attraction to women. This is consistent with Chapman and Brannock's (1987) model, which states that same-sex attraction is present before there is even enough cognitive awareness for confusion or incongruence. As she grew into the age when her peers were interested in boys and in dating, Sarah was aware that she did not share this attraction, but she had no frame of reference to which to connect this awareness. Likewise, she was aware of her disappointment and sadness when her female friends, to whom she did feel connection, chose to spend time with boys. Still this disappointment and sadness was ill-defined. This was probably the beginning of what Gramick (1984) calls *feeling different,* Cass (1979) labels identity confusion, Chapman and Brannock describe as *incongruence,* and what Sophie (1986) and McCarn and Fassinger (1996) refer to as *first awareness* and *awareness* respectively. That awareness would not mean much until later in her life, but Sarah was clearly noticing something. This may be different for some young girls growing up today who have greater access to knowledge about lesbians and may be able to attach their confusion or not fitting in to something more definable. Even now, however, that is likely to be very dependent on the community in which they live and the openness of discussion in their families, schools, and peer groups.

As she explored her lesbian identity, Sarah could remember those earlier feelings about girlfriends that had been confusing at the time. Likewise, even at the time it was occurring, Sarah could recognize that she had to force attraction to men. This was not an intentional effort to deceive; Sarah was simply working as hard as she could to fulfill what she believed was expected of her. A friend once explained to me that if, on an attraction scale of one to ten, all the men you date fall in the minus five range, a two can look pretty good. Such was the case with Jesse. Sarah married him in good faith, expecting to live a comfortable, if not completely fulfilling life with him. This might have happened had Kelly not come into her life.

Sarah's experience once Kelly did enter the picture is in line with the models of lesbian identity development discussed in this chapter. Sarah and Kelly found each other somewhat accidentally; they did not seek each other out for a relationship (although many women do recognize their attraction to women in general and then proceed to seek out someone special). Yet, Sarah recognized that there was something different in her connection with Kelly than there had been with other women and certainly different from her connection to men, even Jesse. At first this was primarily confusing, although Sarah could recognize that confusion as one she had known previously. She experienced some uneasiness in those reflections and could have shut them down, but instead continued to explore them. She also allowed herself to be open to the fantasies she had about kissing Kelly. Cass (1979) described this as *identity tolerance*. Sarah could tolerate the idea of being attracted to women enough to continue to be open to it. Again, such awareness might be so threatening as to necessitate shutting down any exploration of what it means. Once Sarah and Kelly did become involved sexually, they both continued the process of exploration regarding the meaning of this. In keeping with the McCarn and Fassinger (1996) model, this exploration included both personal exploration of their own relationship and efforts to learn about a lesbian community when they were out of town. Also in keeping with virtually all of the models, was an awareness of the dangers that a lesbian identity brought with it. Sarah was acutely aware of the risks to her job and her family should she fully embrace such an identity. As Matthews and Bieschke (2001) point out, adopting a lesbian identity means more than simply transitioning from a heterosexual to a lesbian identity; it means moving from a dominant, privileged identity to a minority, often persecuted identity.

The period of activity with the lesbian community while they were in graduate school, even as returning adults, went along with Cass's (1979) Identity Pride stage and McCarn and Fassinger's (1996) Deepening/Commitment phase. Again, consistent with McCarn and Fassinger, Sarah experienced this deepening of her relationship with Kelly as well as greater involvement in the lesbian community. Over time, Sarah and Kelly both moved somewhat away from this focus on things lesbian. Their lesbian identities continued to be important aspects of their lives, but represented just a part of their lives. They settled into a routine that continued to acknowledge their lesbian identities but did not focus on them. This integration or synthesis of a lesbian identity with a larger, more comprehensive identity represents a final or end stage in virtually all of the models. Being the last stage, however, does not mean that lesbian identity development stops. It can reflect a settling-in of sorts for a short or long period of time, but McCarn and Fassinger (1996) in particular stress that there can be a lifelong cycling back through some or all of the stages as life events unfold and precipitate further self-reflection.

In the present case, social forces led Sarah to again take a look at the ramifications of being lesbian, especially in a society that was fighting against the legitimacy of such an identity. The national debate over gay marriage struck a very personal chord for Sarah, especially since these external forces combined with other developmental issues related to midlife and aging. Suddenly, being lesbian became a more salient aspect of her identity than it had been for some time. While the politicians argued over the legitimacy of what they called *a gay lifestyle,* Sarah felt the ramifications quite personally as she looked at her own future security. This did not occur for Kelly the way that it did for Sarah. Although they had progressed through many of the stages/phases of lesbian identity development together, they were now at an impasse because Sarah was cycling back through some of the identity development tasks, which is quite normal, but Kelly was not. It is hard to tell why the changing social climate affected Sarah more intensely than it did Kelly. Perhaps having been in a heterosexual marriage made Sarah more acutely aware of the privileges she had previously enjoyed and now lacked. Perhaps Kelly was simply at a different point in her midlife development and had not yet begun to think about retirement and later life security. Maybe she was in a state of protective denial concerning the degree to which the national debate affected her personally, or maybe she too was hurt to think that after more than twenty years together Sarah was feeling such a strong need to have their relationship validated. In any event, Sarah and Kelly were at different points in the process, which was generating conflict. Exploring these different reactions will be part of the work they do in counseling. Their counselor will need to have a firm understanding of both typical lifespan development, especially midlife and later life development, and lesbian identity development if she or he is to help Sarah and Kelly understand each other's perspectives and move beyond their current state of feeling stuck in conflict. It will also be important for the counselor to appreciate the impact that a social climate of bias, discrimination, and sometimes outright hostility can have on lesbian identity development.

## Summary

This chapter has presented several models of lesbian identity development and described some of the ways in which familiarity with them is important for counselors. It is important to keep in mind that the whole area of identity development around sexual orientation is quite new. As we can see from this chapter, there are numerous models available; however, there has not been extensive research on any of them. Although each model has its unique perspective, there is clearly a lot of overlap, which perhaps suggests some support for the basic progression. In a culture that presumes heterosexuality, lesbian identity development seems to begin with a sense of confusion around sexual orientation when one's own thoughts and feelings start to feel incongruent with the heterosexual norm. A period of exploration generally follows. When this exploration leads to the conviction that one likely is lesbian, if one can accept that identity one moves into a period of increased focus on that identity. Over time, that focus seems to lessen, with sexual orientation taking an evident but perhaps less prominent role in one's overall identity. As can be seen through the case of Sarah, these models do make intuitive sense. Still, even within these models individual differences play out (e.g., Sophie, 1986). Counselors need to use these models as guides without rigidly imposing them on any given client.

Another important thing to keep in mind is that the client is not the only person in the counseling relationship; the counselor also has a sexual orientation identity, regardless of how the counselor self-identifies. Although most of the work around sexual orientation identity development has focused on lesbians and gay men, and, to a lesser extent, bisexual individuals, Mohr (2002) and Worthington, Savoy, Dillon, and Vernaglia (2002) have recently offered models of heterosexual identity development. They suggest that a counselor's own heterosexual identity development process will influence how she or he works with sexual minority clients. Likewise a lesbian counselor's development of her own lesbian identity will affect her work with lesbian clients. Indeed, Brown (1996) suggests this influence is so strong that it would be ethically problematic for a lesbian or gay counselor to see lesbian or gay clients while in the process of coming out. She suggests waiting at least two years from first beginning the coming out process.

Finally, it is critical for counselors to remember that lesbians represent a hidden minority (Fassinger, 1991). It is vital not to assume that clients are heterosexual until this is explored. Even then, clients in very early stages of development, stages marked by confusion, may have difficulty responding to counselors' probes. It is important to remember that when a counselor assumes a lesbian client is heterosexual, not only are the lesbian aspects of her identity missed, but the assumed heterosexual aspects are incorrectly classified (Whitman, Cormier, & Boyd, 2000). Thus, counselors need to become comfortable with addressing sexual orientation openly with all clients.

## Annotated Bibliography

Brown, L. S. (1996). Ethical concerns with sexual minority patients. In R. P. Cabaj & T. S. Stein (Eds.), *Textbook of homosexuality and mental health* (pp. 897–916). Washington, DC: American Psychiatric Press.
Brown offers some important information with respect to ethical considerations in working with lesbian (and gay male and bisexual) clients. She makes it clear that sexual orientation identity development is a process for both clients and counselors and that there are ethical considerations pertaining to the interaction between the two.

Cass, V. C. (1979). Homosexual identity formation: A theoretical model. *Journal of Homosexuality, 4,* 219–235.
Cass, V. C. (1996). Sexual orientation identity formation: A Western phenomenon. In R. P. Cabaj & T. S. Stein (Eds.), *Textbook of homosexuality and mental health* (pp. 227–251).
Although somewhat dated now, the 1979 article is considered a classic in terms of gay and lesbian identity development. It was the first of the early

models to really take hold and even now is used often in research and practice. It is the model that served as the basis for many later models and should be considered "must" reading from a historical perspective if nothing else. The 1996 article represents a more updated approach to lesbian identity development.

D'Augelli, A. R., & Patterson, C. J. (Eds.). (1995). *Lesbian, gay, and bisexual identities over the lifespan: Psychological perspectives.* New York: Oxford University Press.
D'Augelli, A. R., & Patterson, C. J. (Eds.). (2001). *Lesbian, gay, and bisexual identities in youth.* New York: Oxford University Press.
These two books represent the most comprehensive single sources for information on developmental issues facing lesbians (and gay men and bisexual people). They focus less on development of a lesbian (or gay male or bisexual) identity per se and more on the developmental issues that sexual minorities face at different stages of the lifespan. The 1995 book goes across the lifespan, while the 2001 book focuses on adolescence and young adulthood, which is a critical period for sexual minorities.

Matthews, C. R., & Bieschke, K. J. (2001). Adapting the Ethnocultural Assessment to gay and lesbian clients: The Sexual Orientation Enculturation Assessment. *Journal of Humanistic Counseling, Education, and Development, 40,* 58–73.
Although not a formal assessment instrument, this article does offer an approach to help practitioners determine where clients are in the process of transitioning from a heterosexual identity to a lesbian (or gay) identity. Because virtually all people are raised with the assumption that they are heterosexual, adapting a lesbian (or gay) identity means giving up that majority identity as well as developing a "new" minority identity. This article provides an informal process for assessing client status in making that transition.

McCarn, S. R., & Fassinger, R. E. (1996). Revisioning sexual minority identity formation: A new model of lesbian identity and its implications for counseling and research. *The Counseling Psychologist, 24,* 508–534.
This is the current state of the art with respect to lesbian identity development. Although this chapter presents a brief overview of the model, it is worth reading the entire article to get a sense of its richness. Recognition of the parallel processes that are occurring for the individual at both the individual level and the member-of-a-minority-group level was a major advancement.

# References

American Counseling Association (ACA). (n.d.). *Discrimination based on sexual orientation: History of the American Counseling Association's position.* [Brochure]. Alexandria, VA: Author.
American Counseling Association (ACA) Governing Council. (2004). ACA Governing Council minutes. Retrieved December 16, 2004, from American

Counseling Association Web site: http://www.counseling.org/AM/Template.cfm?section&Template=/search/SearchDisplay.cfm.

American Psychological Association (APA). (1975). Proceedings of the American Psychological Association for the year 1974: Minutes of the annual meeting of the Council of Representatives. *American Psychologist, 30*, 620–651.

American Psychological Association (APA). (2000). Guidelines for psychotherapy with lesbian, gay, and bisexual clients. *American Psychologist, 55*, 1440–1451.

Association for Gay, Lesbian, and Bisexual Issues in Counseling (AGLBIC). (n.d.). Competencies for counseling gay, lesbian, bisexual, and transgendered (GLBT) clients. Retrieved June 25, 2002, from http://www.aglbic.org/competencies.html.

Bieschke, K. J., & Matthews, C. R. (1996). Career counselor attitudes towards gay, lesbian, and bisexual clients. *Journal of Vocational Behavior, 48*, 243–255.

Bradford, J., Ryan, C., & Rothblum, E. D. (1994). National lesbian health care survey: Implications for mental health care. *Journal of Consulting and Clinical Psychology, 62*, 228–242.

Bringaze, T. B., & White, L. J. (2001). Living out proud: Factors contributing to healthy identity development in lesbian leaders. *Journal of Mental Health Counseling, 23*, 162–173.

Brown, L. S. (1996). Ethical concerns with sexual minority patients. In R. P. Cabaj & T. S. Stein (Eds.), *Textbook of homosexuality and mental health* (pp. 897–916). Washington, DC: American Psychiatric Press.

Buhrke, R. A. (1989). Female student perspectives on training in lesbian and gay issues. *The Counseling Psychologist, 17*, 629–636.

Cass, V. C. (1979). Homosexual identity formation: A theoretical model. *Journal of Homosexuality, 4*, 219–235.

Cass, V. C. (1984). Homosexual identity formation: Testing a theoretical model. *Journal of Sex Research, 20*, 143–167.

Cass, V. C. (1996). Sexual orientation identity formation: A Western phenomenon. In R. P. Cabaj & T. S. Stein (Eds.), *Textbook of homosexuality and mental health* (pp. 227–251). Washington, DC: American Psychiatric Press.

Chan, C. S. (1989). Issues of identity development among Asian-American lesbians and gay men. *Journal of Counseling and Development, 68*, 16–20.

Chapman, B. E., & Brannock, J. C. (1987). Proposed model of lesbian identity development: An empirical examination. *Journal of Homosexuality, 14*(3/4), 69–80.

Cochran, S. D., Sullivan, J. G., & Mays, V. M. (2003). Prevalence of mental disorders, psychological distress, and mental health service use among lesbian, gay, and bisexual adults in the United States [Electronic version]. *Journal of Consulting and Clinical Psychology, 71*, 53–61.

D'Augelli, A. R. (2002). Mental health problems among lesbian, gay, and bisexual youths ages 14 to 21. *Clinical Child Psychology and Psychiatry, 7*, 433–456.

D'Augelli, A. R., & Patterson, C. J. (2001). *Lesbian, gay, and bisexual identities in youth.* New York: Oxford University Press.

Dillon, F. R., Worthington, R. L., Savoy, H. B., Rooney, S. C., Becker-Schutte, A., & Guerra, R. M. (2004). On becoming allies: A qualitative study of lesbian-, gay-, and bisexual-affirmative counselor training. *Counselor Education and Supervision, 43*, 162–178.

Fassinger, R. E. (1991). The hidden minority: Issues and challenges in working with lesbian women and gay men. *The Counseling Psychologist, 19*, 157–176.

Gonsiorek, J. C. (1991). The empirical basis for the demise of the illness model of homosexuality. In J. C. Gonsiorek & J. D. Weinrich (Eds.), *Homosexuality: Research implications for public policy* (pp. 115–136). Newbury Park, CA: Sage.

Graham, D. L. R., Rawlings, E. I., Halpern, H. S., & Hermes, J. (1984). Therapists' needs for training in counseling lesbians and gay men. *Professional Psychology: Research and Practice, 15*, 482–496.

Gramick, J. (1984). Developing a lesbian identity. In T. Darty & S. Potter (Eds.), *Women-identified women* (pp. 31–44). Palo Alto, CA: Mayfield.

Greene, B. (1998). "Family, ethnic identity, and sexual orientation: African-American lesbians and gay men," in C. J. Patterson & A. R. D'Augelli (Eds.), *Lesbian, gay, and bisexual identities in families: Psychological perspectives* (pp. 40–52). New York: Oxford University Press.

Grossman, A. H., D'Augelli, A. R., & O'Connell, T. S. (2003). Being lesbian, gay, bisexual and sixty or older in North America. In L. D. Garnets & D. C. Kimmel (Eds.), *Psychological perspectives on lesbian, gay, and bisexual experiences* (2nd ed., pp. 629–645). New York: Columbia University Press.

Herek, G. M. (1995). Psychological heterosexism in the United States. In A. R. D'Augelli & C. J. Patterson (Eds.), *Lesbian, gay, and bisexual identities over the lifespan* (pp. 321–346). New York: Oxford University Press.

Human Rights Campaign (n.d.). Marriage/Relationship Recognition. Retrieved June 19, 2006, from http://www.hrc.org.

Hooker, E. (1996). Epilogue. In R. P. Cabaj & T. S. Stein (Eds.), *Textbook of homosexuality and mental health* (pp. 917–919). Washington, DC: American Psychiatric Press.

Israel, T., & Hackett, G. (2004). Counselor education on lesbian, gay, and bisexual issues: Comparing information and attitude exploration. *Counselor Education and Supervision, 43*, 179–191.

Kitzinger, C., & Wilkinson, S. (1995). Transitions from heterosexuality to lesbianism: The discursive production of lesbian identities. *Developmental Psychology, 31*, 95–104.

Liu, P., and Chan, C. (1996). Lesbian, gay, and bisexual Asian Americans and their families. In J. Laird & R. J. Green (Eds.), *Lesbians and gays in couples and families: A handbook for therapists* (pp. 137–152). San Francisco: Jossey-Bass.

Loiacano, D. K. (1989). Gay identity issues among Black Americans: Racism and homophobia, and the need for validation. *Journal of Counseling and Development, 68*, 21–35.

Martell, C. R., Safren, S. A., & Prince, S. E. (2004). *Cognitive-Behavioral therapies with lesbian, gay, and bisexual clients*. New York: Guilford.

Matthews, C. R., & Bieschke, K. J. (2001). Adapting the Ethnocultural Assessment to gay and lesbian clients: The Sexual Orientation Enculturation Assessment. *Journal of Humanistic Counseling, Education, and Development, 40*, 58–73.

Matthews, C. R., & Bieschke, K. J. (2003, August). *Factors influencing psychologists' affirmative attitudes and behaviors with GLB clients*. Poster presented at the 111th Annual Convention of the American Psychological Association, Toronto, Ontario, Canada.

Matthews, C. R., Selvidge, M. M. D., & Fisher, K. (2005). Addiction counselors' attitudes and behaviors toward lesbian, gay, and bisexual clients. *Journal of Counseling and Development, 83*, 57–65.

McCarn, S. R., & Fassinger, R. E. (1996). Revisioning sexual minority identity formation: A new model of lesbian identity and its implications for counseling and research. *The Counseling Psychologist, 24*, 508–534.

Modricin, M. J., & Wyers, N. L. (1990). Lesbian and gay couples: Where they turn when help is needed. *Journal of Gay and Lesbian Psychotherapy, 1*(3), 89–104.

Mohr, J. J. (2002). Heterosexual identity and the heterosexual therapist: An identity perspective on sexual orientation dynamics in psychotherapy. *The Counseling Psychologist, 30*, 532–566.

Morales, E. S. (1990). Ethnic minority families and minority gays and lesbians. In F. W. Bozett & M. B. Sussman (Eds.), *Homosexuality and family relations* (pp. 217–239). New York: Harrington Park Press.

Parks, C. A. (1999). Lesbian identity development: An examination of differences across generations. *American Journal of Orthopsychiatry, 69*, 347–361.

Pearson, Q. M. (2003). Breaking the silence in the counselor education classroom: A training seminar on counseling sexual minority clients. *Journal of Counseling and Development, 81*, 292–300.

Phillips, J. C., & Fischer, A. R. (1998). Graduate students' training experiences with lesbian, gay, and bisexual issues. *The Counseling Psychologist, 26*, 712–734.

Pilkington, N. W., & Cantor, J. M. (1996). Perceptions of heterosexual bias in professional psychology programs: A survey of graduate students. *Professional Psychology: Research and Practice, 27*, 604–612.

Pope, M. (1995). The "salad bowl" is big enough for us all: An argument for the inclusion of lesbians and gay men in any definition of multiculturalism. *Journal of Counseling and Development, 73*, 301–304.

Reid, J. D. (1995). Development in late life: Older lesbian and gay lives. In A. R. D'Augelli & C. J. Patterson (Eds.), *Lesbian, gay, and bisexual identities over the lifespan: Psychological perspectives* (pp. 213–240). New York: Oxford University Press.

Reynolds, A. L. (2003). Counseling issues for lesbian and bisexual women. In M. Kopala & M. A. Keitel (Eds.), *Handbook of counseling women* (pp. 53–73). Thousand Oaks, CA: Sage.

Ritter, K. Y., & Terndrup, A. I. (2002). *Handbook of affirmative psychotherapy with lesbians and gay men*. New York: Guilford.

Rivers, I., & D'Augelli, A. R. (2001). The victimization of lesbian, gay, and bisexual youths. In A. R. D'Augelli & C. J. Patterson (Eds.), *Lesbian, gay, and bisexual identities and youth: Psychological perspectives* (pp. 199–238).

Rudolph, J. (1988). Counselors' attitudes toward homosexuality: A selective review of the literature. *Journal of Counseling and Development, 67*, 165–168.

Savin-Williams, R. C. (1990). *Gay and lesbian youth: Expressions of identity*. New York: Hemisphere.

Scott. R. L. (Producer) & Reyna, E. (Producer/Director). (1995). *Psychotherapy with gay and lesbian clients: Vol. 3. Coming out* [Motion picture]. (Available from Buendia Productions, P. O. Box 1869, Santa Ana, CA, 92702)

Sevig, T., & Etzkorn, J. (2001). Transformative training: A year-long multicultural counseling seminar for graduate students. *Journal of Multicultural Counseling and Development, 29*, 57–72.

Sophie, J. (1986). A critical examination of lesbian identity development. *Journal of Homosexuality, 12*(2), 39–51.

Sorensen, L., & Roberts, S. J. (1997). Lesbian uses of and satisfaction with mental health services: Results from Boston Lesbian Health Project. *Journal of Homosexuality, 33*(1), 35–49.

Thompson, C. A. (1992). Lesbian grief and loss issues in the coming out process. *Women and Therapy, 12*, 175–185.

Whitman, J. S., Cormier, S., & Boyd, C. J. (2000). Lesbian identity management at various stages of the coming out process: A qualitative study. *International Journal of Sexuality and Gender Studies, 5*, 3–18.

Worthington, R. L., Savoy, H. B., Dillon, F. R., & Vernaglia, E. R. (2002). Heterosexual identity development: A multidimensional model of individual and social identity. *The Counseling Psychologist, 30*, 496–531.

# CHAPTER TEN

# Gay Male Identity Development and Counseling

## John Marszalek and Mark Pope

G ays and lesbians are more visible than ever in the United States. In the November 2006 elections, sixty-seven openly gay/lesbian candidates were elected to local, state, and federal offices, including two reelected to the U.S. House of Representatives (Gay and Lesbian Victory Fund, 2006). It is no longer surprising to see gay characters on television and in the movies, and viable gay communities thrive in large urban areas. Nevertheless, many Americans still consider being gay an abomination, and others, although they tolerate the fact that some people are gay, do not believe gays deserve equal rights under the law. In November 2004, eleven states passed constitutional amendments banning same-sex marriage, in 2006 the president of the United States called for a federal constitutional amendment banning same-sex marriage, and as of 2007, no federal laws had been enacted to ban workplace discrimination based on sexual orientation. Most organized religions consider being gay sinful. Consequently gay men are often unsure when it is safe to come out at work, in their communities, in their churches, and to their families because of these societal messages that indicate that it is not okay to be gay.

When gay men begin developing same-sex feelings that do not match the messages of the environment (i.e., homosexuality is bad), they may disguise their feelings behind a mask of heterosexuality and internalize negative societal messages. As the same sexual feelings are repressed, they experience incongruence between conflicting components of their true selves and their false selves (Beard & Glickauf-Hughes, 1994). This internal battle may be felt in various forms including depression, anxiety, physical symptoms, and internalized homophobia (Beard & Glickauf-Hughes, 1994; Gonsiorek, 1995; Hopke, 1993). It is no surprise, then, that gay youth are more likely than heterosexual youth use to illegal drugs, alcohol, and tobacco at an earlier age and are at a higher risk for suicide (Cochran, Ackerman, Mays, & Ross, 2004; Frankowski & American Academy of Pediatrics, 2004).

Counselors can help gay men by providing gay affirmative counseling to counter the negative societal messages concerning homosexuality that many gay clients have internalized and to affirm individuals' identities as gay men. Helping gay men develop positive identities is important because research confirms that gay identity development is directly related to psychological adjustment (Marszalek, Dunn, & Cashwell, 2002; Miranda & Storms, 1989). In order to help gay men develop a positive gay identity, counselors must be aware of the process of gay identity development.

In this chapter the concept of gay identity is introduced and implications for counseling are discussed. After reading, you should have an understanding of the process of gay identity development and should be able to answer the following questions: (1) What are the stages of Cass's (1979) Homosexual Identity Formation model? (2) What are the styles of Ivey's (1990) Developmental Counseling Therapy (DCT) theory? (3) How is gay identity development related to DCT? (4) How does a person discover that he is gay? (5) How can counselors help gay clients progress through the developmental process? (6) What is gay affirmative counseling?

## Gay Male Identity

James tells his counselor, "What's happening with me? I'm so confused? How can I be having feelings about another man?"

A year later James has "come out" as a gay man. He tells his counselor, "For the first time in my life I feel like I know who I am. It feels so freeing to finally accept that I am gay and to just be myself."

Does this story sound far fetched? It is not as unusual as you might think. But you may be wondering, "How can someone who seemed heterosexual suddenly become confused and then later become certain of being gay and accept this identity?" It is this question that has led

## ABOUT THE CHAPTER AUTHORS

### John Marszalek

During my doctoral program, I read Allen Ivey's (1990) book, *Developmental Therapy*. I had already become familiar with gay identity development models and was astounded to discover that Ivey's DCT theory applied to gay identity development as described by Vivienne Cass. At the encouragement of my dissertation chair, I called Dr. Ivey to see if he would chat with me about his thoughts on how DCT applied to gay identity development. When I was able to track him down on the phone and told him why I was calling, he said something like, "I've been waiting for your call. I wondered when someone would apply DCT to gay identity development."

I'm thrilled to have this chapter included in *Lenses*. I hope that you find the application of Ivey's and Cass's theories to gay identity development and counseling as powerful as I have.

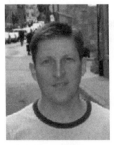

**John Marszalek**

*John Marszalek*, Ph.D., LPC, NCC, LMFT, is an assistant professor of counseling at Xavier University of Louisiana. His research interests include gay identity development and dream interpretation. John has worked with gay men and lesbians in private practice and community agencies. He splits his time between New Orleans and Columbus, Mississippi, where he is the happiest when he is playing the piano, jogging, or going with his family to watch the Mississippi State University Bulldogs play any sport.

### Mark Pope

I teach cultural identity development (both ethnic/racial and gay/lesbian) every semester in my multicultural classes and in my clinical classes. My students love this information because it gives them a simple, shorthand way to understand a complex phenomenon. They seem to be able to apply it quickly (if not always fully) to their practice; it does allow them to have a beginning place to understand other human beings and their identity development processes, and also why it's important.

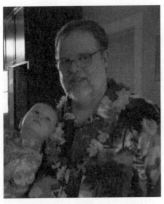

*Mark Pope*, Ed.D., LPC, LP, NCC, MCC, MAC, ACS, is a professor of counseling and family therapy at the University of Missouri– Saint Louis. He is editor of *The Career Development Quarterly* (2005–2008) and a former president of the American Counseling Association (2003–2004), National Career Development Association (1998–1999), and Association for Gay, Lesbian, and Bisexual Issues in Counseling (1975–1977). He is a fellow of a whole bunch of professional societies and has received a whole bunch of awards for his work. He loves his partner, Mario, and work deeply. He is a member of the Saint Francis River Band of Cherokees, and his current career vision is someday to be president of a small liberal arts college.

**Mark Pope and daughter**

theorists to develop models to describe the process of gay identity development: a process in which gay men first become aware of same-sex feelings, accept these feelings, transfer these feelings into behavior, identify with other gay men, disclose these feelings, and integrate these feelings into their overall identities (Cass, 1979; Coleman, 1981/1982; Hencken & O'Dowd, 1977; Lee, 1977; Plummer, 1975; Troiden, 1984, 1988).

The gay identity development process can be a lifelong, complex process and can begin at any age. We have worked with clients who were first considering the possibility that they were gay in their fifties, and we have worked with clients who identified themselves as gay in junior high school. Although the age at which gay men come out to others has decreased, most likely due to increased resources, support, and visibility in the gay community (Ryan & Futterman, 1998), acceptance of self in an often heterosexist environment can be a lifelong process.

## Cass's Homosexual Identity Formation Model

Although more than twenty-five years old, Vivienne Cass's (1979) Homosexual Identity Formation (HIF) is the most frequently cited model in the literature on gay/lesbian identity development and set the groundwork for future gay/lesbian identity development models (Troiden, 1984). Cass's model is one of the most comprehensive models because it integrates both psychological and sociological perspectives of gay/lesbian identity (Levine & Evans, 1991) and applies to both gay men and lesbians across the lifespan (Barret & Logan, 2002). According to Cass (1990), gay identity is viewed as a developmental process in which the individual plays an active role in forming an identity and is affected by interactions with the environment. For example, a gay man who begins to notice that he is having same-sex feelings might meet other gay people who affirm his feelings or he could attend a fundamentalist religion that encourages him to repress his feelings. His progress in forming a gay identity, then, could be affected by the amount of challenge or support in his environment.

Cass (1979, 1984) based her HIF model on her observations of her gay male and lesbian clients and proposed a six-stage model to describe the gay identity process: (1) confusion, (2) comparison, (3) tolerance, (4) acceptance, (5) pride, and (6) synthesis. Prior to stage one, confusion, individuals have not yet even considered the possibility of their being gay. We will describe the stages of the HIF model in more detail below as we compare them to Ivey's Developmental Counseling Therapy (DCT) theory.

## Ivey's Developmental Counseling Therapy Theory

Marszalek and Cashwell (1998) noted that Ivey's (1990) Development Counseling Therapy (DCT) can be applied to gay identity development. In DCT, Ivey applied Piaget's (1965, 1973) childhood cognitive development to adult cognitive development. According to Ivey, adults use four different styles as they process various issues in their lives and make meaning of their environments. Each of the DCT styles parallels the HIF stages (Marszalek & Cashwell, 1998). To explain the DCT model and how it applies to Cass's gay identity development theory, we are going to lead you through an exercise based on DCT questioning strategies (Ivey, Ivey, Myers, & Sweeney, 2005). As you work through this exercise, either record your responses in writing or hold onto to them in your mind. We will return to the exercise several times as we explain DCT and Cass's HIF model.

---

### READER EXERCISE

Think of one early recollection from your childhood or adolescence of a time when you first noticed that you were attracted to or had emotional feelings about someone. Focus on the image in your mind of that early recollection. Try to imagine yourself in that image as if it were happening right now. Ask yourself the following questions as you imagine yourself in this image: What do I see? What do I hear? What am I feeling? What I am sensing in my body?

---

## Early Sensorimotor Style/Pre-Confusion Stage

This first style of DCT is sensorimotor in which one focuses on the five senses and bodily sensations in making meaning of issues and experiences.

---

### READER EXERCISE

Think back on the image you focused on in your mind. You may have felt vague feelings that you could not describe. You may have felt sensations in your body as you focused on the image. You may have recalled a smell or sound or something else from your five senses that you actually experienced as you focused on the image.

---

For gay men, instead of focusing on an image, they would be experiencing a present moment. Early in this stage, termed *pre-confusion* by Cass (1979), they might experience vague feelings but may not know what they are. They may not even recognize that they are having vague feelings. Many gay men can recall feeling different from others around them before they even thought of the possibility of being gay.

James, the client described in the beginning of this chapter, recalled an image of playing soccer with other children in junior high school. He recalled vague feelings of attraction to another player and also feelings of being different from the other boys. Of course, at the time, he was not able to label these feelings or even be aware of what they were. This is an example of the beginning of the process of gay identity development.

---

### READER EXERCISE

Now focus on your recollection again. Put yourself into that image as if you are yourself years ago when you had the experience. What is going through your mind? What do you make of this experience?

---

## Late Sensorimotor Style/Confusion Stage

Evidence of progression from having feelings and sensations to beginning to think about them even if the thoughts are not logical and connected is the late sensorimotor style.

---

### READER EXERCISE

As you focused on your recollection, you may have had random, unconnected thoughts about the experience. You may have been unsure about what you were feeling or how to put your feelings into words.

---

A gay person may become aware of same-sex feelings/thoughts and become confused (Cass, 1979). According to Cass, this confusion is often triggered by an event in one's environment. These events can lead to a conflict inside a gay man because his same-sex feelings/thoughts did not match his belief that he is heterosexual. During this stage, gay men deny these feelings/thoughts or rationalize what they are experiencing.

For example, James recalled noticing in junior high that he could not stop thinking about another boy on his soccer team. He also recalled seeing a gay man in a movie and being fascinated with the character. During counseling, James recalled saying to himself, "Why am I feeling this way? What is happening to me? It will probably go away when I get to high school."

## READER EXERCISE

Now back to your image of an early recollection. Can you still put yourself in the image? This time, look around and describe to yourself what is happening. Who is there? Where are you? What are you saying? What are you doing? What are other people saying and doing? Can you describe what you are feeling?

### Early Concrete Style/Comparison Stage

If you can answer the questions in the previous exercise, you are focusing on the concrete details of your image and developing awareness from an early concrete style that is characterized by concrete, detailed language. You can observe this concrete style of awareness when people describe the details of their days to you or answer your questions in short, single-word responses.

How does this style apply to gay identity development? In this stage, termed *comparison* by Cass (1979), a gay man acknowledges the details of what he is experiencing and compares them to other men in his life. That does not mean, however, that gay men in this style of awareness would acknowledge being gay. For example, a man might rationalize that "I have same-sex feelings or I had sex with someone of the same sex, but I'm still heterosexual." It is possible to acknowledge feelings but not make the connection to one's identity. In addition, Cass stated that a man might think of being gay as a possibility but not commit to a gay identity.

James recalled noticing when he was thinking about Tom, another player on his soccer team, and noticing how he felt when Tom spoke to him. As far as he knew, his experiences of attraction did not compare to other boys around him and the men in his family who he believed were attracted to women. He did not know what to think of his experiences and pushed them to the back of his mind; they felt too uncomfortable.

### Late Concrete Operational Style/Tolerance Stage

When you use logical and if/then causal reasoning, you are using a late concrete operational style (Ivey et al., 2005, p. 141. In a late concrete operational style of awareness, you make the connection that you feel, sense, think, or behave in a certain way in a particular circumstance.

## READER EXERCISE

If you reflect on your early recollection, can you complete the following statement: "When I focus on this image in my mind, I feel _____." For example, you might think: "When I focus on this image I feel happy." In this case you might be feeling the happiness at a sensorimotor style and then make the connection that you feel that feeling when you focus on the image.

When applied to gay identity development, a gay man using a late concrete style in focusing on his identity can use causal thinking to describe his same-sex feelings, thoughts, or emotions. Cass (1979) stated that a man in her *tolerance stage* may tolerate the possibility that he is gay, but not fully embrace it or believe that it is true. He may experiment sexually or emotionally through dating; he may connect with other gay people but still not commit to an identity, continuing to have mixed feelings.

During counseling, James recalled thinking to himself, "whenever I look at Tom, I feel nervous" and "whenever I think about him I feel warm inside." However, James still did not accept the idea that he was gay. Like James, gay man in this stage may rationalize that they have same-sex feelings only with one person or in certain instances.

### Early Formal Style/Acceptance Stage

Gay men using an early formal-operational style begin to recognize the patterns among their same-sex feelings, thoughts, and behaviors. They realize that they are emotionally and physically attracted to members of the same sex in several different instances, a pattern they had not acknowledged prior to this point. Cass (1979) stated that gay men are in a stage of *acceptance* when they acknowledge that they are gay.

What can trigger this realization for a gay man? It can be meeting other gay people, talking to a counselor or friends, or reading about a gay character that reminds him of himself. According to Cass (1979), as men accept their gay identities, they may increasingly connect with other gay people and enter the gay community.

## READER EXERCISE

Now return to the image in your mind. Think of what you've done with the image so far. You've put yourself in it and become aware of your senses, feelings, and thoughts. Then you described to yourself the concrete details of what was happening and what you were feeling. Next you used causal, if/then thinking to connect your feelings, senses, and/or thoughts to details in the image. Now let's move to the next style of awareness. Can you think of another time in your past or even today when you found yourself attracted to someone emotionally or physically? Can you think of a time when you felt similarly to how you did when you explored your first image. Take a moment and focus on this second image. Be aware of your senses, feelings, and thoughts. Describe the details of the image to yourself, especially focusing on what you are doing and what others are doing. Then see if you notice any similarities or any patterns between the two experiences you have recalled. For example, you may have noticed that in both experiences you became nervous and stammered when you were with a person to whom you felt an attraction. In this case you are developing a formal operational style of awareness in which you reflect on your concrete descriptions of events and recognize patterns. You recognize that when you were with that person in your first image, you were nervous. And you were also nervous when you were with another person to whom you were attracted. You see a pattern that you get nervous and stammer when you are attracted to someone emotionally or physically.

For James, meeting other gay men helped him to understand his sexual orientation from a formal operational style. His counselor had encouraged him to attend a support group for those who were struggling with the coming out process or were questioning if they were gay. Meeting other gay men who discussed similar stories helped James to realize that his feelings were not abnormal and that he was gay.

## Late Formal Operational Style/Pride Stage

For a gay man, an awareness of his gay identity at a late formal style would be seeing the pattern of patterns in regards to his being gay. For example, in early formal operations a man might make the connection that his behavior, thoughts, and emotions are gay. He might see another pattern of being treated differently every time someone thought he was gay. Recognizing these patterns might lead to an awareness that "society is going to treat me differently because I am gay and this is something I'll have to deal with the rest of my life."

---

## READER EXERCISE

If you are able, go back to your images of your two recollections of being attracted physically or emotionally to someone. Think about the pattern you identified. Can you think of other times when you experienced the same pattern. I gave you an example before of a pattern of getting nervous and stammering when attracted to someone emotionally or physically. Someone who gets nervous and stammers when they meet someone to whom they are emotionally or physically attracted may realize that they do the same thing when they meet people of importance at their jobs. They may recognize a "pattern of patterns"—a new style of awareness. There is a pattern of being nervous and stammering in situations in which they have to perform. Can you see a pattern of patterns in your experiences?

---

Cass (1979) stated that a gay man enters a *pride stage* when he becomes aware of the dichotomy between his view of his gay identity as acceptable versus society's rejection of this identity. People deal with this dichotomy by directing their feelings of anger at heterosexuals or feeling a sense of belonging with the gay community. For many gay men in a pride stage, sharing their coming-out stories with other gay men is important for understanding how their journeys have been similar and for feeling a shared struggle with the gay community. Gay men see patterns in each others' experiences and feel affirmed.

Over time, James became more involved in the gay community, and he realized that he was feeling a part of a group. He began to experience anger that many in his church considered gay people to be an abomination. He said to his counselor, "Now that I have accepted that I am gay, I can't imagine being straight. If someone offered me a pill that would make me straight, I wouldn't take it. Why can't other people understand that?"

## Early Dialectic Style/Synthesis Stage

Piaget's (1965, 1973) last stage in his child cognitive development model was formal operations. Ivey (1990) theorized that adults are capable of abstract reasoning that extends beyond Piaget's formal-operations stage. He used Plato's concepts of knowledge and intelligence to define this post-abstract thinking of the *dialectic style.* It is possible for people to reach new styles of awareness by understanding that their views of the world are influenced by their dialectic with the environment; in other words, they understand that they do not live in a vacuum and that they cannot avoid being influenced by the environment in which they exist.

A gay man using a dialectic style to contemplate his gay identity would already have acknowledged and accepted a gay identity. He would have become a part of the gay community. And now he would, as Cass (1979) described in her *synthesis stage,* integrate his gay identity into his overall identity. He would think about how various aspects of his identity can be intertwined and how his environment has

---

### READER EXERCISE

Now one last time, can you return to your images of your recollections of being attracted physically or emotionally to others? Think about the patterns you identified and the pattern of patterns of which you became aware. What do you make of it all? How do you put it all together? How has your family and/or your environment influenced you? We gave you an example before of a person recognizing a pattern of getting nervous and stammering when he is attracted to someone emotionally or physically. Then he might recognize a pattern of being nervous and stammering in situations in which he has to perform. Now going a step further, he might realize that he grew up around perfectionistic people; that no matter what he did, it was never good enough. He always felt like he was performing. He realizes that his experience with his family has impacted the way he views the world today and that the world is a place in which one has to perform. Is it possible for you to see how your environment has influenced you?

influenced his identity development. For example, James had a deeper understanding of how society and his family had influenced his gay identity development. He could reflect on how his gay identity was related to and affected aspects of his overall identity such as his gender identity and spiritual identity.

According to Ivey (1990), as adults develop in a dialectics style, they realize that their knowledge and understanding of their experiences is constantly fluctuating in a process that Ivey (1990) termed *dialectic deconstruction*. Knowledge or beliefs that previously seemed fixed are deconstructed, leading to new points of view. New perspectives may lead to the beginning of another cycle through development, because this new knowledge is initially processed at less complex cognitive styles. Consequently, for those individuals who are capable of thinking at a late dialectic style, higher styles of thinking lead to new insight. This newfound insight is frequently reprocessed at pre-operational and concrete thinking styles before individuals process it at a more abstract style (Ivey, 1990).

James, as with other gay men, had experiences that challenged his thinking. For example, one night James was sitting outside a coffee shop frequented by gays and lesbians in the community. Several men drove by the shop and threw a bucket of paint at the people sitting at the café tables and yelled homophobic slurs. James felt a sense of helplessness and an intense anger. He realized that he had become so comfortable in the gay community that he forgotten how much hatred toward gays and lesbians existed in this country. It reminded him that people hated him who did not even know him. He felt so angry that his stomach hurt and for a brief moment he thought that all heterosexuals could not be trusted. In the next instant he realized that he was sitting with one of his best friends, Cheryl, who was heterosexual and to whom he could always turn when he needed support. He realized that there could be other heterosexuals at work or in his neighborhood that could also be like Cheryl but that he shut out because of his fear of the hatred. In a mater of moments, James had cycled through the developmental styles of DCT and had developed deeper insight into himself.

## Counseling Implications

Understanding the process of gay identity development is one of many essentials involved in providing gay affirmative counseling to gay clients. Gay affirmative counseling includes counselors being aware of

TABLE 10.1    Parallels Between Ivey's Developmental Counseling
Therapy (DCT) and Cass's Homosexual Identity
Formation (HIF) Model

| Ivey's DCT | Cass's HIF Model |
| --- | --- |
| **Sensorimotor Style** | |
| Early sensorimotor | Pre-Stage One |
| Late sensorimotor | Stage One: Confusion |
| **Concrete Operational Style** | |
| Early concrete | Stage Two: Comparison |
| Late concrete | Stage Three: Tolerance |
| **Formal Operational Style** | |
| Early formal | Stage Four: Acceptance |
| Late formal | Stage Five: Pride |
| **Dialectic/Systemic Style** | |
| Early dialectic | Stage Six: Synthesis articulation |
| Dialectic Deconstruction | |

their own strengths and weaknesses in working with gay clients, being
able to use a variety of counseling interventions, countering the negative societal messages concerning homosexuality that many gay clients
have internalized, affirming individuals' identities as gay men, viewing homosexuality as an alternative sexual orientation identity to
heterosexuality, not viewing homosexuality as a disorder to be cured,
and understanding major issues for gay men that may arise during
counseling (Harrison, 2000; Maylon, 1993). These major issues include

## READER EXERCISE

As you worked through this mental exercise, did you develop any
new understandings about yourself? Did you develop any new
perspectives on what a gay man experiences in becoming aware
of and accepting his sexual orientation?

the impact of negative societal attitudes toward gay men and lesbians, discrimination in the legal, societal, and religious arenas, same-sex relationship dynamics, the effect of AIDS on the gay community, and identity development issues (Fassinger, 1991; Hall & Fradkin, 1992; Maylon, 1993; McHenry & Johnson, 1993).

Gay affirmative counseling approaches have been proposed to promote positive identity and psychological adjustment among gay men and lesbians (Browning, Reynolds, & Dworkin, 1991; Fassinger, 1991; Gumaer, 1987; Hall & Fradkin, 1992; Kauhlwein, 1992; Marszalek & Cashwell, 1998; Shannon & Woods, 1991). These approaches have not developed new techniques or counseling theories but have advocated integrating identity development and others issues specific to gay men that may arise during counseling with gay clients. Gay affirmative counseling approaches have usually involved applying specific techniques or specific theoretical schools such as Self-Psychology (Beard & Glickauf-Hughes, 1994) or cognitive therapy (Kauhlwein, 1992) to identity development issues. For example, a counselor might use cognitive therapy to help a client recognize how his negative, internalized belief that being gay is a sin leads to self-hate and leads him to isolate himself from the gay community.

Identity development issues include those issues that arise during each stage of identity development, as we described in the previous section. However, also included is the impact of additional identity development issues for double and triple minorities, those individuals who have two to three minority statuses based on race, gender, and/or sexual orientation (Gonsiorek & Weinrich, 1991). In addition to developing a gay identity, then, gay minorities also develop second and third identities (e.g., gender identities, ethnic identities). A major issue for gay minorities is moving through several developmental processes in order to develop positive gay and minority identities. In developing an identity with one minority group, minorities may believe that they are risking the acceptance of another group. They may feel the need to make a choice between their racial/ethnic identities versus their gay identities (Lowe & Mascher, 2001). For example, Loiacano (1989) said that some Black gay men and lesbians are afraid to come out due to fear of being ostracized in the Black community. Understanding this process can help counselors to determine when clients' presenting issues are developmental rather than pathological and help them to support clients as they proceed through the developmental process.

## Using DCT to Provide Gay
## Affirmative Counseling

We described the gay identity development process through an integration of Cass's HIF Model and Ivey's DCT theory. In addition to being a theory of adult development, DCT is also a counseling theory (Ivey et al., 2005). We have used DCT in counseling with diverse gay men in private practice, groups, and inpatient substance abuse settings. We have found it effective with our clients because of the intentionality in providing interventions based on a client's style and because of its applicability to Cass's (1979) HIF model. In addition, in an empirical study conducted with seventy-eight gay men, Marszalek, Cashwell, Dunn, & Heard (2004) found a relationship between their HIF stages and their DCT styles.

Using a DCT approach, counselors can assess the DCT style at which a client is presenting for a particular issue and provide an appropriate counseling intervention based on the client's style. Counselors can use a structured approach by leading clients through the Standard Cognitive/Emotional Developmental Interview (Ivey, Ivey, & Rigazio-DiGillio, 2005) or a more unstructured approach by integrating DCT interventions into the counseling session. One way counselors can provide an intervention is to match a client's preference for a particular cognitive style both to facilitate rapport and to expand horizontal development (or development within a style).

DCT allows the counselor to draw from a variety of theories and integrate them into the DCT framework. For example, clients who prefer to function in the sensorimotor style may benefit from an approach that involves the senses, such as relaxation, biofeedback, or Gestalt techniques. Clients who prefer the concrete style may benefit from problem solving, reality therapy, or rational emotive behavior therapy approaches. Formal operational clients respond well to client-centered methods and psychoanalytic approaches, and dialectic clients are best matched with systemic and multicultural approaches and techniques (Ivey et al., 2005).

The goal is to assist clients in experiencing as many DCT styles as possible related to a particular issue. DCT researchers have noted that clients who can use all four DCT styles have less physiological and psychological distress (Rigazio-DiGillio, Ivey, & Locke, 1997). Consequently, another way that counselors can provide an intervention is to mismatch the preferred style of the client to promote vertical development (development from one style to another). For example, when James was operating from a concrete operations style (Cass's tolerance stage) in his awareness of his gay identity, he would describe his attraction to a male friend but not make the connection that his same-sex attractions were connected to a deeper gay identity. His counselor at first worked from a concrete style using a cognitive therapy approach to help James understand how his thoughts were connected to his feelings and behaviors. Later his counselor used a person-centered and Jungian approach to place more focus on James's *inner self* and to encourage movement to a formal style.

What we find particularly valuable about DCT is that it helps us be aware of our own preferred style in counseling and the preferred style of our clients. Like many counselors, our preferred style is formal operational. If we counsel a client who operates predominantly from a formal operational style, we develop a strong relationship but can tend to overintellectualize issues unless we encourage growth in other styles such as sensorimotor. On the other hand, if we counsel a client who tends to present issues in a concrete style, we may struggle to build rapport if we attempt to push the client into a formal style too early.

## Jeff: Learning to Be Himself

The following case is written in the first-person by John Marszalek, the first author of this chapter.

Jeff, a twenty-five year old White male, called me for an appointment after seeing my advertisement in a local gay newspaper. At the time, I had a counseling private practice in a large metropolitan area in the southeast and volunteered at the local gay, lesbian, and bisexual community center. In our initial conversation on the phone, Jeff stated that he was seeking counseling for depression. He did not reveal his sexual orientation but stated that he had seen my advertisement in the local gay newspaper. We set a time to meet the following week.

At the time of our appointment, I opened my office door to find Jeff sitting in my waiting room. He was casually, though neatly, dressed and of average height and weight. I noticed that he was nervously flipping through a magazine. When I introduced myself to him, he shook my hand politely, and followed me into my office. I asked him what had brought him to counseling, and he began to tell his story. He spoke rapidly with few pauses and with good grammar.

> "I've been feeling really depressed lately. I moved here about three months ago to take a job as an accountant. I just finished my

degree in the spring and spent a lot of the summer goofing off and looking for jobs. I had really planned to stay in Buffalo, but I ended up taking the job here. Now I'm wondering if I made the right decision, and I miss my family so much. I keep thinking about all of the things they're doing that I'm missing, and I just get more depressed. (A few tears were evident in Jeff's eyes). I really could have stayed in Buffalo if I wanted to, but I really didn't look very hard. The truth is I really didn't know what I wanted to do. I was feeling confused and just needed to get out of there. But now I'm wondering if I made the right decision."

"Because you miss your family so much and are feeling depressed?" I asked.

"That's part of it. (He looked down at the floor and his voice lowered). I've been so depressed and lonely. And whenever I felt that way in the past I would go running. It seems to pick me up a little. Anyway, I had been running in a park near my apartment, and I kept seeing another guy running after work every day. A couple of weeks ago he came up to me when I had stopped at the water fountain, and we started talking. I ended up going to his house, and you know. . . ." (He looked embarrassed. He continued looking at the floor).

There was a long pause, and then he looked back at me.

"So you went to his house. . . ."

(Jeff let out a breath.) "I don't know why I did it. Tom was someone to talk to. I've been so lonely. And it was nice to just do something besides go to work, go home, and then start over again. He asked me if I wanted to go with him to his house to have a drink and then it just kind of happened. . . ."

(He paused.)

"We kind of . . . had sex."

"And how do you feel about that?" I asked.

"I'm so embarrassed . . . (Pause) . . . I can't even believe I'm telling you this."

"It's not okay to talk about having sex with another man?" I asked.

"No . . . I don't know . . . I've never talked with anyone about it before."

"It's okay to talk about it here," I said.

"I know . . . Okay . . . (Jeff's eyes were teary and he paused). I kept calling him every day after work. We would get together and do things. Not just sex. Talk and go to movies. Go running together. And then last week, he said that he needed some space.

I fell apart. He said I was a nice guy, but he wanted to be with
someone who had already come out. He gave me the newspaper
and showed me your ad."

"And you're feeling sad and hurt."

"I'm just so damn lonely. And I don't know what all this means.
I mean, am I gay?"

"What do you think?" I asked.

"I guess I've wondered for a long time but I've never really let
myself even think that."

"Because?"

"Because I'm not supposed to be gay."

"You're not supposed to be?"

"I was always the perfect one in my family. I almost became a
priest for God's sake."

"So being gay would not be okay for you."

"No . . . I don't know . . ."

"Well, you don't have to decide whether you're gay or not today.
Or even if it's okay or not today. But to help me get to know you
better, I'd like to hear more about your life. What brought you
to where you are today."

Jeff then proceeded to tell me his story.

Jeff felt very close to his parents and spoke to them frequently
on the phone. His mother was a nurse and involved in a nearby
Catholic church. He described his mother as loving, high-energy,
and very talkative.

"She has an opinion on everything. When I talk to her about
things that are bothering me, she tries to solve them and then
bugs me if I don't do what she suggested. I love her, but it drives
me up the wall sometimes. If she knew I was here, she would want
me to tell her what was wrong."

Jeff's father was a business man, and Jeff described him as a strong,
quiet man who anchored his mother. Jeff felt close to him, although
he had never felt that he fully lived up to his father's expectations.

"I'm the oldest child. My brother Frank is three years younger
than me. My father has always been a sports fanatic, and I was never
really as good in sports as Frank. I made the highest grades, and the
teachers liked me. Frank didn't do bad, but he was more of an average student. But he was popular in school because he was on the
football team. I just never got into sports like Frank and my father
did. I remember sitting across the room from them on Sunday after-
noons watching NFL football and wondering what the big deal was."

Jeff compensated by being "perfect" at everything else, especially academics and religion. Jeff's family regularly attended mass
at a Catholic church, and their priest was a friend of the family
who often came to their home after dinner. Jeff looked up to Father
Mark and was one of his altar boys at church. Jeff also developed
close relationships with the sisters who ran the parochial school.

"I always felt so calm and accepted when I was with Father
Mark. And the sisters made me feel special because I did so well
in school."

Jeff went to high school at a local Catholic boys' school and afterward entered a seminary run by an order of priests he wished to join.
He felt like he belonged there and felt a sense of brotherhood with the
other seminarians. During his second year in the seminary, he began
having a sexual affair with Bob, another seminarian with whom he had
developed a close friendship. Jeff said that Bob initiated the sex, and
Jeff went along with it because he felt close to Bob. However, after a
few months, Bob began avoiding him. When Jeff confronted him, Bob
told him that they had had fun and now it was time to focus on their
future ordinations. Jeff confided in his spiritual director about what
had happened and how it made him doubt whether he should become
a priest. His spiritual director instructed him to go to confession and
avoid any future contact with Bob. Jeff missed Bob, and he felt that he
had failed in someway. He found himself increasingly doubtful about
whether or not to be he should be in the seminary, and he could not
understand how Bob acted like nothing had happened.

I asked Jeff how he felt at that time.

"I don't know. . . . I was so pissed at him. He made it seem like
there was something wrong with me because I wanted to be with
him. It got hard to be around him but I felt so depressed when I
wasn't."

"It sounds like you really cared about him," I said.

Jeff seemed taken by surprise and sucked his breath in to hold
back his tears, "I guess I did . . . maybe I still do. . . ."

During his time in the seminary, Jeff was extremely confused and
could not understand how he could be having feelings for another man.
He had always assumed that one chose to be gay, and he simply could
not believe that God wanted him to be gay. Consequently, he did not
know what to do with his feelings and thoughts about Bob. Sometimes

he wondered if he was just lonely and had had sex with Bob like men did in a prison when there were no women around. Other times, he entertained the idea that he might be gay. During these times he felt the most guilt and depression. The thought of being gay brought him a profound sense of loneliness. He felt guilty because being gay did not match with being perfect nor what the church wanted of him. He did not know what to do with his feelings for Bob or the anger he felt when Bob began avoiding him. Against the urging of his spiritual director, Jeff left the seminary and returned to Buffalo, telling his family that he had decided that he was not meant to become a priest. He never told anyone about the confusion that he felt inside.

Jeff settled into life near his family and began taking classes at a nearby college, majoring in accounting. He blocked out his feelings and thoughts about his sexuality by throwing himself into his work. His social life focused around his family and a close friend from high school, Barbara. Although his family suspected that they were dating, his relationship with her remained platonic. From his description of her, Barbara was too passive to ever press Jeff on why their relationship never moved beyond friendship. Jeff also made some friends at college.

Near the end of his senior year, Jeff went to a gay bar with another student, Steve. They had become friends while taking classes together, and one day after class Steve invited Jeff to go out on the weekend with some of his friends and him. Jeff was surprised when they went to a gay bar and was stunned to see all of the men together in a bar.

> "What was that like for you?" I asked.
>
> "All of the guys there seemed to be having a good time talking and hanging out together. I kept wondering how they could be so happy."
>
> "It seemed surprising that gay men could be happy?"
>
> "Yea . . . I guess I figured it was the alcohol. I mean how could they be happy being gay?"

When Steve asked Jeff if he was gay, Jeff said that he had a girl-friend but that it was okay with him if Steve was gay. Nevertheless, going to the gay bar made him question himself again. One part of himself thought that if he met the right girl he would be sexually attracted to her. Another part of himself thought that even if he were gay he should be celibate as his church taught.

Any brief urges to explore his sexuality were frightening to him because he lived so close to his family. He was petrified that someone would find out that he was not perfect. And in his eyes, being gay would be an imperfection. On the other hand, he found himself drawn to the gay bar and sometimes fantasized about moving away to a place where he would not have to worry about his family finding out about his feelings.

> "The weekend would come, and I would get lonely. I'd find myself thinking about being at that bar. A couple of times I drove down to the area, but I was afraid to go in by myself."
>
> "You didn't feel comfortable talking to Steve?" I asked.
>
> "I don't know. I wasn't sure what to say. And I didn't see him around at school as much as when we had a class together."
>
> "And it didn't seem okay to talk to Barbara or your family?"
>
> "No! I can't imagine telling them. Barbara is so into church, and I don't know what my family would think. Just the thought of them finding out freaks me out."

As he grappled with these feelings, he found himself becoming irritable with his family. Family functions had been a major part of his social life, but he began to resent them. As he wrapped up his senior year and began applying for jobs, he found out that he was near the top of his class. He signed up for a job fair through the career center on campus, and several accounting firms from outside the area encouraged him to apply for positions.

> "It was exciting to have them actively recruiting me. Plus I kept fantasizing about being in a place where I could be on my own."
>
> "What did you fantasize?" I asked.
>
> "That I lived in a big city where no one knew me and I made friends like Steve's."
>
> "What was it about Steve's friends that made you want to know other people like them?"
>
> "They were nice. . . . They had all finished college, had places of their own, and just seemed happy."
>
> "What did you imagine made them happy?" I asked.
>
> "They were all friends with each other. They talked about the things they would be doing over the weekend and trips they took together. They hung out together all the time."
>
> "And that's what you wanted?"
>
> "Yea. I just wanted people to hang out with that were exciting. I love Barbara and my family, but it's not exciting to be with them. It's different."

"Tell me about the excitement."

"What do you mean?" Jeff asked.

"I'm curious about your feeling of excitement. Let's look at it a little. Sometimes when you have feelings you can feel them in your body. If you imagine yourself when you've felt excited, where do you feel it in your body?"

"Oh . . . You mean like when I get depressed and feel like there's a lump in my throat?" Jeff asked.

"Yes, that's it. When you feel excited where do you feel it in your body?"

". . . . I feel it in my chest. . . . Like there's something in there I'm trying to grab."

"Something in there you're trying to grab." I said.

"Yea — it's hard to explain."

"Tell me about a time when you felt that feeling of excitement and felt it in your chest."

"Well . . . when I was with Steve's friends, and they were talking about a trip they were going to take together to Toronto. I felt that feeling."

"That feeling of excitement."

"Yes."

"What was going through your mind?" I asked.

"I was imagining what it would be like to go with them to Toronto. How nice it would be to hang out with them."

"So if you imagine that you are there with them in Toronto, what do you see?"

"I see us all having dinner together on Yonge St."

"Anything special about Yonge St.?"

"It's a cool area of Toronto where you see all sorts of people, and you can just be yourself."

"So in your imagination, you are sitting with friends in a restaurant and being yourself?"

Jeff paused and began to tear up a little. "I guess that is what I want. It's just so scary."

## Jeff's Process of Gay Identity Development

I think that Jeff had probably vacillated between Cass's (1979) confusion and comparison stages for years. He recalled noticing in high school that he was not attracted to girls as were his other male friends. He was aware that he felt a strange feeling when he was around certain boys (that he later identified in counseling as being an attraction), but in high school he did not label the feelings. Jeff did go to school dances with girls; however, he was always the perfect gentleman. He rationalized that he was not attracted to them because he was planning to be a priest.

## Late Concrete Style/Tolerance Stage

By the time Jeff entered counseling with me he had begun working on Cass's (1979) tolerance stage evidenced by his wondering out loud if he were gay. He was not ready to wholeheartedly embrace this identity, and it was so hard for him to believe that "someone like me could be gay." He still wondered if he could make himself be attracted to women. In addition, he could not imagine ever telling his family that he was gay, and that thought alone made him feel depressed.

## Early Formal Style/Acceptance

Over time Jeff began to notice a pattern of having certain feelings when he was attracted to another man, and he realized that he had been having these feelings since he was an adolescent. He began to commit to the reality that he was a gay and had been as long as he could remember; however, he had hidden that reality behind the false self that he felt he was expected to be by society, his church, and his family.

I encouraged Jeff to go to a gay male coming-out group at the local gay community center in which I often volunteered. Another counselor led the group, and I knew that he was an effective group leader. He was a retired counselor and an openly gay man in a long-term relationship. He was a good role model for the members, and they admired him. Jeff agreed to meet with him to find out more about the group, and eventually he did join it.

As I have found with other clients with whom I have worked, the group served to speed up Jeff's progress in terms of his identity development. He heard other men's stories concerning their struggles with coming out to themselves, friends, families, and co-workers. Coincidently, another member had been a former priest, and Jeff connected with him regarding their experiences in the Catholic Church. During our sessions, Jeff would talk to me about his experiences in the group and how many of the stereotypes he had about gay men were being challenged.

After each group, many of the members would go out to dinner together. After about a month, Jeff started joining them and seeing them in other social situations. His depression began to lift as he made friends. However, he continued to feel anxious about how he was going to tell his family that he was gay and if he should. This issue was one that was discussed frequently in the coming-out group, along with how open one should be about their sexual orientation at work. Over time, Jeff seemed to be more accepting of himself but still feared how others would react if they discovered he was gay. He talked about living two lives: one in which he hid himself and one in which he could be himself. Being able to be himself in the group and with me made him feel energized because he did not have to put so much work into hiding himself. He described feeling as if he had been holding his breathe for a long time and could now release it.

I continued using a person-centered approach to help Jeff focus on his feelings. I also continued to help Jeff notice the patterns between how he felt today and how he had felt in the past; how he reacted to events today and how he had in the past. I remember asking him, "How do you imagine people would react if they knew you were gay?" He replied that they would be horrified and would reject him. He had a fantasy in his mind of his mother gasping and running out of the room as if he were a monster. He remembered feeling that way in the seminary when he worried about someone finding out about his affair with Bob. Jeff and I also talked about (as he did in the group) the reality that many people would not accept his being gay and could even be discriminatory. My challenge was to help him protect himself and be realistic about people's reactions while at the same time not assuming that everyone would react negatively. I wanted to help him develop a sense of when it was okay to come out to other people.

## Late Formal Style/Pride Stage

Over time Jeff did come out to a few co-workers whom he knew to have gay friends. He continued attending the group and along with a few other members volunteered occasionally at the community center. He became particularly close with a female volunteer who was a member of PFLAG and who had a gay son. Jeff began moving from an acceptance to a pride stage as he became more comfortable with himself but would focus on others' negative views about gays and lesbians in society.

For example, around the time I was meeting with Jeff a large fundamentalist church was causing waves in South Florida as the minister called for a repeal of nondiscrimination and domestic partnership laws in the area. After one particular coming-out group, Jeff expressed furor about the minister "saying things about me and other gay people that aren't true. How can he hate? I don't understand how someone could hate me just because I'm gay."

Talking about this minister in the coming-out group triggered Jeff's anger regarding his own experiences with his church. He expressed anger that the church expected him to be celibate because he was gay and that if he had a relationship someday the church would not recognize it. We spent many sessions helping Jeff express his anger in productive ways. I used interventions appropriate for a formal style (i.e., object relations, DCT questioning, person centered) to help Jeff identify patterns of feeling guilty and "less-than" for having same-sex feelings. Identifying these patterns helped Jeff to express his anger and to realize that he had internalized negative feelings about being gay from society and his church.

## Dialectic Style/Synthesis Stage

About a year after I had first met Jeff, he met Ron at a community center function. The two of them began dating, and Jeff and I spent time talking about relationship issues. As the dating progressed into a relationship over our second year, Jeff would revisit previous stages when he would wonder what people would think when Jeff and Ron went out on a date. He also grappled with what he would tell his family if they moved in together at some point. He eventually did tell his family, and to his surprise, they reacted well. His brother told him his family had suspected he was gay for sometime, especially after he started talking about his "friend" Ron so often.

Several events helped Jeff synthesize his identity as a gay man. One was his family's acceptance of his relationship with Ron. When the two eventually moved in together, his family sent them house warming gifts and referred to them as a couple. This support helped Jeff to be able to embrace both the gay community and his family. Another event that helped Jeff synthesize his identity was joining a local church with a gay-affirming minister and congregation. Finally, his continued friendships with people he had met in the gay community, including heterosexual volunteers, helped him.

From a DCT dialectic style or what Cass (1979) described as a synthesis stage, Jeff was able to think about how his being gay fit into his overall identity and into his place in his community. He could reflect on his own gay identity development process and understand how his view of himself as a gay man was continuing to evolve. He also understood over time how his relationship affected who he was.

## Counseling Goals

Early in the counseling process, my initial goal was to focus on the counselor–client relationship and not push Jeff to make a commitment to being gay or not. It was obvious to me that he was struggling through the gay identity development process, but I knew that pressuring a client could lead to what Cass (1979) termed *identity foreclosure*. I wanted to provide enough support so that Jeff could develop at his own pace; however, I also wanted to provide enough challenge so that Jeff did not grow too comfortable in a stalled development.

I used a DCT approach to assess Jeff's developmental style and to determine the most appropriate interventions. I realized that Jeff was using a late concrete style because he could use causal reasoning to recognize that he had had same-sex feelings for Bob and Tom; he was in an HIF tolerance stage because he tolerated the possibility of being gay but not making a commitment to it. Matching his late concrete style, I used a cognitive behavioral approach to encourage horizontal development and to challenge his irrational thoughts about the possibility of being gay and about gay people. Challenges would come up naturally during our sessions.

> For example, Jeff might state that "gay men are promiscuous and that just isn't me."
>
> I might respond by asking, "So you believe that all gay men are promiscuous?"
>
> He would then respond, "Well, I don't know about all gay men."
>
> "So you've known gay men who were not promiscuous."
>
> "Yes. Like one of the guys I work with who's been with someone over ten years. I know he's not promiscuous."
>
> "And it doesn't seem that if you were gay that you would be one of those men who are not promiscuous?"

To encourage vertical development, I would also use interventions appropriate to a formal style such as object relations' focus on the transference and on his "true self" versus "false self." For example, we would discuss who he thought he needed to be when he was with me and how that related to who he felt he had to be with other people in his life. I would also work to help him see patterns in his life by using questions from the DCT Standard Cognitive Developmental Interview (Ivey et al., 2005), such as "can you think of another time in your life when you've felt the way you feel right now." Using these questions to help Jeff identify patterns also entailed helping Jeff be aware of bodily sensations and feelings at a sensorimotor style that he had in various situations in the present and past.

## Comments

I did not hear all of Jeff's story the first session but over many sessions. Our work together did not proceed as smoothly as I have portrayed here, and I have described only the highlights of our work together over those two years. In addition, we discussed many other issues than his gay identity. When he first came to see me, his presenting issue was his confusion about being gay. However, over time other issues invariably surfaced. For example, Jeff's depression was not only caused by his struggle with being gay but was also a product of his need to be perfect. He put tremendous pressure on himself in many aspects of his life, and we often focused on his need to be perfect and on teaching him ways to place less pressure on himself.

Jeff was fortunate because his family reacted well to his disclosure that he was gay. This outcome is unfortunately not always the case. Many clients face alienation from their families when they disclose their sexual orientations. In addition, many clients live in rural areas where it can be more difficult to find a support network. Others have jobs in which disclosing one's sexual orientation can affect job stability or potential for promotion. One of the counselor's roles in these cases is to help clients find resources in their communities or nearby communities. Another of the counselor's roles is to help clients learn when it is okay to come out to other people. Counselors can help clients protect themselves and be realistic about people's reactions to their sexual orientation and, at the same time, not assume that everyone will react negatively.

As I noted earlier, Jeff and I worked several years together. We were fortunate that we did not have a time limit, because he was able to pay my sliding scale fee and we did not have a set termination date. Although brief counseling models are in vogue in today's managed care environment, identity development cannot be rushed. Few clients will be able to move from identity tolerance to identity synthesis in ten sessions or less, and attempts to rush clients can lead to identity foreclosure (Cass, 1979). My practice is to let clients make the determination of how long they want to work with me, although we do discuss what they are getting out of counseling at various points in the process. In addition, when clients are ready, I do encourage them to attend a coming-out group if one is available in their communities. The group process is invaluable in helping clients realize that other gay men have gone through and are going through what they are, in providing them with another level of support, and in providing a conduit for applying gains in individual counseling to life outside counseling.

## Summary

In this chapter, we described the concept of gay identity development, one component of an overall identity (Chickering & Reisser, 1993). Gay men frequently repress their gay identities for fear of being rejected, abandoned, or facing physical harm. However, being able to accept one's identity and express this identity to others is related to positive psychological adjustment (Marszalek et al., 2002; Miranda & Storms, 1989).

Gay identity development models have been developed to outline the process through which gay men become aware of and express their identities to others. In particular, we outlined Cass's (1979) six-stage HIF model and discussed how it may be applied to the styles of Ivey's DCT theory to form the following consolidated styles/stages: (1) early sensorimotor style/pre-confusion stage, (2) late sensorimotor style/confusion stage, (3) early concrete style/comparison stage, (4) late concrete style/tolerance stage, (5) early formal style/acceptance stage, (6) late formal style/pride stage, (7) dialectic style/synthesis stage. To help the reader better understand DCT and how it can be applied to gay identity development, we led the reader through an early recollection and visualization exercise.

Next, we explained that gay affirmative counseling approaches have been proposed to promote positive identity development and psychological adjustment with gay men. Counselors can use gay affirmative counseling approaches to help counter the negative societal messages concerning homosexuality that many gay clients have internalized and to affirm individuals' identities as gay men. Because DCT is both a theory of adult development and a counseling practice theory, we proposed using DCT as a gay affirmative counseling approach to help gay clients progress through the stages of gay identity development, as outlined by Cass (1979).

We concluded with John's case study of Jeff, a client with whom John worked as he progressed through the gay identity development process. Jeff had struggled to understand his same-sex feelings and thoughts for years but was not able to make a commitment to a gay identity until he recognized his pattern of hiding his true identity behind a mask of heterosexuality. John's use of DCT to integrate theories such as object relations, cognitive behavioral, and person-centered theories worked well with Jeff; that is not to say that it would work well with all clients. You can integrate other theories into the DCT framework by assessing the style of the client and using a theory that is appropriate for that style. You can also use theories that will challenge a client to process experiences and issues at other styles. The goal is to assist clients in experiencing as many DCT styles as possible related to a particular issue, because clients who can use all four DCT styles have less physiological and psychological distress (Rigazio-DiGillio et al., 1997). It is important to note, however, that not all clients will be able to use a dialectic style in processing issues (Ivey et al., 2005) and some gay men may not reach a synthesis stage of development (Cass, 1979). As a counselor, though, you can help your gay clients progress through the gay identity development process as far as they are able; and with your help, your clients can learn to be who they are.

## Annotated Bibliography

Association for Gay, Lesbian & Bisexual Issues in Counseling (AGLBIC) website: http://www.aglbic.org/
AGLBIC is a division of the American Counseling Association. AGLBIC's website provides resources for both members and nonmembers, including the Competencies for Counseling Gay, Lesbian, Bisexual, and Transgendered (GLBT) Clients and an extensive bibliography on counseling issues for GLBT clients.

Barret, B., & Logan, C. (2002). *Counseling gay men and lesbians: A practice primer.* Pacific Grove, CA: Brooks/Cole.
In addition to dedicating a chapter to gay and lesbian identity development, Barret and Logan provide information on issues specific to counseling lesbians, gay men, bisexual, and transgendered clients. Clinical examples and "tips for practitioners" are integrated into each chapter.

Cass, V. C. (1979). Homosexual identity formation: A theoretical model. *Journal of Homosexuality, 4*, 219–235.
In this article, Cass introduced her theory of gay and lesbian identity development. It is one of the most frequently cited articles on the coming-out process and set the groundwork for future models.

Cass, V. C. (1984). Homosexual identity formation: Testing a theoretical model. *The Journal of Sex Research, 20*, 143–167.
Cass described her study of 178 males and females to test the validity of her six-stage model. This is an important source for researchers interested in conducting empirical research on gay and lesbian identity development.

Isay, R. A. (1996). *Becoming gay: The journey to self-acceptance.* New York: Henry Holt.
Isay's describes his patients' and his own experiences with gay identity development, including identity issues for gay adolescents, older gay men, married gay men, and gay men with HIV or AIDS. Isay also describes his struggle to make being gay acceptable in the psychoanalytic community. It is a follow-up to his book *Being Homosexual: Gay Men and Their Development.*

Ivey, A. E. (1990). *Developmental therapy.* San Francisco: Jossey-Bass.
In this classic book, Ivey describes his Developmental Counseling Therapy (DCT) theory. It is a must read for counselors and researchers who want an in-depth understanding of DCT as a model of human development and a counseling theory.

Ivey, A. E., Ivey, M. B., Myers, J. E., & Sweeney, T. J. (2005). *Developmental counseling and therapy: Promoting wellness over the lifespan.* Boston: Houghton Mifflin.
Ivey and his colleagues provide case studies, transcripts, and exercises to help practitioners and students learn how to apply DCT, wellness theory, and positive psychology to the practice of counseling. This book covers developmental issues across the lifespan and includes a chapter on multicultural counseling.

Marszalek, J. F., III, Cashwell, C. S., Dunn, M. S., & Heard, K. (2004). Comparing gay identity development theory to cognitive development: An empirical study. *Journal of Homosexuality, 48*(1).
This article provides more detail on the proposed integration of Ivey's DCT and Cass's HIF model described in this chapter. In addition, the authors describe an empirical study providing initial evidence that gay identity development can be categorized by DCT concrete and abstract frames of reference.

Perez, R. M., Debord, K. A., Bieschke, K. J. (2000). *Handbook of counseling and psychotherapy with lesbian, gay, and bisexual clients.* Washington, DC: American Psychological Press.
This book is an important reference for counselors of sexual minorities. Contributors to this edited book provide chapters on gay identity development, counseling with diverse groups of gay clients, and research.

# References

Barret, B., & Logan, C. (2002). *Counseling gay men and lesbians: A practice primer.* Pacific Grove, CA: Brooks/Cole.
Beard, J., & Glickauf-Hughes, C. (1994). Gay identity and sense of self: Rethinking male Homosexuality. *Journal of Gay and Lesbian Psychotherapy, 2*(2), 21–37.

Browning, C., Reynolds, A. L., & Dworkin, S. H. (1991). Affirmative psychotherapy for Lesbian women. *The Counseling Psychologist, 19*, 177–196.

Cass, V. C. (1979). Homosexual identity formation: A theoretical model. *Journal of Homosexuality, 4*, 219–235.

Cass, V. C. (1984). Homosexual identity formation: Testing a theoretical model. *The Journal of Sex Research, 20*, 143–167.

Cass, V. C. (1990). The implications of homosexual identity formation for the Kinsey Model and scale of sexual preference. In D. P. Charter, S. A. Sanders, & J. M. Refinish (Eds.), *Homosexuality/heterosexuality: Concepts of sexual orientation* (pp. 239–266). New York, NY: Oxford University Press.

Chickering, A. W., & Reisser, L. (1993). *Education and identity.* San Francisco: Jossey-Bass.

Cochran, S. D., Ackerman, D., Mays, V. M., & Ross, M. W. (2004). Prevalence of non-medical drug use and dependence among homosexually active men and women in the US. *Addiction, 99*, 989–999.

Coleman, E. (1981/1982). Developmental stages of the coming out process. *Journal of Homosexuality, 7*, 31–43.

Fassinger, R. E. (1991). The hidden minority: Issues and challenges in working with lesbian women and gay men. *The Counseling Psychologist, 19*, 157–176.

Frankowski, B., & American Academy of Pediatrics: The Committee on Adolescence (2004). Sexual orientation and adolescents. *Pediatrics, 113*, 1827–1832.

Gay and Lesbian Victory Fund. (2006, November). Gay candidates win in record numbers across U.S. *News.* Retrieved from http://www.victoryfund.org/index.php?src=news&prid=183

Gonsiorek, J. C. (1995). Gay male identities: Concepts and issues. In A. R. D'Augelli & C. J. Patterson (Eds.), *Lesbian, gay, and bisexual identities over the lifespan: Psychological perspectives* (pp. 24–47). New York: Oxford University Press.

Gonsiorek, J., & Weinrich, J. (1991). *Homosexuality: Research implications for public policy.* Newbury Park, CA: Sage.

Gumaer, J. (1987). Understanding and counseling gay men: A developmental perspective. *Journal of Counseling and Development, 66*, 144–146.

Hall, A. S., & Fradkin, H. R. (1992). Affirming gay men's mental health: Counseling with a new attitude. *Journal of Mental Health Counseling, 14*, 362–374.

Harrison, N. (2000). Gay affirmative therapy: A critical analysis of the literature. *British Journal of Guidance and Counseling, 28*, 24–53.

Hencken, J. D., & O'Dowd, W. T. (1977). Coming out as an aspect of identity formation. *Gay Academic Union Journal: Gai Saber, 1*, 18–22.

Hopke, R. H. (1993). Homophobia and analytical psychology. In R. H. Hopke, K. L. Carrington, & S. Wirth (Eds.), *Same-sex love and the path to wholeness.* Boston: Shambhala.

Ivey, A. E. (1990). *Developmental therapy.* San Francisco: Jossey-Bass.

Ivey, A. E., Ivey, M. B., Myers, J. E., & Sweeney, T. J. (2005). *Developmental counseling and therapy: Promoting wellness over the lifespan.* Boston: Lahaska.

326 CHAPTER TEN

Ivey, A. E., Ivey, M. B., & Rigazio-DiGilio, S. (2005). The standard cognitive/emotional developmental interview. In A. E. Ivey, M. B. Ivey, J. E. Myers, & T. J. Sweeney, *Developmental counseling and therapy: Promoting wellness over the lifespan* (pp. 408–418). Boston: Lahaska.

Kauhlwein, K. T. (1992). Working with gay men. In A. Freeman & F. M. Dattilio (Eds.), *Comprehensive casebook of cognitive therapy* (pp. 1–19). New York: Plenum.

Lee, J. A. (1977). Going public: A study into the sociology of homosexual liberation. *Journal of Homosexuality, 3,* 49–78.

Levine, H., & Evans, N. (1991). The development of gay, lesbian, and bisexual identities. In N. Evans, & V. Wall (Eds.), *Beyond tolerance: Gays, lesbians, and bisexuals on campus.* Washington, DC: American College Personnel Association.

Loiacano, D. (1989). Gay identity issues among Black Americans: Racism, homophobia, and the need for validation. *Journal of Counseling and Development, 68,* 21–25.

Lowe, S. M., & Mascher, J. (2001). The role of sexual orientation in multicultural counseling: Integrating bodies of knowledge. In J. G. Ponterotto, J. M. Casas, L. A. Suzuki, & C. M. Alexander (Eds.), *Handbook, of multicultural counseling* (2nd ed., pp. 755–778). Thousand Oaks, CA: Sage.

Marszalek, J. F., III, & Cashwell, C. S. (1998). A parallelism of Ivey's developmental therapy and Cass's homosexual identity formation model: Promoting positive gay and lesbian identity development. *Journal of Adult Development and Aging: Theory and Research, 1,* 13–31.

Marszalek, J. F., III, Cashwell, C. S., Dunn, M. S., & Heard, K. (2004). Comparing gay identity development theory to cognitive development: An empirical study. *Journal of Homosexuality, 48*(1), 103–123.

Marszalek, J. F., III, Dunn, M. S., & Cashwell, C. S. (2002). The relationship between gay and lesbian identity development and psychological adjustment. *"Q": The Journal of the Association of Gay, Lesbian, and Bisexual Issues in Counseling, A Division of the American Counseling Association* [Online journal], *2*(1). Available at http://www.aglbic.org/Q/Vol2Num1

Maylon, A. K. (1993). Psychotherapeutic implications of internalized homophobia in gay men. In C. Cornett (Ed.), *Affirmative dynamic psychotherapy with gay men* (pp. 77–92). Northvale, NJ: Aronson.

McHenry S., & Johnson, J. W. (1993). Homophobia in the therapist and gay or lesbian client: Conscious and unconscious collusions in self-hate. *Psychotherapy, 30,* 141–151.

Miranda, J., & Storms, M. (1989). Psychological adjustment of lesbians and gay men. *Journal of Counseling and Development, 68,* 41–45.

Piaget, J. (1965). *The moral judgment of the child.* New York: The Free Press.

Piaget, J. (1973). *The child and reality: Problems of genetic psychology.* New York: Grossman.

Plummer, K. (1975). *Sexual stigma: An interactionist account.* London, UK: Routledge & Kegan Paul.

Rigazio-DiGillio, S. A., Ivey, A. E., & Locke, D. C. (1997). Continuing the post-modern dialogue: Enhancing and contextualizing multiple voices. *Journal of Mental Health Counseling, 19*, 233–255.

Ryan, C. C., & Futterman, D. (1998). *Lesbian and gay youth: Care and counseling.* New York: Columbia University Press.

Shannon, J. W., & Woods, W. J. (1991). Affirmative psychotherapy with gay men. *The Counseling Psychologist, 19*, 197–215.

Troiden, R. R. (1984). Self, self-concept, identity, and homosexual identity: Constructs in need of definition and differentiation. *Journal of Homosexuality, 10*(3/4), 97–109.

Troiden, R. R. (1988). Homosexual identity development. *Journal of Adolescent Health Care, 9*, 105–113.

# CHAPTER ELEVEN

# Black Racial Identity Development

## Dafina Lazarus Stewart

Our readers may be wondering why we have devoted an entire chapter to Black racial identity development. You may even be wondering if this focus is not in fact creating segregation and difference where none actually exists. Indeed, if all humans are governed by the same general patterns of identity development, then how does it help the cause of inclusion for us to pull out and discuss specific groups of people? Does such an enterprise overemphasize our differences at a time when we should be concentrating on our similarities? Does this focus on African Americans imply a culturally regressive or deficient orientation that suggests that African Americans are inferior to other racial or ethnic groups, particularly White European Americans? Moreover, are we overlooking the individual distinctiveness of the people within these groups by attempting to discuss general group patterns and identity issues? Lastly, there are some readers who may be asking us why we are focusing on race, when there really is no biological basis for such distinctions (see Renn, 2004, for an excellent discussion of this point). The answers to these questions lie in the realities of the social consequences of race discussed below.

Given the societal conditions in which we live in the United States, such questions are not unreasonable, and do point to legitimate and authentic issues for multiculturalism and diversity both as counselors and as members of the global human community. Neither should such questions be ignored or discarded as irrelevant. However, the following points must be made. Although it is true that there is no such thing as a sustainable biological racial construct, race is a social and cultural reality across the globe. For instance, throughout history, groups of people worldwide have been objectified, ridiculed, ostracized, and marginalized based on differences in skin color, facial features, hair texture, and eye color. This societal oppression has created an intense and unavoidable need to theoretically, philosophically, and sociologically deal with the concepts of race and racism in societies over time and across multiple contexts. Indeed, studying Black racial identity development does not imply an inferior position for African Americans relative to Whites or any other population. Neither does it imply that African Americans compose a cultural monolith any more than Chickering's theory of identity development (see Chickering & Reisser, 1993) overrides possibilities for individual expression among college students. However, it would demonstrate the most egregious form of objectification and marginalization not to take into account the impact of social conditions on the psychosocial development of individuals and groups within a society. Therefore, it is not only necessary but appropriate that we focus in this text on African American, Latino, non-heterosexual, women's, and bicultural peoples' identity development.

With this in mind, please consider the following questions as you read this chapter.

1. How does the experience of societal oppression impact the development of value orientation, worldview, and political stance, which are part of identity development?
2. What is the relationship between social movements and theory development?
3. How can learning about the identity development of a particular group give us better insight into the identity development of all groups?
4. As members of an increasingly multicultural and multiracial society, what is our responsibility as counseling professionals to marginalized members of that society?

## Overview

The discussion of the pathways toward identity development in Americans of African descent has been the subject of literary, sociological, and popular discussion since the turn of the twentieth century. Some significant examples are W. E. B. DuBois's *The Souls of Black Folk* (1903/1994); the film *Imitation of Life* (1934); and Ellison's, *The Invisible Man* (1947/1995).

## ABOUT THE CHAPTER AUTHOR

### Dafina Lazarus Stewart

Writing about African American (Black) racial identity development has been an interesting process for me, mostly because I was
able to see myself in the various stages in development. I remem-

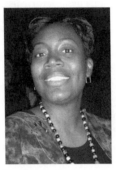

ber experiencing the personal significance
of race when I entered college—pumping
my fist in the air and shouting "Black is
beautiful!" across campus to fellow Black
students. And now, hopefully, I am abiding
in a place where my race is one of many significant facets of my identity—not insignif-
icant but no longer blocking out other
facets of self. I hope that this chapter on
Black racial identity development will be
helpful to you as you assess your personal

**Dafina Lazarus
Stewart**

journey or those of others with whom you
work and counsel.

*Dafina Lazarus Stewart*, Ph.D., is an assistant professor of higher
education and student affairs at Bowling Green State University.
Her professional interests include identity development, spirituality, and African American college students. Dr. Stewart has
presented at local, regional, and national conferences, seminars,
and symposia. She lives in Bowling Green, Ohio, where she enjoys
spending time with her daughter, going for walks, and minister-
ing at her local church.

Human development theory entered this ongoing conversation during the
height of the Black Power movement of the late 1960s and 1970s and in
the wake of integration and desegregation efforts across the United States
as slogans such as, "Black is beautiful" and "Black Power!" and the soul-
ful sounds of James Brown singing, "I'm Black and I'm proud!" (Ellis &
Brown, 1968, track 5) were at their height in the voices of African Americans in this country. Such literary and popular culture artifacts provided
tangible, albeit anecdotal, examples of African Americans' struggles to
develop racial and cultural identity even before empirical research was done
to support and describe these struggles through theoretical lenses.

In light of this background, it is critical to understand the following about this discussion of what we are calling Black racial identity

development. First, the theories that attempt to chart the course of the identity development of African Americans in the United States cannot be separated from the historical context and sociological conditions of people of African descent in the United States that birthed these theories. Each of the theories in this area has its foundation in the collective assumption that the experience of oppression in the United States impacts the identity development of members of marginalized and oppressed groups. As such, this body of theory does not claim to speak to some innate or biologically inherent difference in Black people, but rather points to the implications of differences that have been sociologically imposed and nurtured. This constructionist approach grounds these theories in their historical context and thus inherently highlights the interaction between people and their environments.

Second, it is important to understand the term *Black* racial identity development is meant to refer to a specific group, particularly people of African descent living in the United States. When the progenitor of these theories was first introduced, the Cross model of Psychological Nigrescence, the term *Black* was gaining acceptance as a self-referent within the African American community, as the term *Negro* was falling into disfavor. Currently, there are some who use the term *Black* as a pan-African descriptor, encapsulating all peoples of African descent both in the African Diaspora and continental Africa. However, please keep in mind that this body of theory is not necessarily pan-African in nature or application but speaks rather specifically to the unique experience of people of African descent living in the United States under conditions of social, economic, and educational segregation. Consequently, this body of theory has come under recent criticism for lacking relevance to African Americans who grew up and assimilated into White environments and also for failing to speak to the differing experiences of immigrants of African descent in the United States who have not been raised with a critical consciousness of race and racial identity formed by societal oppression. This is not to say that this body of theory cannot speak to or illuminate the development of these disparate groups, but to encourage the reader to keep in mind the heterogeneity of Black communities in the United States, recognizing the ways that individuals and subcommunities of Black people (speaking pan-Africanly) differently experience race in the United States' social context as well as globally.

However, despite these two caveats, it remains that this body of theory still addresses the same fundamental questions that all identity development theories seek to address: "Who am I?" and "How do I come to know myself in context and in relationship with others?" The primary difference is that this body of theory centers the answers to these questions in the context of the lived experiences of Black oppositional racial difference in the United States.

## Black Racial Identity Development Theories

As discussed in the previous section, this body of theory attempts to explain how the development of a Black racial lens impacts an individual's response to the core identity questions of "Who am I, and what does that mean to me?" and "How do I come to know myself in context and in relationship with others?" Most of the theories in this body of research situate the context of this development in the traditional college years, in keeping with the focus of general psychosocial development theorists such as Arthur Chickering and James Marcia (see Chickering & Reisser, 1993; Marcia, 1967, 2002). However, some theorists studying Black racial identity development posited a lifespan development approach that may or may not begin during the traditional college years and more importantly, does not end during those years nor sees full resolution until later in life (for instance see Parham, 1989; Myers et al., 1991).

Despite the idiosyncrasies of the individual models, the following *basic assumptions* apply:

- *There is a need for the individual to recognize and accept a positive self-concept about his or her Black racial identity in opposition to the negative portrayals taught by the dominant society.* A healthy self-image has been posited to be an important foundation for successful resolution of identity development issues.

- *Maturation along this developmental trajectory includes an ability to work across racial differences with others in her or his environment.* It is important to note that the successful resolution of racial identity requires the individual to move beyond a limited group identification toward more holistic understandings of the relationship between the individual and a multifaceted global society.

- *Continued maturation results in the balancing of positive racial self-concept with other aspects of identity, such as gender, social class, personality, and sexuality.* No individual can be fully described or understood using only one facet of identity. It is critical that the multilayered nature of individual identity always be emphasized.

- *Awareness and activism on behalf of the African American community increases as a client develops his or her Black racial identity.* These theories suggest that a natural outcome of continued racial identity development is advocacy or the tangible demonstration externally of one's internal framework.

What follows is an in-depth summary of the theories that constitute this body of knowledge. As you read, the above assumptions will become more relevant to you.

Prior to the 1970s, most of the studies that produced the theories and models discussed elsewhere in this text were done with predominantly White and male student populations. These findings were initially assumed to be generalizable to women, people of color, and nonheterosexuals. However, the 1970s saw the emergence of work done by and about these marginalized groups and demonstrated that the foundational theories had not told the whole story of identity development. On the heels of the civil rights movement and the resurgence of Black nationalism, militant activism, and virulent campus racial disturbances, understanding African American life through the perspectives of African American people became critically important. Several researchers, some noted here, moved to fill this gap and frame the discussion of African American racial identity development as an important element of general psychosocial development. William E. Cross Jr. was among the scholars examining the concept of psychological nigrescence (Evans, Forney, & Guido-DiBrito, 1998). Nigrescence is the process of transformation from a non-African–centered identity to an African-centered one. Cross's Model of Psychological Nigrescence describes this process as a positive one, with first three (1971) and then five sequential stages (1991). As Cross said about his model in *Shades of Black* (1991):

> [W]hile nigrescence is not a process for mapping the socialization of children, it is a model that explains how *assimilated* Black adults, as well as *deracinated*, *deculturalized*, or *miseducated* Black adults are transformed by a series of circumstances and events into persons who are more Black or Afrocentrically aligned." (p. 190, emphasis in original)

His work was the foundation upon which the majority of the theories of racial identity as well as other theories of identity development for other marginalized groups development have been built (see Table 11.1).

Cross's Nigrescence Model, or the Negro-to-Black Conversion Model, as it was first named, was developed through self-analysis and participant observation studies. Observations were conducted in his hometown of Evanston and in neighboring Chicago during the Black Power phase

TABLE 11.1   Cross Model of Psychological Nigrescence

| Stage | Description |
| --- | --- |
| Pre-Encounter | Clients in this stage give little salience to their racial identity, placing value in other things—religion, family status, social status, or profession. As long as these things continue to provide meaning and fulfillment, the client will probably not need to continue in this identity development process. |
| Encounter | A set of experiences, which are then personalized, require the client to reevaluate and redefine their prior worldview and value orientation. These experiences may be either positive or negative but result in the client seeking new information in order to determine if a change in identity perspective is needed. |
| Immersion-Emersion | A period of transition during which the old identity is competing with an emerging, new identity. During this transitional phase, the client may exhibit very aggressive and anxious displays of Blackness and a harsh rejection of White cultural values and norms, as well as White people. Rage, guilt, and pride may be the emotional markers of this transitional period. In the emersion period that signals the coming end of this transition, the client matures in her and his understanding of Blackness and begins to see a more complex relationship between identity in context and in relationship with others. |
| Internalization | The new identity in Blackness is fully internalized, resulting in protection from psychological insults, a sense of belonging and anchorage, and a foundation from which to relate to people, cultures, and situations beyond Blackness. The client in this phase is much calmer and relaxed about his and her Black identity, and the racial anxiety from the previous stage becomes racial pride steeped not in hatred of Whiteness but in self-love and deep connection to Blackness and the Black community. |
| Internalization-Commitment | In this phase, the client's internalized Black identity seeks to be translated into a plan of action and investment in the future and potential of the larger Black community and in other oppressed communities s well. A sustained interest and commitment marks clients in this phase of Black racial identity development. |

Based on Cross's discussion of his work in *Shades of Black* (1991).

## ABOUT WILLIAM E. CROSS JR.

Dr. William E. Cross Jr., Ph.D., is the progenitor of Black identity development theory for late adolescence and adulthood. Following the research done by Kenneth Clark on the impact of prejudice and segregation on the self-concept and self-esteem of Black children, Cross provided the next major theoretical model by directly addressing the psychosocial development of Black people in the United States. He is considered to be one of the leading experts on the study of African American identity and his text *Shades of Black: Diversity in African-American Identity* (1991) is a classic in the field.

Dr. Cross was born and raised in the midwest, in Evanston, Illinois. He completed his undergraduate studies at Denver University in Colorado and graduated in 1963. In 1976, he received his doctorate in psychology from Princeton University. He has taught in the area of African American studies and psychology at such esteemed schools as Cornell University, The Pennsylvania State University, and the University of Massachusetts-Amherst. Currently, Dr. Cross serves as professor and coordinator of the social-personality doctoral program in the department of psychology at the Graduate Center of the City University of New York (CUNY). Dr. Cross is also a consultant to the government, education, and industry on the business and educational implications of America's changing demographics (Brown University, 2004).

of the Black social movement. His interactions with close friends and associates as they and he together developed a new Black identity helped him to construct his Nigrescence Model. Further expansion of the model came as a result of student activism at Princeton in the fall of 1971, and produced an advanced undergraduate seminar on Black issues the following spring, with Cross as the instructor. Through class discussions with these students, Cross expanded his model and recognized that diversity within the Black experience is natural and should not be pejorative. His work in *Shades of Black* seeks to discuss nigrescence theory with a revised perspective on Black identity that rejects both overly pejorative and overly romantic discourses for one centered on diversity and complexity in Black psychological functioning (Cross, 1991).

This model on African American identity development has been the focus of numerous essays, countless empirical studies, and scholarly debate within the fields of psychology and African American Studies. Although Cross's work highlights the African American experience, it has been extremely influential to scholars theorizing and researching Jewish, Asian American, nonheterosexual, and White ethnic-group identity development models.

## Stages in Cross's Nigrescence Model

In its first stage, *Pre-Encounter*, African Americans either viewed their racial identity as irrelevant and inconsequential or as a sign of deficiency. Whiteness can be viewed as a preferred racial status, and the attitudes of African Americans in this stage may not differ significantly from those of White racists. An individual in pre-encounter may believe that racism does not exist and may agree with societal stereotypes that depict African Americans as lazy or violent.

The second stage, *Encounter*, involves an experience or a series of experiences that causes disequilibrium and challenges the individual's previous views about race and the significance of race in the person's life. These experiences can be either positive or negative. Reflection upon the experience causes the person to look at the world through a different lens. For example, a student may begin college in a predominately White setting and for the first time confront racist attitudes and beliefs personally directed at him or her. Trying to understand these unwarranted attacks causes the person to accept that racism is real and that it is necessary for him or her to seek validation and affirmation as a Black person.

The *Immersion-Emersion* stage is a period in which the old identity is discarded and the new Afrocentric world view is taken on in full force. Initially, the individual may express a hatred for all things White or non-Black and adopt many superficial markers of Black identity, such as changing hairstyles, manner of dress, or learning an African language, for instance. As the individual progresses through this stage toward *Internalization*, dualistic conceptions of blackness versus whiteness are replaced by more nuanced and less emotionally charged interpretations.

In the Internalization stage, this new identity is rooted more firmly within the self and is reflective of inner security and self-confidence about being African American. Individuals in this fourth stage are more ideologically flexible and open to other perspectives. This may be portrayed by developing interracial friendships with people of different races and ethnicities or joining multiracial groups. One's identity as

Black is no longer reliant on superficial appearances, such as hairstyles and clothing, although these may remain the same as in the Immersion-Emersion stage.

This openness is increased in the fifth and final stage, *Internalization-Commitment*, as the ideology of the new identity gets translated into action on behalf of African American and other oppressed groups. In this final stage of development, a collective "we" voice begins to emerge, replacing the previous egocentric perspective (Cross, 1971, 1991; Evans, Forney, & Guido-DiBrito, 1998). Such individuals may actively participate in grass-roots movements focused on inner-city youth and support issues that reach beyond the Black community, such as immigration, domestic partnership insurance, or gender equality.

It is important to note that Cross makes a distinction between personal identity or general personality and reference group orientation. The latter was the focus of the Nigrescence Model, such that Cross posits that African Americans both enter and leave the model with their fundamental personalities largely intact and unaffected by their integration of a new Black identity. Consequently, there is room and need to use both the Cross model and other models of general personality or personal identity development, such as those provided by Chickering and Marcia to more fully assess, evaluate, and counsel African Americans.

Thomas Parham (1989) has critiqued and expanded upon the work of Cross (1971) and Wade Nobles (1980, see below) in the development of psychological nigrescence for African Americans. Whereas previous models characterized movement across a series of sequential stages in response to pressures in the social environment and other life circumstances, Parham (1989) discussed three alternatives to resolving identity. In other words, Parham claimed that racial identity development did not neatly progress in an orderly fashion, nor was the length of time a person took to move from one stage to the next fixed. Rather, individuals may revisit previous stages of identity (recycling) and may linger over a certain stage for an extended period of time (stagnation). Due to these alternative resolutions, racial identity development should not be perceived as being begun or completed during the college years, and several cycles of development may occur throughout a person's lifetime (Parham). Accordingly, the Cross model was meant to discuss identity change within the context of a social movement, not as a lifespan evolutionary process (Parham). Models of nigrescence then can be viewed as processes of self-actualization under conditions of oppression, in a developmental process that is subject to continuous change during the life cycle (Parham). Similar to Keniston (1971), Parham said that young adults were seeking ways to define themselves in relation to their social environment and they began to look for their reflections within that external environment. Parham (1989) said that the core of Black people's personalities was essentially African in nature. Going further, he said that African American students faced a dilemma of inclusion and exclusion, being a part of yet apart from American society as they were exposed to two different value systems, one rooted in African values and traditions and the other in European and American values and traditions (Parham). Within the context of racial identity development then, movement between racial identity stages may represent an attempt to balance—African American and European American values within one's own life space (Parham).

Joseph White and Parham (1990) continued the themes noted above. Building from earlier work by Nobles as well as work by Erikson and DuBois, White and Parham (1990) also assert that the personality, consciousness, and core identity of Black people are African in nature. Further, they also highlight communal orientation as a fundamental "self-extension orientation" of African people (White & Parham, p. 43). These authors discussed the development of a culturally centered identity, which has five characteristics: (1) an understanding of a collective or extended self; (2) an understanding and respect for the sameness in self and others; (3) a clear sense of one's spiritual connection to the universe; (4) a sense of mutual responsibility for other Black people; and (5) a conscious sense that deviance is defined as any act in opposition to oneself (White & Parham, pp. 44 –45). However, referencing the writings of James Baldwin, the authors also pointed out that this development was often mitigated by oppression and racism (White & Parham). White and Parham also repeated the theme noted by DuBois (1903/1994) and Parham (1989) that Black identity developed in the midst of a set of dualities that were challenged by oppression and racism. Despite this, interrelatedness, connectedness, and interdependence were viewed as the unifying philosophic concepts in the Black experience base (White & Parham, 1990). Developmentally, these concepts may impact an individual's approach to and interpretation of developmental goals such as autonomy, self-concept, and mature interpersonal relationships.

Later, Robert Sellers (1997) and Janet Burt (1998) produced reconceptualizations of African American identity that build upon theories by Erikson, Marcia, and Cross. Sellers' model, the Multi-dimensional Model of Racial Identity, has four components: (1) racial salience; (2) racial centrality; (3) racial regard; and (4) racial ideology (1997). Racial salience described the extent of which race was a relevant part of African Americans' self-concepts at a specific moment in time. Racial centrality dealt with the extent to which African Americans normatively define themselves with respect to race. Racial regard represented the dynamic relationship between the individual's affective and evaluative judgments of African Americans and the individual's perception of other's affective and evaluative judgments of African Americans. Lastly, racial ideology constituted a person's attitudes, opinions, and beliefs about how they feel that African Americans should collectively behave.

Janet Burt's (1998) African American Identity Model includes family socialization and sociohistorical consciousness in the development of racial identity for African Americans. The four components in her model were family socialization, racial consciousness, cultural connectedness/collective thought, and self-concept. Burt asserted that the socialization process within the family structure impacts the racial identity formation of an individual. Racial consciousness was the extent to which a person understands the impact that race, history, and culture have on the individual and collective experience of African Americans. The other two components constituted the degree to which a person had adopted African American cultural norms and values and had a healthy and positive sense of self when functioning both within and outside the African American community and culture (Burt, 1998).

These two models by Sellers (1997) and Burt (1998) and the culturally centered identity model presented in White and Parham (1990) differ from most of the models presented above in that they are not stage theories. Individuals did not move from one stage to another in linear progression. Rather, each component had its own growth cycle, and the dynamic relationship among the components constitute racial identity development in the individual, similar in structure to Heath's (1968) maturational development theory. In working with clients, these models contribute to building a more holistic understanding of the multiple components that may contribute to a person's racial identity structure. Failure to understand the degree of centrality a person attaches to race or the impact of how the family socialized her or him to consider race would probably lead to inappropriate interventions and inadequate resolutions of internal conflicts.

## A Different Mirror

The majority of research in this body of theories concerning the development of Black racial identity situates the discussion in the oppressive context of an assumed racist society and/or college campus. Notably, however, two scholars have rejected that starting point, seeking instead to understand the development of Black identity development from a more positive ethnocultural base.

In the wake of Cross' initial research, Wade Nobles (1980) asserted the need for a Black psychology that was based on a Black cultural ethos. According to Nobles, culturally relevant Black psychology would be the foundation of theories concerning the psychological development and mental health of African Americans. Like Cross, Nobles' work was also rooted in the nigrescence movement of the 1970s. He argued that a Black psychology based on a Black ethos needed to be fundamentally different from a White psychology based on a White cultural ethos. African philosophical traditions, largely rooted in West Africa, provided the base of the Black cultural ethos to which he referred. Nobles justified this orientation by saying that White ethnographers who argue the "intra-distinctiveness" of West African societies may be allowing racist assumptions to blind them to "the underlying similarities in the experiential communality of African peoples" (1980, p. 24). This common ethos, or collective unconsciousness (Bynum, 1999), has two characteristics: (1) human unity and harmony with nature; and (2) an emphasis on community survival (Nobles, 1980). Therefore, Black psychology would not be derived from the negative aspects of Black life in America, but rather from the positive features of a basic African philosophy.

His relevance to Black racial identity development theory is in the tenets of his Afrocentric psychology, which follow (Nobles, 1980). First, to be human meant belonging to the whole community. The egocentric I is replaced by a collective We: "Only in terms of other people does the individual become conscious of his own being" (Nobles, p. 30). This is the concept of collective responsibility and is further articulated as whatever happens to one happens to all and whatever happens to the group happens to the individual. Nobles makes no distinction between act and belief or between the spiritual and the physical in his theory of Black psychology. Instead, everything is seen as functionally connected. Further, the uniqueness of a person's environment determines the parameters of that person's existence. Finally, "[B]lack psychology needs to concern itself with rhythm, orality, the soul, the extended self, and the natural orientation to ensuring the survival of the tribe" (p. 35). This has developmental implications for the inclusion of spirituality in our assessment of African American clients as well as the connection to family, friends, and other personal networks.

Within the last fifteen years, cultural psychology has emerged with a specific focus on multicultural counseling and research into multicultural identity development. Moreover, certain researchers and counselors in this field have sought to integrate what they call a more "optimal" perspective in the study of theories of development to counteract the fragmented and suboptimal worldview, which they say is represented in much of the developmental theories reviewed above. Myers et al. (1991) discuss identity development as a process of continuous integration and expansion of one's sense of self. They use Optimal Theory (OT) as the foundation for what they suggest is a more inclusive "pancultural" model of identity development. They critiqued current models of racial–ethnic identity development as limited and reflective of a suboptimal worldview and suggested the possibility of a more optimal framework along the following four dimensions. First, the authors said that a unified developmental model across oppressed people is possible due to a common worldview. Second, that this universal worldview could be the foundation for such a model and thus applied panculturally. Third, that concurrent assessment of the multiple ways in which human beings experience oppression would yield a more accurate reflection of that individual and their experiences. Finally, the individual and his or her meaning-making was a central player in the development of identity. The authors suggested that previous models of racial–ethnic identity development had not considered these factors. Moreover, previous models may have been reflective of the particular periods in which they initially emerged (i.e., the civil rights, women's, and gay pride movements), rather than a more universal process.

Fundamental to the optimal identity development process that the authors introduced was an understanding of the presence of conflicting conceptual systems. In this culture, the authors suggested that the maintenance of a positive sense of self, or identity, was made increasingly difficult because oppressed peoples were defined as those who allow their power to be externalized and therefore must rely on external validation for their self-worth (Myers et al., 1991). Any self-worth that was achieved under this system was by definition vulnerable and insecure because self-worth in this culture was related to certain criteria determined a priori as making some group of people better than another (Myers et al.). Those criteria were most notably White skin and male sex characteristics (Myers et al.). Such a material foundation was determined to be insufficient to achieve or maintain a grounded sense of self.

According to an optimal model of identity development, "self-knowledge [was] the process of coming to know who and what we are as the unique expression of infinite spirit" (Myers et al., 1991, p. 55). Such knowledge then made possible the integration of all the material manifestations of being, such as race, gender, class, age, color, and ethnicity, into a whole sense of self (Myers et al.). The resultant identity development model, grounded in research interviews and counseling sessions, was identified as Optimal Theory Applied to Identity Development (OTAID). The OTAID describes a seven-phase process that is sequential but neither linear nor categorical. Therefore individuals may or may not move through all the phases of the model in one lifetime, nor is there a predictable amount of time that an individual may spend in a phase. The OTAID was described instead as an "expanding spiral" in which the end of the process looks similar to the beginning. At the beginning, Absence of Conscious Awareness, individuals experience themselves as connected to all life but are lacking in self-knowledge. At the end of the process, Transformation, through self-knowledge individuals again become aware of their connection to the universe and all life. Through each phase, the individual comes to know her- or himself in a fuller, more complete way and begins to understand that individual identities as raced, gendered, classed, or aged are actually interrelated and interdependent (Myers et al.). Moreover, the intervention of the surrounding suboptimal culture provides opportunities for the individual to continually redefine and expand his or her self-knowledge (Speight et al., 1991). Gradually, the individual comes to appreciate him or herself and others as integrated wholes and unique expressions of infinite spirit.

## Cynthia and Her Co-Workers: Personality Conflicts or Racial Hostility in the Workplace?

I am a counselor associated with the HR department in a large company with several divisions. Typically, the employees I see have been referred to me by their supervisors for work stress issues or for being in danger of termination because of poor work performance that is suspected to be due to some mental health or addiction issue. The company sees my office as the last opportunity for corrective intervention before the person is fired. Reviewing my case notes from my client sessions today, I came across my entry for Cynthia, an African American female in her early thirties. This was her fifth session after delaying seeing someone for about six months because she wanted to try to "handle it" herself. Realizing that she wasn't making progress on her own, she came to see me because of the recommendation of a friend of hers in the company. She stood out to me because unlike most of my caseload, Cynthia came in on her own, not by supervisor referral.

My notes from my first session with her indicate that Cynthia seemed very guarded at first and very slow to open up. Her primary complaint at that time was that she didn't fit in with the rest of her co-workers, where she works as a member of a marketing team. This had become problematic because her team supervisor confronted her with being "distant and unsociable." These characterizations didn't hold with what Cynthia had come to know about herself, and she's worried that this false perception will have an impact on her advancement in the company.

In the second session, Cynthia talked about her family background and education. I learned that she was born and raised in New York City and attended a predominantly White, upper-class high school on scholarships and heavy financial assistance and then came to the Midwest for college and graduate school, both also in predominantly White environments and much smaller towns than New York. When I asked her to describe her college experience, she responded with two words, "anger" and "struggle." When I probed deeper, Cynthia revealed that the campus was a hotbed of racial tension, especially during her tenure there, which saw the Rodney King trial and verdict, the ensuing civil disturbances in Los Angeles, and then numerous campus feuds and disputes, which were perceived to be racially motivated.

Cynthia further revealed that she went through a major transformation in college. Cynthia described herself as she began her undergraduate years as a young woman with very long chemically-straightened hair, who was naïve about race relations given that her high school was very welcoming and open-minded despite its lack of numerical racial and ethnic diversity. She also identified then as a Republican and an ardent Boston Celtics basketball fan in deliberate opposition to the "norm" for Black folks from New York City, who were either Knicks or Lakers fans. Thanks to the campus flare-up over the first nonguilty Rodney King verdict and a very Afrocentric and militant boyfriend her sophomore year, Cynthia decided that she needed to completely reinvent how she presented herself to others. While she was in Washington, D.C., for a government internship, she cut her hair down to a very short natural style, decided to change her major from international studies to sociology so that she could become a teacher and be more "relevant" to the Black community, and changed her political party affiliation to Independent, disavowing both the Republicans and Democrats as disinterested in the plight of Black peoples across the United States and African peoples across the globe.

When she returned to campus that summer, she took Swahili and ended her study of Russian and served as president of the campus Black student group three times in the next two years. One of her major successes was helping to open up a theme house on campus for students interested in the serious study of Black history and cultural life. Despite the break-up with her militant boyfriend less than a year after they started dating, Cynthia maintained her newfound Afrocentric identity and continued to keep her hair and her politics "natural," as she called it. When one of the Black administrators on campus, whom she greatly admired, was fired and the position itself eliminated the summer following her graduation, Cynthia wrote a very angry and passionate letter to the college renouncing her financial support until the position was reinstated and the college made demonstrable efforts to increase the Black and minority student populations on campus and improve the campus climate for those students.

Following this session, I realized that Cynthia presented a very clear example of someone who had gone through the Pre-Encounter, Encounter, and Immersion-Emersion phases of the Cross Black racial identity model. I decided in the third session to see if she had dropped out in the Immersion-Emersion phase or if situations continued to mature her development into the Internalization and Internalization-Commitment stages.

The third session revealed that Cynthia had continued to develop her racial identity after college and during graduate school and early employment positions. My notes attributed this development to her acknowledgement that she realized that "all White people aren't crazy" and meeting and developing mutually enriching personal friendships with a few White friends and professional colleagues. Her organizational commitments still have a heavy focus on African American issues, but she also speaks very passionately about social class and gender issues due to classes she took in graduate school. Cynthia also revealed that she rediscovered her spiritual foundation, which she says she lost sight of in college because of narrow, traditionalist beliefs about women's roles and her own inability at the time to balance an Afrocentric philosophy with her Christian religious views.

After this session, it still wasn't clear to me why she was having such problems with her co-workers perceiving her as "distant and unsociable." She appeared to be neither to me now that I had spent more time with her. So in the fourth session, I asked her about her work situation more specifically. Cynthia revealed that she works in a small team of about five people most of the time and that there is a lot of what she called "extracurricular" socializing, meaning that people often got together for drinks and meals after work and on the weekend, and partners/spouses were often included. Cynthia confessed that she didn't normally attend these gatherings. I asked her why and her first response was, "White people have fun differently than Black people do and I don't find what they do to be fun at all." At first, I wasn't sure how to take this comment. Had Cynthia regressed back into the dualistic Immersion-Emersion stage, in which she saw all White people negatively? I realized that it was possible that Cynthia experienced a new Encounter when she began her job at this company and found herself the only person of color in her team and only one of three people of color in her division. So I decided to probe deeper.

**Dafina:** "Hmm, that's interesting. Do you socialize with your friends who are White?"

**Cynthia:** "Well . . . yes. We usually go to movies or the zoo. I know that sounds incredibly corny, but we have a lot of fun. We also go out to eat a lot. We have some favorite restaurants that we like to visit. And I love jazz, so sometimes we go out to a jazz restaurant and just listen to music for hours. I never thought about that before—I do have a lot of fun with them."

**D:** "So, are those times different from when you spend time with other African Americans?"

**C:** "Well, a group of Black people do different things, you know. I mean, we're not likely to hang out at the zoo. And the movies we would go to would be different. I mean, I saw *Last Holiday* with my girls, not with my White friends."

**D:** "So what do you make of that?"

**C:** "Yes, it's different but it's still fun and I do have fun with both sets of friends. But you know the reality is that I don't spend a lot of time socializing with anybody."

**D:** "Why is that?"

**C:** "Well, I really don't have a lot of free time. I work late hours and then Sundays and two evenings a week, I'm at church. When I find myself with free time, mostly I just prefer to hang out at home alone and sleep. I guess you would say that I'm an introvert."

**D:** "Well, you do seem to exhibit a lot of those traits."

**C:** "Yea, well, I'm an introvert and I'm comfortable with that. But most of the people on my team at work are definitely extraverts."

**D:** "What makes you say that?"

**C:** "Oh my goodness, they talk *all* the time! All their thoughts are processed outside their heads. They love being around noise and lots of people. Their ideal social event is to go to a club with blaring music where you have to scream in order to be heard. They love that kind of stuff. I can't stand it. They never seem to want to be alone—everything they do, they have to do with somebody else. I don't need that. I work perfectly fine and better, mind you, on my own. I mean there's nothing wrong with getting together to brainstorm every once in a while, but that seems to be all these people do all day, every day. It's amazing we get anything done!"

Now, things made more sense to me. I jotted down in my notes: personality style conflict NOT racial one. Yet there still seemed to be something more. I asked Cynthia if she liked the people she worked with. Cynthia replied that they seemed all right, a little too chipper in the morning sometimes and inclined to talk too much, but generally they seemed to be nice enough people. In response to what she did for fun, Cynthia was generally nondescript since she has so little time for "fun" in general, but she stated that writing poetry, watching movies, and having good conversations about social and political issues were fun for her. She also expressed a desire to attend some of the talks that the local college sponsors but that the times usually conflicted with either a work or church commitment.

At this point, it dawned on me that I didn't know much about her personal life. I inquired and Cynthia got a really sour look on her face and answered that she was currently single and had been for two years. Her last relationship ended when she realized that the man she was seeing was constantly borrowing money from her and that they argued more than anything else. I jotted in my notes: She's single, they're not—not much in common in personal lives to talk about. It was time for the session to end, but I decided to ask more about her co-workers and why she didn't think she would have "fun" socializing with them if she thought they were nice people in our next session.

Today, Cynthia burst into my office crying and blurted out,

*Cynthia:* "I think they're going to fire me. It's because I don't go out drinking with them and I'm going to sue these people for discrimination! You can't require that I go out drinking with people in order to keep my job!"

*Dafina:* "Cynthia, whoa, what happened?"

*C:* "What happened is what's been happening every day since I've been here. Susie and John complained to our team leader, Amy, that I'm not contributing to the group on this project we've been working on. I can't believe it! I've worked my butt off on this project!"

*D:* "Okay, so what makes you think you're going to be fired?"

*C:* "It all started last Wednesday evening. It was after 5 and we were in a team meeting going nowhere—as usual—and Susie suggested that we go around the corner to Charlie's Bar and Grill. She said maybe the change of scenery would spark some new ideas. For crying out loud, we had a million ideas on the table already! Well, Wednesday nights I teach a class at church and I need to be there by 6:30 so that I can start class at 7. So I told them I couldn't go. Susie looked at me really funny and John told me that I needed to get my priorities straight. Next thing I know, Amy is telling me that only team players get promotions and salary raises and that it was important for the team to be able to feed off each others' creative energies. She basically threatened my job if I didn't go to a bar every time they think we need to!"

*D:* "Cynthia, you seem really agitated and frustrated. Let me see if I've got this straight. From what you've told me the team wanted to go after hours to a bar in hopes of generating more ideas for your project but you couldn't go because you had to be at church. Then, some day after that, Amy called you into her office and emphasized the importance of team work to success with the company. Is that a fair recounting of what happened?"

*C:* "Yes, mostly."

*D:* "Okay, what did I miss?"

*C:* "It's obvious that Susie and John told Amy that I wouldn't go out with them and made it seem like I wasn't a team player. That had nothing to do with it! I had a schedule conflict. I can't just back out of my class at the last minute like that. Other people are depending on me too!"

*D:* "Of course, it's perfectly reasonable that you couldn't change your plans at the last minute. Would you like some water?"

*C:* "Yes, thank you." *I gave Cynthia a bottle of water and some time to drink some of it before I continued.*

*D:* "Cynthia, despite what you think Amy was implying, she can't fire you that easily. There is a process that any team leader has to follow if they think an employee is not working out."

*C:* "Really?"

*D:* "Really."

*C:* "But that's not all she said."

*D:* "What else did she say?"

*C:* "I'm the only Black person on my team. I think she was saying that I have a problem working with White people and that I needed to be more multicultural. What nerve! She has no idea who I am and what kind of work I've done in diversity and social justice issues!"

*D:* "Let's step back a moment, Cynthia. What exactly did she say that gave you the impression that she thinks you have a problem with White people and you need to develop a more multicultural perspective?"

*C:* "I don't remember exactly. She made some ignorant comment about me coming across as 'too aggressive and militant' and that 'the world isn't as black and white as it used to be.'"

*D:* "I can see how that would upset you."

*C:* "You better believe I'm upset!"

*D:* "Did Amy directly say that your job was on the line?"

*C:* "No, she didn't." (This reassured me but I was still concerned that Amy didn't speak to Cynthia about seeing the staff counselor, me, to resolve the situation if termination was indeed that much of a possibility. That seemed odd to me since Amy has referred other people from different work teams for various problems, including issues involving teamwork.)

*D:* "I still believe that this situation with your marketing team and your team supervisor can be resolved without you losing your job." (Cynthia gave me a suspicious look but I continued since she had calmed down somewhat.) "From what you've told me during our last few sessions, I think the main issue here might be that you don't enjoy the main social activity that takes place during these extended brainstorming sessions—drinking—because your spiritual beliefs are more conservative. How am I doing so far?"

*C:* "That makes sense."

*D:* "Okay, I also think that your being an introvert and the rest of your team being extraverts is creating some strain also. It seems that you all really don't understand how you all work best."

*C:* "Okay, yea, I can see that. I definitely don't understand how they can think in the midst of so much noise and confusion."

*D:* "Sure. If you don't mind, may I ask you another question I've been thinking about?"

*C:* "Hmm, okay."

*D:* "Do you feel out of place at all when the team does socialize together and their significant others and spouses are along?"

*C:* ". . . Yea . . . I am really tired of being alone everywhere I go. I mean, I even get tired of hanging out with my friends at church too because of that. I mean, I really appreciate everything you're saying. It certainly casts a different light on things. But I still think race is an issue."

*D:* "Okay, why is that?"

*C:* "No one on the team speaks to me when we're in the office. Not even in casual conversation. When work-related conversations come up, they don't include me even when it's relevant for all of us. I feel like such an outsider. I don't think I've ever been accepted as a member of the team."

This last confession by Cynthia, which hadn't come up before, caused me to consider if there may indeed by racial conflict issues here. I also realized that perhaps this was a new Encounter experience for Cynthia in learning about working relationships with non-African Americans. However, with proper management at this stage, it would be possible to prevent the self-segregation that would come with Cynthia progressing through another Immersion-Emersion phase. I thought the chances for successfully integrating this new knowledge with new resolution skills at the Internalization stage were pretty high, given that Cynthia realized that her previous generalization of White people's socializing preferences was unwarranted given her other relationships. I remembered the importance of relationships and community to African American identity that I had learned in graduate school, so the involvement and cooperation of her whole team as well as her team supervisor would be necessary.

A light bulb went off in my head, and I thought I had an idea for an action intervention strategy. At the close of this session, Cynthia seemed more at ease and not so defensive. I suggested that the two of us postpone our next session for four weeks, during which time I would implement my intervention strategy. Cynthia left my office curious but confident that she would be vindicated at the end of all this.

The next morning I received a call from Cynthia's team supervisor, Amy, about Cynthia. Amy expressed a great deal of concern about the way her conversation with Cynthia went the previous day, not knowing that Cynthia had been in counseling with me for the last five weeks about the situation in her marketing team. Amy felt that Cynthia may have misunderstood what she was saying to her in their evaluation meeting the previous day and asked for my advice. What a great opening! I asked Amy why she thought she was misunderstood, and she told me that Cynthia stated that her comments were discriminatory. She continued to say that she felt that Cynthia was oversensitive and that she really needed to work on her people skills. I suggested that a more appropriate intervention might be for the team to come together for a workshop the following week, during office hours to discuss teamwork and cultural sensitivity issues. Amy was convinced that the problem lay with Cynthia alone, but agreed to make the time for the workshop to take place the following week.

Using workshop design skills I learned in graduate school, I designed a six-hour workshop. Because I knew that identity was composed of multiple facets and not limited to race and culture, but included personality styles also, I made sure those were addressed my design. The first three hours would be spent using the Myers-Briggs Typology theory to bring out and work to resolve the personality issues in the team. The sixteen personality type preferences in Myers-Briggs would help the team to see what unique contributions could be made to the team's work using everybody's style preferences, not just those of one or two dominant people. Then, the team would have lunch together but in pairs, working through a dialogue activity to help the team get to know each other on a more personal basis. This would help begin the process of building community and relationships for Cynthia with the rest of her teammates as well as for the teammates to get to know Cynthia better. The second half of the day would begin with the dialogue dyads introducing each other to the rest of the team. After that, I decided to do a short presentation about cultural sensitivity, highlighting some general cultural differences in socializing, followed by a group dialogue about how the team could work better for everyone. This would allow me to introduce issues of race in a nonthreatening manner, recognizing that both Cynthia and her White co-workers had something to learn about each other's cultural styles of communication.

The day of the workshop, Amy related her hope that this would work since she really valued Cynthia's work and didn't want to lose her. I asked Amy if she had ever said that to Cynthia. Amy looked at me in a stunned manner and admitted that she should have. There was a great deal of tension in the room. It was obvious that the team really didn't know what to do. It was also painfully obvious that the only person not talking to anyone else was Cynthia. The first half of the workshop went really well. The team really seemed to connect to the Myers-Briggs and were able to self-identify the personality differences and conflicts among the team. Even Cynthia and Amy agreed on how difficult it was for Cynthia to be one of only two introverts in the group. Moreover, Susie confessed that she actually prefers introversion as well, but has worked really hard to develop the extraverted side of her personality. This caused Cynthia to realize that she had extraverted moments, too. The next activity, which required the team to break into two groups to build a tower out of an erector set, also illuminated some things for the team members about group dynamics and personality styles.

The success of the morning session spilled over into lunch. I intentionally had Susie and Cynthia do their dialogue dyad together. They came back from lunch realizing that they had more in common than they thought—they even both loved jazz! The break before the beginning of the second half showed a marked difference in the group's interactions. Cynthia was actually engaged in conversation with Shawn and John and at several points actually had the attention of the entire group as they asked her about her church and the class that she taught.

I was feeling really great about the progress the group had made. Then I began the cultural sensitivity presentation and noticed that the mood in the room changed a little. Some of the earlier tension was back, and some of the White team members noticeably became uncomfortable. However, I used my skills to continue to work through the tension. Once people realized that they weren't being put into boxes, they relaxed and began to see that simple issues weren't necessarily that simple for people from other races and ethnicities.

When the time came for the group to come up with some ways to improve their effectiveness as a team, I was pleasantly surprised by what emerged. They asked Cynthia what kinds of things she would like to do as social activities and came up together with the idea of only doing monthly social activities and rotating the responsibility of organizing the gatherings among the team members. The team also decided to make better use of Cynthia's and Peter's MBTI types as judgers and put them in charge of keeping the group on task and on-time in group brainstorming sessions.

At my next session with Cynthia, about three weeks after the daylong workshop, I asked her how things were going.

*Cynthia:* "I can't believe it, it's like I'm working in a whole new place. Susie and I actually get along really well now. She's even coming to church with me next Sunday!"

*Dafina:* "Wow, it sounds like things have definitely improved. How have you changed since our last session?"

*C:* "How have I changed? Hmm, I didn't expect that question." After pausing for a minute or so, Cynthia continued, "I think I've realized that I don't have to be so guarded at work. I used to think that if I let people know how involved I was at church that I would get a lot of criticism. I realized also that my spirituality is much more important to me now as a way of making meaning of things in my life than my race is. But I've still got a serious commitment to social justice issues—it just doesn't dominate my life anymore."

*D:* "That's a big insight, Cynthia. How did you come to realize all this?"

*C:* "Actually, it started with that interview thing you had me and Susie do at lunch the day of the workshop. I was thinking later about how I answered the questions she asked me and realized that I talked a lot more about God and my spiritual beliefs and how they affected my life than I did about being Black. Being African American is still important to me, but like I said, it's just not the only thing in my life anymore."

The smile on Cynthia's face let me know that things were going to continue to improve for Cynthia. I encouraged her to come back anytime. She agreed to do so and thanked me for my help.

I sat back in my chair and put my feet up on the desk with a gratified smile. Another person on their way to successfully resolution thanks to my broad knowledge of counseling theories and ability to apply them to practice. Job well done, counselor!

## Relevance to Scholars and Practitioners

Gaining an in-depth understanding of Black racial identity theories is an essential tool for building multicultural competence in counseling professionals. Due to the reality of socially constructed meanings of race and societal and institutional racism, African Americans have long had to deal with what DuBois (1903/1994) termed *double consciousness.* The competing pulls to be both American and African result in psychological stress and anxiety and may underlie other issues that African American clients present as their reasons for seeking counseling services. Moreover, it should be understood that counseling is not often seen as a preferred option for African American clients because it has traditionally been seen as a sign of weakness and an inability to handle one's own life issues. Therefore, it is essential that a counselor, especially one who may be of a different race/ethnicity than the client be able to demonstrate competency with the issues of double consciousness and Black identity that may be presented by African American clients in the counseling setting.

## Gender

Issues of gender, though, should be considered as well when seeking to apply a Black racial identity development framework to our work with African American clients. The complex interaction of race and gender cannot be dismissed as irrelevant to our applications of the Cross model or any other model to African American female clients.

Brown-Collins and Sussewell's (1986) study of African American women's emerging selves pointed to the complexity of the integration of race and gender. Their research also showed, like Gilligan (1977), Belenky and her colleagues (1986), and later Josselson (1987), that an African American woman perceived her notion of self through relationships to other people (Brown-Collins & Sussewell). The study's conclusions identified multiple self-referents for African American women: the psychophysiological, an African American referent, and what was termed *myself*. The psychophysiological referent spoke to the Black woman's knowledge of herself as a woman. The second referent involved self-knowledge of social and political realities, in which knowledge obtained and understood about the self was a collective-affective experience. The myself referent reflected self-knowledge that was unique to one's personal history and a by-product of both her blackness and her femaleness and needed to be studied simultaneously (Brown-Collins & Sussewell).

This emphasis on self-knowledge was carried on in Diane Goodman's (1990) work to include the voices of African American women in theories of women's development. Goodman sought to address the deficiency in feminist research by explicitly focusing on the experiences of African American women and considering the interaction of sex and race. Goodman addressed identity development in African American women as a result of the interaction of the following two factors. First, she ascribed an Afrocentric worldview to most African American women that defined the self as positively dependent on others, defined through relationship with others, and tied to the welfare of the larger community, akin to Nobles's (1980) enunciation of an Afrocentric cultural ethos. This was coupled with the family socialization of African American women to be both independent and self-reliant and to define their existence in relationship to African American men.

These interacting factors resulted in three areas of self through which Goodman's respondents spoke about themselves and their identities

(Goodman, 1990). Those areas were sense of self, sense of self in relationship, and sense of being in the world, or ontology. As Goodman talked with these women, the role of spirituality was clearly interwoven into their stories of self and relationships with others. Religion and spiritual beliefs play an important role in the process of change and personal growth experienced by these women, as reflected in the case study with Cynthia. Another conclusion of these findings was that the capacity for self-reflection was related to those with the most integrated self-concept and those most seriously preoccupied with moral and spiritual issues (Goodman).

In light of this, counselors should be able to discern the different ways that pre-encounter, encounter, immersion-emersion, internalization, and internalization-commitment may present in African American women. For instance, body image issues and self-perceptions of beauty may be the primary external markers of an African American woman's movement through the Cross model. For an African American male, these external markers are less likely to revolve around body image and beauty, though emphasizing "manhood" issues of respect, autonomy, and being able to provide for oneself and one's family.

## Practice Considerations

It is important to remember that this body of theory was principally developed for late adolescents and adults. Although work has been done (see William Cross and Peony Fhagen-Smith, 1996 and 2001) on Black racial identity development from infancy throughout the lifespan, elementary and secondary school counselors should be very cautious in their applications of the tenets of these models to children. Recall from earlier in this chapter that this body of theory presumes the basic personality and characteristics of individuals have been formed and are largely set *prior* to dealing with issues of racial identity and the formation of a new Black or Afrocentric identity. What may appear to be a youth struggling with an encounter experience may in reality be an issue of balancing peer group relationships alongside a growing sense of personal autonomy.

Nevertheless, in light of the realities of continued racial segregation at the primary and secondary grade levels nationally, a growing number of African American children are entering predominantly White environments for the first time prior to leaving for college. Therefore it would be wise for school counselors to familiarize themselves with the Cross model and particularly the earlier stages of pre-encounter and encounter, as well as with those models that discuss issues of adaptation, acculturation, and assimilation, such as those by Parham and Jewelle Gibbs (1974) and George DeVos (1980) (see the annotated bibliography).

The most relevant and applicable use for this theory in practice likely would be in counseling centers on predominantly White college campuses and predominantly White employment settings. On college campuses, African American students may be entering a predominantly White environment as both resident and student for the first time. Consequently, the environment may pose numerous encounter experiences and opportunities. Moreover, the balkanization of many college campuses easily feeds into the extremism of the immersion-emersion transition for students. As such, learning to manage emotions such as disappointment, frustration, rage, guilt, and anomie would be vital for these students and may require the assistance of on-campus counseling professionals through individual counseling or programmatic strategies.

In predominantly White work environments, African Americans who attended predominantly White colleges, as we saw in Cynthia's case study, may recycle through new experiences of encounter, immersion-emersion, internalization, and internalization-commitment as they discover new facets of their social roles and identities and are exposed to new philosophical perspectives and world views. For African Americans who attended historically Black colleges and universities, remained in highly diverse multiethnic environments in community colleges, or immediately entered the workforce after high school, the workplace environment may be the first encounter experience that prompts the consideration and possible development of a new Black identity in the individual. The encounter experience may involve much more complex issues, requiring resolution by a number of units within a company, including human resources and even legal affairs. Moreover, unlike the college campus, the workplace is not necessarily a hospitable or safe environment for adopting the new performances of self and voice that typically mark the immersion-emersion phase of Black identity development. Consequently, African American employees progressing through the model for the first time or repeating it may need assistance in working through the emotions, concepts, and beliefs with which they are now confronted, and may not have other acceptable outlets to express, depending on the nature of the work environment and their position and responsibilities within it.

## Validity of the Theory and Potential Shortcomings

Although the Cross model has become a classic in identity development and African American Studies, questions have been raised about
its applicability to African Americans who are not in predominantly
White contexts and whether it sets up one standard of Black identity
as the only authentic choice for African Americans.

I believe that it is important to recognize that African American students attending predominantly Black or highly diverse colleges may
not develop a Black racial identity along the same path as those in predominantly White settings. Further research needs to be done in this
area to compare racial identity development in these two very different environments. Also, there is a danger in situating identity always
in the context of opposition as the Other. As pointed out in the models advanced by Wade Nobles (1980) and Linda James Myers and her
colleagues (1991), using an Afrocentric framework as the beginning
point instead of the endpoint may be more empowering and may result
in healthier modes of adaptation and persistence in the face of societal
racism for African Americans.

I would like to emphasize, also, that Cross acknowledges that there is
diversity within Black identity and that individuals may choose not to
progress beyond the pre-encounter phase or adopt an Afrocentric value
orientation if other structures in their lives (religion/spirituality, family,
etc.) are sustainable as guiding frameworks (Cross, 1991; Cross & Fhagen-
Smith, 1996). Such "dropping out" may also happen during the immersion-
emersion transition. Cross and Fhagen-Smith acknowledge that this can
indeed be a healthy choice and is a part of the diversity of the Black
community and of Black identity development. Consequently, counseling
professionals should be wary of pushing an Afrocentric perspective on their
clients, allowing them as individuals to define what is important and sustainable for them as meaning-making tools in their lives.

# Summary

In conclusion, it is important to keep in mind the four basic assumptions of Black racial identity development theory that were discussed
at the beginning of this chapter:

1. Due to racist messages about self-image, self-worth, and cultural value
   that are prevalent in U.S. society, it is necessary for African Americans
   to develop a positive self-concept that recognizes and accepts the positive contributions of their African racial and cultural heritage.

2. As individuals mature in this development, they will develop an increasing capacity to work with others in multicultural settings.
3. The development of other aspects of identity, such as gender, social class, sexuality, and spirituality, can be balanced with their racial identity development; however, this integration will usually not occur until racial self-concept issues have been adequately resolved.
4. Community activism and service are seen as necessary indicators of maturity and resolution of racial identity conflicts.

These fundamental tenets shape the body of theories that were discussed in this chapter. It is also crucial to keep in mind the diversity of Black identity. Not all individuals reflect their racial identity development in the same patterns, nor do all individuals enter or leave the models at the same points. Gender differences between Black men and women must be considered because different life situations and circumstances may impact and cause the individual to show their racial identity development in different ways that reflect, in part, the general gender differences in our society at large.

Moreover, the historical and sociological underpinnings of these theories cannot be dismissed. The emergence of the civil rights and Black Power movements were critical in shaping not only the racial identity development of African Americans then and now, but also in shaping how theorists thought about the racial identity development of African Americans. The very idea of a "Negro-to-Black conversion experience" is deeply and inextricably rooted in ideas about self-determination, cultural resistance, and racial pride that found new voice in the racial struggles of the 1960s and 1970s. Granted, these themes had been aired before, especially in the post-Reconstruction era into the early decades of the twentieth century through the voices of DuBois, Marcus Garvey, and Ida B. Wells, to name just a few. Nevertheless, the positioning of more and more African Americans in doctoral programs and faculty positions across the nation's colleges and universities, thanks to the Supreme Court's 1954 *Brown* decision, allowed the reemergence of these themes in the sixties and seventies and for them to find serious analysis and contemplation in academic scholarship, not solely in literary and popular culture circles.

This body of theory regarding the racial identity development of African Americans is very important to practicing professional counselors. Its import lies mainly within the counselor's need to be multiculturally competent in his or her dealings with a diverse range of clients and life experiences. African Americans and other people of color in this society often deal with pressures and situations that involve racial and cultural conflict, as well as basic psychological tasks. Therefore, a counselor must be skilled in recognizing and analyzing cause and effect, and correlations, and in identifying needed resolutions at multiple levels, which may fall outside their own realm of personal experience.

The case study involving Cynthia and her co-workers is a good example of the ways that multiple aspects of an individual's identity can be at play in a counseling scenario. If the counselor stopped only at the apparent personality conflicts between Cynthia and the rest of her marketing team, the very real problems of lack of cultural sensitivity and racial exclusion and segregation would have been missed. Such an incomplete counseling intervention can leave clients with feelings of mistrust, feeling silenced, and hesitant to seek counseling in the future. Also important, others involved in the situation, in this case Cynthia's supervisor and co-workers, would be left to continue to behave and think in ways that dehumanize and offend others.

Lastly, I would encourage students and other readers of this chapter to continue to develop a clear understanding of this body of theory by reading the works cited in the annotated bibliography and through examining case studies of African American clients' experiences. Your professional practice and possibly even your own personal development will be greatly enhanced by doing so.

# Annotated Bibliography

Asante, M. K. (1988). *Afrocentricity*. Trenton, NJ: Africa World Press.
  Modern models of Black racial identity development typically reject a cultural deprivation orientation and espouse varying degrees of Afrocentricity in their grounding framework and discussions of how individuals are said to progress through the model. Therefore Asante's classic piece on the philosophy of Afrocentricism, though not without criticism, would provide an important context for understanding the Cross model and others that have followed.

Clark, K. B. (1955). *Prejudice and your child*. Boston: Beacon Press.
Clark, K. B., & M. P. Clark (1939a). The development of consciousness of self and the emergence of racial identification in Negro pre-school children. *Journal of Social Psychology, 10*, 591–599.
Clark, K. B., & M. P. Clark. (1939b). Segregation as a factor in the racial identification of Negro pre-school children: A preliminary report. *Journal of Experimental Education, 8*(2), 161–163.
Clark, K. B., & M. P. Clark. (1940). Skin color as a factor in racial identification of Negro pre-school children. *Journal of Social Psychology, 11*, 159–169.

Clark, K. B., & M. P. Clark. (1947). Racial identification and preference in Negro children, In T. M. Newcomb and E. L. Hartley (Eds.), *Readings in social psychology* (pp. 169–178). New York: Holt.

Clark, K. B., & M. P. Clark. (1950). Emotional factors in racial identification and preference in Negro children. *Journal of Negro Education, 19*, 341–350.
Taken together, these works by noted psychologists Kenneth and Mamie Clark set the groundwork for the Black racial identity development theories that later followed in the 1970s and thereafter. This scholarship was central in helping mainstream psychology and counseling to understand that the social condition of racial oppression in the United States created an oppositional context of development African American children. These works also stand as the first major scholarship done by African American researchers on African American people. They rejected models of cultural deprivation and deficiency, a rejection that became a fundamental aspect of later nigrescence models.

Cross, William E. (1991). *Shades of Black: Diversity in African American identity.* Philadelphia: Temple University Press.
This book presents the revised version of the Cross model of Nigrescence as well as a copious review of the literature on earlier Black racial identity development models. It has become a classic in the field of psychology and African American Studies.

DuBois, William E. B. (1994). *The souls of Black folk.* New York: Dover. (Original work published in 1903)
Although this is primarily a sociological text, DuBois's discussion of the conflicted nature and identity of African Americans helps to underpin the philosophical orientation and outlook depicted in models of identity development that appeared at the opposite end of the twentieth century. In this book, DuBois also argues for the appropriateness of the Black experience as a subject of serious scholarly inquiry.

Helms, J. E. (Ed). (1993). *Black and White racial identity: Theory, research, and practice.* Westport, CT: Praeger.
Second only to Cross, Janet Helms is a major figure in the discussion of racial identity development for both Caucasians and African Americans. This text helps counseling professionals see the interrelationships between Black and White racial identity development, as well as the mutual impact of oppression and racism on both the oppressor and the oppressed.

Parham, Thomas (Ed.). (2002). *Counseling persons of African descent: Raising the bar of practitioner competence. Multicultural Aspects of Counseling Series 18.* Thousand Oaks, CA: Sage.
This is an important text for counseling professionals because it discusses in-depth the counseling needs for people of African descent and takes a pan-African look at these issues. Parham also presents scholarship not commonly discussed that comes from a uniquely and wholly Afrocentric perspective, rooted in the cultural perspectives, traditions, and worldviews of African peoples.

Riggs, Marlon (Producer/Director). (1987). *Ethnic notions* [Motion picture]. (Available from California Newsreel, Order Department, P. O. Box 2284, South Burlington, VT 05407; http://www.newsreel.org).

In this film, Riggs poignantly and authentically portrays the development of racial stereotypes used against African Americans. This film will help viewers to better understand why theorists, such as Cross, promote the need for African Americans to adopt an Afrocentrically based reference group orientation as part of their identities.

Tatum, Beverly D. (1997). *"Why are all the Black kids sitting together in the cafeteria?" and other conversations about race.* New York: Basic Books.

Like the earlier work of Kenneth Clark, Tatum helps us to better realize the need for psychic safety that many African Americans experience when functioning in predominantly White social environments. Using the work of Cross and Clark, Tatum also seeks to explain the development of Black racial identity, especially in the context of secondary education. Unlike many of the other authors highlighted here, Tatum also devotes a chapter to the identity development issues that exist in multiracial families.

DeVos, George (1980). Ethnic adaptation and minority status. *Journal of Cross-Cultural Psychology, 11*, 101–124.

Feagin, J., Vera, H., & Imani, N. (1996). *The agony of education: Black students at White colleges and universities.* New York: Routledge.

Fleming, Jackie (1985). *Blacks in college.* San Francisco: Jossey-Bass.

Gibbs, Jewelle (1974). Patterns of adaptation among Black students at a predominately White university: Selected case studies. *American Journal of Orthopsychiatry, 44*, 728–740.

Hughes, M. (1987). Black students' participation in higher education. *Journal of College Student Personnel, 28*, 532–545.

Pounds, A. W. (1987). Black students' needs on predominately White campuses. In D. J. Wright (Ed.), *Responding to the needs of today's minority students* (pp. 23–38). San Francisco: Jossey-Bass.

The above set of articles is useful for counselors who want to gain a general understanding of the issues faced by African American college students in predominantly White environments. Because this was the environment that produced the Cross model, it would be most helpful to really understand the oppositional nature of these environments and why and how they might produce encounter experiences for African American college students.

# References

Belenky, M. F., Clinchy, B. M., Goldberger, N. R, & Tarule, J. M. (1986). *Women's ways of knowing: The development of self, voice, and mind.* New York: Basic Books.

Brown-Collins, A. R., & Sussewell, D. R. (1986). The Afro-American woman's emerging selves. *The Journal of Black Psychology, 13*, 1–11.

Burt, J. M. (2000, April). *African American identity model.* Roundtable paper discussion presented at the American Educational Research Association Annual Meeting, New Orleans, LA.

Chickering, A., & Reisser, L. (1993). *Education and identity.* San Francisco: Jossey-Bass.

Cross, W. E., Jr. (1971). Toward a psychology of Black liberation: The Negro-to-Black conversion experience. *Black World, 20*(9), 13–27.

Cross, W. E., Jr. (1991). *Shades of Black: Diversity in African American identity.* Philadelphia: Temple University Press.

Cross, W. E., Jr., & Fhagen-Smith, P. (1996). Nigrescence and ego identity development: Accounting for differential Black identity patterns. In P. B. Pedersen, J. G. Draguns, W. J. Lonner, & J. E. Trimble (Eds.), *Counseling across cultures* (4th ed., pp. 108–123). Thousand Oaks, CA: Sage.

Cross, W. E., Jr., & Fhagen-Smith, P. (2001). Patterns of African American identity development: A lifespan perspective. In C. L. Wijeyesinghe & B. W. Jackson III (Eds.), *New perspectives on racial identity development: A theoretical and practical anthology* (pp. 243–270). New York: New York University Press.

DeVos, G. A. (1980). Ethnic adaptation and minority status. *Journal of Cross-Cultural Psychology, 11*, 101–124.

DuBois, W. E. B. (1994). *The souls of Black folk.* New York: Dover. (Original work published in 1903)

Ellis, A., & Brown, J. (1968). Say it loud, I'm Black and I'm proud [Recorded by J. Brown]. On *Say it live and loud—James Brown live in Dallas 8/26/68* [CD]. Dallas: Universal Motown Records Group.

Ellison, R. (1995). *The invisible man* (2nd internat. ed.). New York: Random House. (Original work published in 1947)

Evans, N. J., Forney, D. S., & Guido-DiBrito, F. (1998). *Student development in college: Theory, research, and practice.* San Francisco: Jossey-Bass.

Gibbs, J. T. (1974). Patterns of adaptation among Black students at a predominately White university: Selected case studies. *American Journal of Orthopsychiatry, 44*, 728–740.

Gilligan, C. (1977). In a different voice: Women's conceptions of self and of morality. *Harvard Educational Review, 47*, 481–517. Reprinted in B. Puka (Ed.), *Caring voices and women's moral frames: Gilligan's view.* New York: Garland.

Goodman, D. (1990). African-American women's voices: Expanding theories of women's development. *SAGE, 7*(2), 3–14.

Heath, D. (1968). *Growing up in college.* San Francisco: Jossey-Bass.

Josselson, R. (1987). *Finding herself: Pathways to identity development in women.* San Francisco: Jossey-Bass.

Keniston, K. (1971). *Youth and dissent.* Orlando, FL: Harcourt Brace Jovanovich.

Marcia, J. (1967). Ego identity status: Relationship to change in self-esteem, "general maladjustment," and authoritarianism. *Journal of Personality, 35*(1), 118–134.

Marcia, J. (2002). Identity and psychosocial development in adulthood. *Identity, 2*(1), 7–28.

Myers, L. J., Speight, S. L., Highlen, P. S., Cox, C. I., Reynolds, A. L., Adams, E. M., et al. (1991). Identity development and worldview: Toward an optimal conceptualization. *Journal of Counseling & Development, 70*(1), 54–63.

Nobles, W. W. (1980). African philosophy: Foundations for Black psychology. In R. L. Jones (Ed.), *Black psychology* (pp. 23–36). New York: Harper & Row.

Parham, T. A. (1989). Cycles of psychological nigrescence. *The Counseling Psychologist, 17*(2), 187–226.

Renn, K. A. (2004). *Mixed race students in college: The ecology of race, identity, and community on campus*. New York: State University of New York Press.

Sellers, R. M. (2000, April). *Multi-dimensional model of racial identity*. Roundtable paper discussion presented at the American Educational Research Association Annual Meeting, New Orleans, LA.

Speight, S. L., Myers, L. J., Cox, C. I., & Highlen, P. S. (1991). A redefinition of multicultural counseling. *Journal of Counseling & Development, 70*(1), 29–36.

Stahl, J. (Director). (1934). *Imitation of Life* [Film]. (Available from Universal Studios, Hollywood, CA).

White, J. L., & Parham, T. A. (1990). *The psychology of Blacks: An African American perspective* (2nd ed.). Upper Saddle River, NJ: Prentice Hall.

# CHAPTER TWELVE

# Defining Latino Identity Through Late Adolescent Development

## Vasti Torres and Edward Delgado-Romero

For many people, their first experience with independence comes during the college years and late twenties. This life marker makes late adolescent and the college context attractive for theorists who focus on identity. Many counselors and theorists view this period of the lifespan as marked by decisions that impact and eventually mold an individual's identity. Erikson (1968) viewed this late adolescence time in a person's life as one in which conflict between identity and identity diffusion occurs and the resolution of this conflict influences identity.

To consider only Erikson's view of identity development would fail to highlight the importance of culture and the conflicts that emerge as an individual attempts to resolve the differences between the cultures. One of the key reasons cultural or ethnic differences are salient in development is due to the need to negotiate between the collective behaviors some cultures value and the individualistic behaviors valued by other cultures, particularly that of the majority in the United States. For individuals balancing these differences, the goal of identity development can focus on interdependence rather than independence. Consequently ethnic minority adolescents in the United States may struggle with conflicting ideas regarding identity development. Ethnic identity theories attempt to address this gap by considering the specific issues

## ABOUT THE CHAPTER AUTHORS

Our chapter on Latino identity attempts to provide both context for Latinos in the United States and consideration of the diversity among Latino cultures. We present a variety of theories and apply them to nontraditional case studies that highlight some of the issues relevant to a diverse group such as Latinos. Our chapter expects the reader to understand that part of the struggle to self-identify as a minority is the understanding of how oppression influences those who are minorities. There are two reasons we chose college students to situate the case in this chapter. First, both of us have worked on colleges campuses for many years. And second, Latinos continue to lag behind in college educational attainment. There is a need to better understand the conflicts Latino college students' experience.

### Vasti Torres

*Vasti Torres* is associate professor of higher education and student affairs administration in the W. W. Wright School of Education

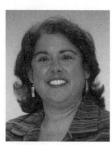

**Vasti Torres**

at Indiana University. Prior to coming to Indiana University in 2003, she was a faculty member at The George Washington University Graduate School of Education and Human Development in Washington, D.C. She teaches courses in student affairs administration and college student development theory. Prior to joining the faculty, she had sixteen years of experience in administrative positions, most recently serving as associate vice provost and dean for enrollment and student services at Portland State University in Portland, Oregon. Dr. Torres' research focuses on how the ethnic identity of Latino students influences their college experience. Her work evolved as a result of not seeing her experiences represented in the college student development literature. She was the principle investigator for a grant investigating the choice to stay in college for Latino students, which incorporates identity and environmental issues in understanding the experiences of these students. She has been honored as an Emerging Scholar and

Diamond Honoree by the American College Personnel Association, Program Associate for the National Center for Policy in Higher Education, Outstanding Faculty by the NASPA Latino Knowledge Community, and SACSA Scholar from the Southern Association of College Student Affairs. Dr. Torres holds a Ph.D. in counseling and student affairs administration from The University of Georgia.

## Edward Delgado-Romero

*Ed Delgado-Romero* is an associate professor in counseling psychology at the University of Georgia. Prior to coming to the Uni-

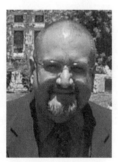

**Edward Delgado-Romero**

versity of Georgia, he was an assistant professor in counseling and educational psychology at Indiana University and the assistant director for the University of Florida Counseling Center. He teaches courses in counseling and counseling psychology and supervises doctoral students in their clinical work. He is a licensed psychologist in Georgia. His areas of research include race and racism in psychotherapy process, burnout of faculty of color, and the general area of Latino psychology. He is a founding member of the National Latina/o Psychological Association. He has been honored for his research, teaching, and mentorship of graduate students by the University of Florida division of Student Affairs, the school of education at Indiana University, the Society for the Psychological Study of Ethnic Minority Psychology, and the Counseling Psychology Student Association at the University of Georgia. Dr. Delgado-Romero holds a Ph.D. in counseling psychology from the University of Notre Dame.

that arise as a result of the convergence of the culture of origin, acculturation to the majority, and identity development.

This chapter focuses specifically on the identity development of Latinos in the United States and uses the late adolescent years to explore the development, establishment, and conflicts that may emerge for Latinos. There are two reasons for concentrating on the late adolescent years and the college context. First, this time is seen as critical to the identity development by members of the majority culture and as a time to develop independence (Chickering & Reisser, 1993; Erikson, 1968). Second, while there is research on the development of identity among Latino children (Aboud & Doyle, 1993; Bernal, Knight, Ocampo, Garza, & Cota, 1993), it is not until the late adolescent years that commitment to an identity is likely to occur. For this reason and because of access to the population, research on Latino identity is more likely to occur in the context of late adolescence or college years. In order to provide an overview of existing theories and emerging theories, we present definitions of critical terms, introduce the assumptions that connect these theories, explain the research on the theories, and organize an overview of all the theories.

## Definitions and Assumptions

The term *Latino* is complex and controversial. It encompasses people from more than twenty countries of origin, each with distinct cultures. The label *Latino* is mainly used to describe individuals who are descendants of or were born in Spanish-speaking countries in South and Central American or certain Caribbean countries and who now live in the United States. It is the context of living in the United States that provides the central focus for the study of Latino identity. The term *Latino* is also a panethnic term that may gloss over marked differences among those who are so identified (McConnell & Delgado-Romero, 2004), and therefore the theories presented all address within-group differences to some extent. This is the first assumptions that must be understood about the Latino identity development literature presented in this chapter: it pertains to those living in the United States and not to those who remained in their countries of origin (Torres, Howard-Hamilton, & Cooper, 2003).

The next assumption that connects each of the theories presented is that some element of acculturation to the majority culture in the United States is considered as part of the definition of ethnic identity. Early acculturation studies tended to focus on the assimilation of new groups into the host (majority) culture (Berry, 1980); this is a simplistic view that assumes the weakening of the culture of origin as the assimilation to the host culture occurs. More recent research on acculturation focus on multidimensional models of acculturation that recognize the acceptance of new cultural values varies greatly by the trait and does not

## Latino Countries of Origin

The 2000 U.S. census confirmed what had been predicted for several years; Latinos are the largest minority group in the United States. While growth of non-Latino White people in the United States grew by 5.9% since 1990, the Latino population increased by 57.9%. This increase impacts the nature of counseling work by bringing into prominence a group that has been previously overlooked.

The generic label of *Latino* can mislead counselors, and therefore it is important to understand the diversity among Latinos. The theories presented focus on the experiences of people from over twenty countries (including the Spanish-speaking Caribbean countries of Cuba, the Dominican Republic, and Puerto Rico; the Central, Northern and Southern American countries of Argentina, Belize, Bolivia, Brazil, Chile, Colombia, Costa Rica, Ecuador, El Salvador, Guatemala, Guyana, Honduras, Mexico, Nicaragua, Panama, Paraguay, Peru, Suriname, Uruguay, and Venezuela), who are in the United States for a variety of reasons. As a result, they find themselves managing their identity in the context of the U.S. majority Anglo (White) culture. The important aspect to understand about this balancing of cultures is that Latinos make choices about the two cultures. To understand their identity it is imperative for a counselor to understand the process of choosing between cultures.

The context of college is specifically highlighted because of the low completion rates of Latinos in higher education. While institutions of higher education can not change preexisting characteristics that may affect students' performance, they can make a difference by creating environments where Latino identity is valued and understood. This desire to create welcoming environments should be at the heart of every counselor's work.

necessitate the weakening of the culture of origin. For example, immigrants may prefer American food at the same time they have a strong attachment to the language of their ancestors. The language trait is preserved while other traits, like choice in food, are highly acculturated to the majority culture. These models consider the complexity of acculturation and how the individual makes choices that influence his level of acculturation (Berry, Kim, Minde, & Mok, 1987; Phinney, 1995). So part of the focus of understanding Latino identity needs to include an understanding of the choices an individual makes between the culture of origin and the American culture in which they reside (Torres, 1999, 2003). Variables such as the timing and context of immigration, region of the United States, and generational status impact acculturation for Latinos.

The final assumption is not clearly articulated by all of the theorists, but is generally accepted as an element in ethnic and racial identity theories. This element is the fact that there is a dominant group that functions in the United States and that those in the dominant group determine power, authority, and social order (Adams, 2001; Spring, 2001; Tatum, 1997). As a result of the existence of a dominant group, individuals who are not from the dominant group experience oppression in overt or subtle ways (Torres, et al., 2003). Consequently, minority groups learn to denigrate minority culture and aspire to be part of the majority culture (Hardiman & Jackson, 1997), which can lead to internalization of prejudice. In simple terms, those from minority cultures (like Latino cultures) feel pressure to assimilate into the dominant culture by giving up their minority culture. Furthermore, within the Latino ethnic group there is also an internalized hierarchy that Shorris (1992) refers to as *racismo,* the discrimination that exists within and between the Hispanic groups. Shorris explains that due to the effects of internalized racism, self-rejection, or the need to project unintegrated parts of the self onto others, Latinos have developed a hierarchy of racism based on national origin and race. Consequently the issue of dominance is multifaceted. These three assumptions contribute to how Latino identity is understood in the context of the United States.

## Latino Identity Theories

In general there is a lack of theoretical and empirical work regarding Latino identity development. The majority of the work in understanding identity development has been in comparing Black and White groups (e.g., Cross, 1971; 1995; Hardiman, 1982; Helms, 1990, 1995). Latinos have often either been ignored or been fit into generic minority identity models that group multiple minority cultures together—for example, Atkinson, Morten, and Sue's Minority Identity Development Model (1989); Sue and Sue's Racial/Cultural Identity Model (1999); and Phinney's Adolescent Ethnic Identity Development (1993). These multigroup theories may gloss over factors specific to being Latino as well as differences among national groups (Delgado-Romero, 2001). Consequently we have chosen three Latino identity theories for this chapter. The first is focused on Mexican Americans, who compromise the largest (58.6%) percentage of U.S. Latinos (U.S. Census Bureau, 2001). The second has a larger application to all Latinos and was developed in the 1990s and is clinically relevant. The final theory is an emerging theory based on a longitudinal study of Latino college students.

The case studies provided at the end of this chapter can be used as examples for these theories. The following descriptions are succinct and highlight important aspects of the models or theories. These descriptions are considered broad introductions. The reader should consider the original source if one particular research study is of great interest.

## Susan E. Keefe and Amado M. Padilla's Research

In the 1980s Keefe and Padilla (1987) conducted a research study among Mexican Americans with the goal of establishing a "theoretical framework for interpreting Mexican American ethnicity and sociocultural change" (p. 23). Recognizing the diversity among the Mexican American population, great care was given to the multidimensional nature of ethnicity and identity. While the participants in this study varied in ages, this classification of Latino identity is one of the first to shed light on the issue of Latino ethnic identity. This three-phase study used both survey and interview data that resulted in a cluster analysis to identify five cluster types that offer insight into the relationship between acculturation and ethnic identity. Below is the description of each of the cluster types:

*Type I: La Raza* This type had high scores on both cultural awareness and ethnic loyalty. These individuals maintain a high identification with Mexican culture and prefer it to the American culture.

*Type II: Changing Ethnics* This type had high scores on cultural awareness and average scores on ethnic loyalties. Individuals in this group tend to see ethnicity has having little consequence and are indifferent to distinctions between the Mexican and American cultures.

*Type III: Cultural Blends* This type had average scores on cultural awareness and ethnic loyalty. The individuals in this cluster type tended to be equally comfortable in both the American and Mexican cultures.

## ABOUT SUSAN E. KEEFE AND AMADO M. PADILLA

Susan E. Keefe is professor of applied anthropology at Appalachian State University. She received her Ph.D. from the University of California at Santa Barbara. Keefe's current work is focused on Appalachian communities and their ethnic diversity.

Amado M. Padilla is a professor of psychological studies in education at Stanford University. He received his Ph.D. in experimental psychology from the University of New Mexico. He was on the faculties of the University of California at Santa Barbara and UCLA prior to moving to Stanford. He has published extensively in the area of acculturation, Latino mental health, and second-language learning. He is currently most excited about his work on the academic resilience shown by high-achieving Latino students. He is the editor of the book *Hispanic Psychology: Critical Issues in Theory and Research*.

*Type IV: Emerging Americans* This type had moderately low scores on cultural awareness and ethnic loyalty. Individuals in this cluster type maintain some of the Mexican cultural values but increasingly recognize the adaptation to the American culture. These individuals tend to not recognize racism and feel a strong attachment to the American culture.

*Type V: New Americans* This type had very low scores on cultural awareness and moderately low scores on ethnic loyalty. For individuals in this group, ethnicity has a minor role in their lives and they make little effort to maintain the Mexican culture.

Other interesting factors that emerged from this study are that *familialism* was found to be pervasive regardless of an individual's level of acculturation. Familialism was defined as a family orientation that also includes an extended network of individuals that are seen as kin (Keefe & Padilla, 1987). In addition, Keefe and Padilla found that in later generations (second and third generations in the United States) the cultural awareness diminished, but the level of ethnic loyalty of Mexican Americans in California remained at a fairly constant level. These findings indicate that familial attachment is a fairly consistent trait among all Mexican Americans and that while knowledge of the culture of origin (language, music, or food) may diminish, cultural connections and pride are maintained in later generations.

This model is categorical and does not provide insight into how individuals came to their own understanding of cultural choices. While the Keefe and Padilla (1987) model framed many of the issues associated with Latino identity, it was not as clear on how the development of identity occurred.

## Aureliano S. Ruiz's Model of Ethnic Identity

Ruiz's (1990) Chicano/Latino model of ethnic identity addressed the shortcomings of general models of racial and ethnic identity and development, as well as the process variables of enculturation and acculturation. The model described the development, transformation, and resolution of ethnic identity conflicts based on case histories with Chicano, Mexican American, and other Latino college students. The model is based on four assumptions: marginality correlates highly with maladjustment; negative experiences of forced assimilation are destructive to the individual; pride in one's ethnic identity is positively correlated to mental health; and pride in one's ethnic identity results in freedom to choose, especially in the acculturation process. Ruiz posited five stages:

*Causal (stage 1)* During the Causal stage messages from the environment and important others ignore, negate, or denigrate Latino heritage. The person may experience humiliating and traumatic experiences related to being Latino and fail to identify with Latino culture.

*Cognitive (stage 2)* During the Cognitive stage three erroneous belief systems are incorporated as a result of negative or distorted messages: group membership as a Latino is associated with poverty and prejudice; assimilation into dominant (White) society is seen as the only viable means of escape; and one-way assimilation (into the dominant culture) is the only road to success.

*Consequence (stage 3)* In the Consequence stage the fragmentation of Latino identity intensifies, especially when confronted with social injustice; the individual may actively reject her Chicano/Latino heritage. Some may seek to escape their despised ethnic self-image by assuming an alien ethnic identity (e.g., changing one's name, hiding dark skin).

*Working Through (stage 4)* The Working Through stage begins with the integration of a healthier Chicano/Latino identity. In this stage the individual is no longer able to cope with ethnic conflict and realizes that an alien ethnic identity is not acceptable. This stage is characterized by an increase in ethnic consciousness and reclaiming, reintegrating, and reconnecting with an ethnic identity and community.

---

### ABOUT AURELIANO S. RUIZ, MFT

Aureliano Ruiz has been a counselor in Counseling and Psychological Services at California State University–Pomona for over thirty years. He received his or B.A. and M.S. from California State University at Fullerton.

---

*Successful Resolution (stage 5)* The final stage is the Successful Resolutions stage, which is characterized by the individual's greater acceptance of self, Latino culture, and ethnicity; improved self-esteem; and a belief that a Latino identity is positive and promotes success.

Ruiz developed his model from case histories derived from counseling sessions. He did not provide methodological information for the development of his model, which leads one to question the process of formal qualitative analysis in the formation of the model. Ruiz stated that his model was different from other models because it dealt with the contributing factors to ethnic identity conflicts and fragmentation. In addition his model provided counseling interventions and addressed language, defense mechanisms, and culture-specific techniques.

## Vasti Torres's Research on Latino College Students

As a result of doing research on college students, I (first author) found that little research had focused on the identity development of Latino college students. Because of my desire to better understand the process of development for Latino college students and a need to help counselors and administrators in college understand the increasing number of Latino students attending college (many of whom were dropping out), I began a series of studies about the college experience of Latino students.

The first study validated the Bicultural Orientation Model (Torres, 1999), which placed Latino college students into four quadrants based on their responses to an acculturation (Marin, Sabogal, Marin, Otero-Sabogal, & Perez-Stable, 1987) and ethnic identity measure (Phinney, 1992). The goal of this validation study was to operationally define the choices Latino students make between their culture of origin and the American culture. Three methods were used to validate the model. First, the model placement was compared with each student's self-identified cultural orientation. Second, a comparison was made with the Bicultural/Multicultural Experience Inventory (Ramirez, 1983) in order to validate the construct of bicultural orientation. And finally a MANOVA was run to test that the measures distinguished among the cultural orientations. The four cultural orientations are:

*Bicultural Orientation* These individuals had high scores on both the acculturation and ethnic identity measures. These students felt comfortable in both the American and Latino culture.

*Latino Orientation* These individuals had low scores on the acculturation measure and high scores on the ethnic identity measure. These students preferred the Latino culture and preferred to interact with more Latinos than Americans.

*Anglo Orientation* These students had high scores on the acculturation measure and low scores on the ethnic identity measure. Overall these students preferred the Anglo (American) culture to the Latino culture.

*Marginal Orientation* These students had low scores on both the acculturation and ethnic identity measures. While college students were not expected in this quadrant, the students identified as Marginal were more likely have spent less time in the United States and more likely to have parents who did not speak English. These factors may impact their ability to feel comfortable in either culture.

Two additional findings are of interest in this study. The first is that students who came from areas where there was a critical mass (more than 35%) of Latinos in the greater community had lower acculturation scores than those who came from majority White areas, but there was no significant difference with the ethnic identity scores. This would indicate that while students who do not have constant reminders of their ethnicity are more likely to adapt to the American culture, they maintain pride in their ethnicity at the same level as those that live in areas with a critical mass of Latinos (Torres, Winston, & Cooper, 2003).

The second finding is that there was no statistically significant difference between the cultural orientations on a measure of stress. This indicates that there seems to be no greater amount of stress, or advantage, associated with any of the orientations. One conclusion that could be made is that among the orientations it truly is about individual choices between the Latino and Anglo cultures rather than outside college stressors. Like other identity theories, this model seems to indicate that Latino college students must resolve the choice between the two cultures and that it is the process of this resolution that is more important than which choices they make (Torres, 2003).

Understanding that the model only placed Latino students into categories, I began a longitudinal study to look at the process of development.

I interviewed Latino college freshmen at seven institutions and continue to follow the same students over time. The findings in this ongoing study indicate that there are four conditions that help situate Latino identity while they are freshmen college students. These conditions help identify the influences that help a student make the choices about their own cultural orientation (Torres, 2003; Torres, 2004; Torres & DeSawal, 2004). It is critical that these conditions be seen as interrelated and that all should be considered together. To only consider one condition would not provide a true understanding of the whole person. The conditions are:

*Environment Where They Grew Up* This condition is described by a continuum that ranges from diverse to Latino majority environments to majority White environments. Individuals who grow up in diverse environments tend to have a strong sense of ethnicity. The individuals who grow up in areas where Latinos are the majority are likely to have a strong sense of ethnicity but take their ethnicity for granted because there is little ethnic challenge. On the other end of the continuum are individuals who come from majority White environments and are more likely to associate or make choices consistent with the majority culture.

*Family and Generational Status in the United States* This condition describes a variety of issues dealing with family influences. First, individuals' families are most likely to influence how they self-identify in their freshmen year. The label used by the parents is likely to be the label used by the student. In addition, the generational status of the family has a strong influence on how freshmen situate their identity. Students with more acculturated parents are likely to take for granted the intermingling of the two cultures, while students with less acculturated parents are more likely to experience conflict between the two cultures. These individuals are expected to balance the expectations of parents with the expectations of the majority group. These expectations can cause conflict and illustrate the nature of cultural conflict.

*Self-Perception of Status in Society* This condition focuses on how Latino students see themselves in relationship to the greater social structures. This condition impacts students' ability to recognize racism and their ability to cope with it. Students who are better able to recognize racism are less likely to perceive any privilege and are open to other cultures. Those students who see themselves as possessing some privilege are more likely to believe negative stereotypes, but they believe these negative images do not apply to them. While most Latinos do not see themselves as privileged, there are intergroup differences and socioeconomic differences that can differentiate the Latino population.

TABLE 12.1    Overview of Existing Theories Dealing with Bicultural
Latino Identity

| Keefe & Padilla, 1987 [Research Based] | Torres, 1999 [Research Based] | Felix-Ortiz de la Garza, Newcomb, & Myers, 1995 [ResearchBased] | Ferdman and Gallegos, 2001 |
|---|---|---|---|
| Type I: La Raza | Latino Oriented | Latino Identified Group | Latino Identified Sub-group Identified |
| Type II: Changing Ethnics | | | |
| Type III: Cultural Blends | Bicultural Oriented | Highly Bicultural Group | Latino Integrated Latino as Other |
| Type IV: Emerging Americans | Possible Anglo Oriented | Possible American Identified Group | Undifferentiated/ Denial |
| Type V: New Americans | Anglo Oriented Marginal Orientation | American Identified Group Low-Level Bicultural Group | White Identified |

Note. Ruiz' model is sequential rather than categorical in nature and is therefore not included.

*College Environment* This condition focuses on the level of dissonance the college environment creates for an individual. The dissonance is between the environment they grew up in and the environment they face while in college. The greater the dissonance the stronger the potential conflict they will experience. Students coming from majority Latino environments to predominantly White colleges will experience greater levels of cultural conflict and vice versa.

These conditions provide insight into the individual differences among Latino students in college (Torres, 2003; Torres, 2004). By understanding the conditions that influence how students situate their Latino identity, counselors and practitioners can begin their conversations with culturally appropriate questions that provide insight into how the students see themselves within the context of the college environment as well as the greater social structure.

Other models of bicultural orientation exist, yet we find the four presented in Table 12.1 to be most applicable and least repetitive for counselors. In an effort to assist in understanding the possible relationships among the various bicultural models, the table summarizes them and their possible relationships to each other.

## Connection to Counseling Practice

Recent calls to the profession of counseling emphasize the need to address multicultural issues in counseling (e.g., APA, 2003; Arredondo et al., 1996). The impetus for this call to action was the concern that traditional counseling theory and practice was based on the experiences of a specific population (e.g., White males) and as such was culturally encapsulated (Wrenn, 1962). Thus the issues of culture, race, ethnicity, language, and other important aspects of identity were essential to address in counseling in a sensitive and competent manner. Thus multicultural competence is essentially an ethical matter for counselors.

The concern about multicultural competence in counseling and counseling research is also fueled by the reality of a rapidly diversifying U.S. population. Nowhere is this more clearly visible than in the case of Latinos who have, through the twin engines of immigration and high fertility rates, become the largest minority group in the United States The Latino population has dramatically increased over last twenty years, from fifteen million in 1980 to nearly thirty-five million in 2000 (U.S. Census Bureau, 2001). The U.S. Latino population overall is the youngest population in the United States, and millions of Latino youth are currently or will shortly be in late adolescence. Evidence suggests that Latinos struggle to attain the same level of success as their White peers, especially in the educational realm where Latino youth drop out of the educational pipeline at all stages in record numbers. Consequently it is important for counselors to understand the relationship between Latino identity development and success in college.

Keefe and Padilla (1987) made a significant contribution to the counseling literature in several ways. First by focusing on a specific national and ethnic group—Mexican Americans—Keefe and Padilla (1987) were able to focus on the unique dynamics that influence ethnic identity. Mexican Americans lived in the United States before there was a United States and have a long history of exploitation by White European immigrants (Griswold Del Castillo & De Leon, 1996; Spring, 2001). At the same time, Mexican Americans are the largest group of U.S. Latinos (nearly 60%) and have a history of social and political activism (e.g., the Chicano movement) that has shaped much of the Latino experience in the United States. Consequently it is important to not lose the uniqueness of the Mexican American experience when it is subsumed under the general term *Latino*. Keefe and Padilla (1987) were able to describe the heterogeneous nature of the Mexican American community at the individual and community level. This model explicitly aided counselors by providing a conceptualization of ethnic identity where extremes of Mexican American identity could be normalized and understood in a developmental framework rather than as pathological identities.

However, while Keefe and Padilla (1987) as well as other theorists (e.g., Felix-Ortiz de la Garza et al., 1995; Ferdman & Gallegos, 2001) advanced an understanding of Latino identity with descriptions of identity that are categorical and static, they offered limited information to counselors on what to do with a client who was placed in one of the stages and little guidance on how counselors could help clients develop their ethnic identity to the point where ethnic identity would be a source of pride and empowerment rather than shame. It was Ruiz who furthered this research by considering this process from a counseling prospective.

Ruiz (1990) proposed a model that could guide Latino ethnic development from mentally unhealthy stages to healthier ones. Ruiz proposed the radical (at the time) notion that a healthy Latino identity was a possible and desirable outcome of the counseling process. Ruiz, like other like-minded scholars (e.g., Atkinson, Morten & Sue, 1989; Cross, 1971, 1995; Helms, 1990, 1995; Phinney, 1993), reenvisioned the role of the therapist as someone who could facilitate cultural development and empowerment. Ruiz suggested ways in which the counselor could match the stage of ethnic identity development using stage and culturally appropriate interventions. For example, during the Causal stage, where the client has internalized negative beliefs about Latino culture, the counselor may work to confront negative self-statements and replace them with positive (culture affirming) statements and participation in events that reflect cultural pride.

Pizarro and Vera (2001) say that Ruiz provided a much needed conceptualization of Latino ethnic identity. However they pointed out that the limitation of the model was a simplistic condensation of identity development that focused on specific (ethnic) conflicts while excluding other potentially salient conflicts (e.g., racial). In addition, the model is limited by the minimal empirical support for the model. Ruiz (1990) based the model on case histories derived from counseling sessions and provided no methodological information on how the model was constructed. In the twenty-four years since the model was proposed, it has been used in case studies as a model of Latino ethnic identity development in therapy (e.g., Delgado-Romero, 2001), but we could find no empirical studies based on the model. Thus the first two models have their strengths and limitations. Keefe and Padilla (1987) provide useful, research-based descriptions of different types of ethnic identity, but minimal developmentally or clinically relevant information. Ruiz (1990) provides a clinically grounded model that traces a progress of ethnic identity, but one with little empirical validation. Therefore we offer the bicultural identity model (Torres, 1999) and the subsequent understanding of the conditions that influence how students situate their Latino identity (Torres, 2003, 2004). It is a model that is grounded in research and includes the strengths of the two earlier models while addressing the limitations of both.

Torres' model is clinically relevant because it situates Latinos on both the dimensions of acculturation and of ethnic identity as a way to consider the extent to which a client accepts mainstream U.S. culture and the dynamic relationship between that acceptance and the maintenance of ethnic identity. Both of these are important to address in therapy. Torres points out that the context (numbers of Latinos in their hometown) under which acculturation takes place is important in understanding the challenges of ethnic identity formation. In an innovative way, Torres, Winston, and Cooper (2003) addressed one of the central myths of acculturation—that acculturation to U.S. norms is an advantage in dealing with stress. Like Ruiz (1990), Torres points out that a strong identification as Latino can help the client negotiate the stress inherent in college-aged adolescence. However, unlike Ruiz, Torres explicitly allows for the fact Latino students can have a bicultural orientation. The ongoing nature of Torres' work also allows development to be considered from a longitudinal perspective. In later work, Torres points out the need to consider the cognitive development of college students as a way to better help them transform negative ethnic images to positive images that can empower them (Torres & Baxter Magolda, 2004).

Taking information from each of these theorists, counselors can better understand the nuances and conditions that can influence Latino ethnic identity development. There is no one blueprint that applies to all Latino adolescents. Counselors must be prepared to ask culturally appropriate questions that can provide insight into how Latino identity is situated and what interventions need to be created to help a Latino work through the potential conflicts she can encounter. What these identity theories illustrate is that there is a need for counselors to understand why Latino identity can differ from other racial/ethnic groups.

## Jimena: "I don't belong here"

Jimena is an eighteen-year-old college sophomore at a large urban university with a growing Latino population. She is Mexican American and her family has been in the United States for four generations. Jimena grew up in a large midwestern city and attends a college close to home. She has always been a strong student and her education, to this point, has been completed in schools where Latinos were a critical mass. Jimena is the first person in her family to go to college, and although she preferred to attend a more diverse school in another state, her parents insisted that she stay close to home and attend the local university where there was limited diversity. She was brought to the university counseling center by the faculty advisor of her Latina sorority (who herself is Latina) because she is failing all of her classes and seems exhausted and depressed. Jimena only agreed to come to counseling if her advisor would go with her and would be present to meet the counselor. For Jimena, this is not an issue of language. Like most U.S. Latino college students, born in the United States or outside the United States, Jimena speaks English perfectly.

> Jimena's advisor said, "I'm completely shocked to find out Jimena is failing all of her classes because she is such an outstanding sister in the sorority. If anything needs to be done, she does it and she is always on top of things. I just assumed that she was doing well in classes. I just don't know what to say! I feel like I should call her parents to come get her and take her to the doctor, but Jimena asked me not call them yet. I wanted her to see the psychiatrist but they said I had to meet with you first."

The counselor recognizes the parental dynamic that is occurring, yet does not want to show lack of respect for the advisor. The counselor has replaced the parents in this case. The counselor thanks the advisor for bringing Jimena in and suggests that the advisor wait in the lobby so that Jimena and the counselor might discuss her problems. The counselor reassures the advisor that they will come get her in a little while. The advisor reluctantly agrees.

> Jimena begins talking, "I really let her [advisor] down, just like I let down the sorority and my parents. Everyone is shocked because I was the one person that everyone thought had it together. I guess I fooled everyone."

"I just don't belong here at college. I hate my major and I hate my classes. The only thing I like about being here is my sorority because it's the only place I fit in. In high school I had lots of friends and we hung out together. Most of them got jobs or went to the local community college, but my parents made me come here. I hate it here. In my classes I'm the only Mexican, and I'm sick of answering stupid questions about my name and telling people that I'm in the United States legally. It gets on my nerves. Luckily I found my sorority, which is a Latina sorority, and the other sisters are just like me. Without them I would have gone home after the first semester, but since you had to have a 2.5 to pledge I decided to go to class. It wasn't too hard because these were my general education classes. Then I wanted to major in Latino studies but my parents freaked out and said I had to be a lawyer or a doctor. I started in pre-law, but I hate my major. I'm doing terrible in every class, so I spend all of my time working on things for the sorority. I guess my advisor found out that I wasn't going to class, and she freaked out, too. I guess you are going to tell me how I need to shape up, too. It doesn't matter because if I fail out then I can't be in the sorority and without them I'm not staying here."

## Jose: Passing for Cuban

Jose is a twenty-year-old junior in college. He approached a counselor from the university counseling center at a Hispanic Heritage Month event and asked if he might come by the office to talk about his major, psychology. The counselor, who is active in the local Latino community and therefore is widely perceived by students as someone who could be trusted, immediately agreed. Previous experience indicated that Latino clients often take an indirect route to counseling, so the counselor invited Jose to come by the office. This invitation gives Jose the indirect route he is seeking out.

After talking about psychology as a major and chatting about university life, Jose asked if he could talk about something that is bothering him. The counselor agreed.

Jose began talking: "I grew up in Miami. My parents moved there when I was in the first grade. My parents are Mexican, but once I went to school I found out that everyone else was Cuban. I really wanted to fit in so I started to tell people that I was Cuban, too. Besides I had watched enough TV and heard enough people talk about Mexicans to know that I didn't want to be Mexican. I changed my accent, and it was pretty easy to fit in actually. I think some of my friends knew I wasn't really Cuban but they didn't care. In Miami if you are Cuban, you are in the majority. So I went all through school being part of the majority. My parents would tease me that I was their Cuban son."

"I wanted to go to a really good college so I came 'up north' to go to school. At first it was really fun, just like high school only better. A lot of my friends came with me and the other students didn't really care if I was Cuban or not, it just seemed like we all got along. But I started noticing little things, like my White friends would make fun of Latinos around me and try to get me to go along with the joke. For a while I did, I even thought it was funny that my nickname was 'spic.' Other than the jokes things didn't really bother me too much. Then some things started to happen that really started bothering me. The first was that some of the students from the Mexican American Student Association called me to see if I wanted to go to a meeting. I was really mad, why did you call me I said? They apologized and said that they thought my last name, Ochoa, was a Mexican name (which it is). I felt like someone had figured out my big secret and I don't want people to treat me like I'm Mexican, because people around here hate Mexicans. I've been feeling like everyone I know lately has been looking at me and thinking that I'm a dirty Mexican."

"To make things worse last week there was an incident where someone spray-painted 'Spics go home' on the side of the Latino cultural center. I know it didn't have anything to do with me, but it made me feel unsafe. Like I said, I grew up in Miami and I've never felt like a minority before, and suddenly after three years of college I suddenly feel like a minority and a fake minority, at that, because I'm not even Cuban. I don't know if you can understand what I'm talking about and it may sound stupid, but it's really bothering me. I feel angry all of the time and really on the edge."

## Working with Jose and Jimena in Counseling

Jose and Jimena are both composite characters based on several Latino clients the authors talked and worked with over the years. Their problems are representative of a broad range of problems that bring Latino clients (directly or indirectly) to counseling. In this section we explore how using ethnic identity development theories (e.g., Padilla & Keefe, 1987; Ruiz, 1990; and Torres, 1999, 2003) can help guide the counselor throughout the course of therapy. In these cases we have assumed that the counselor is familiar with Latino ethnic identity development and that the counselor has invested some time in outreach to the Latino community. However, we do not assume that the counselor is herself Latino or bilingual.

Jose's case is complex because Jose is navigating his identity both within the broad group of Latinos and the cultural differences between Latinos and majority White culture. He has chosen what he perceives to be a higher status identity by saying he is Cuban rather than Mexican, and he is negotiating the conflicts between the Latino cultural group and White majority culture. Jose has been able to find a comfortable position in his life in which he seeks to isolate himself from racism and prejudice by "fitting in" or "passing" as a member of a dominant Latino group. However, he is beginning to be confronted by various disconfirmations of assumed ethnic identity both personal (prejudicial teasing by peers) and in general (racist graffiti directed towards all Latinos). Jose is consistently reminded that his identity is not authentic, and consequently he begins to doubt his relationships with others and experience anger.

Jose does not neatly fit into Keefe and Padilla's (1987) typology because although he is Mexican, he chooses instead to identify as Cuban. He might be thought of as belonging to the *Emerging American type* that had moderately low scores on cultural awareness and ethnic loyalty. Individuals in this cluster type maintain some of the Mexican cultural values but increasingly adapt to the American culture. They tend to not recognize racism and feel a strong attachment to the American culture. This is consistent with Jose's desire to "fit in." Consequently the counselor can understand how Jose identifies himself relative to acculturation and ethnic identity, and can normalize the new experience of racism and lack of authenticity that Jose is experiencing.

According the Ruiz (1990), Jose exhibits characteristics of the first two stages of Latino ethnic identity development. He has internalized negative messages regarding Mexican ethnicity and does not identify as Mexican (stage 1), and his ultimate goal seems to be assimilation (stage 2), be it as a Cuban or a White person. Using the Ruiz framework, the counselor can work with Jose to work through the growing realization of social injustice (stages 3 and 4) and develop cultural pride (stage 5).

Jose illustrates the Self Perception of Status in Society condition (Torres, 2003) and the potential issues involved when an individual believes negative stereotypes. In conjunction with other conditions, a counselor can understand that the environment where Jose grew up influences his perceptions of Mexican American identity and therefore this dimension needs to be explored in order to help Jose find congruence within his ethnic identity. All of these issues come together because of the dissonance Jose is experiencing between his previous environment and the college environment he is presently experiencing.

In the case of Jose, the counselor must be very intentional about considering how much challenge and alternative interpretations one can offer Jose in order to transform his negative images into more healthy congruent images (Ruiz, 1990; Torres & Baxter Magolda, 2004). The rate and path taken by the counselor will be very important in helping Jose develop a healthy identity that will help him manage future conflicts.

Jimena presents a situation entirely different than Jose's, but she does share some similarities. They are both attempting to mediate ethnic identity with the stress of college achievement and normal adolescent development. They both find college a confusing place where their identities have been challenged. Both have employed cultural coping mechanisms to survive. Jimena has chosen an opposite coping mechanism to Jose. Rather than deny her cultural background, Jimena has chosen to fervently embrace it and use it (as expressed through affiliation with her Latina sorority) as a way to deal with an oppressive environment.

Keefe and Padilla (1987) would typify Jimena as being in the La Raza category of identity—that is, she maintains a high identification with Mexican culture and prefers it to the American culture. Jimena does not fit into the Ruiz (1990) model in many ways. She has ethnic consciousness and embraces her Latina culture while devaluing Anglo culture. Ruiz's model does not account for Latinos who have a strong ethnic identity to begin with. However, Jimena does fit in with Ruiz's conceptualization in the sense that she has equated her ethnicity as incompatible with her education. Jimena sees a dichotomous choice between being Latina and being a successful student. Consequently she is stuck, and her educational prospects are not good. It is no surprise that Jimena did not self-refer to counseling. Her conceptualization of the problem is an external one, and she most likely does not trust people outside of her social circle. Thus the role of the advisor in getting her to counseling is a critical one, and the counselor should make sure to reassure the advisor and engage her in supporting the student, while at the same time respecting the confidentiality of the client.

Jimena does illustrate the condition of Familial Influences and Generational Status in Torres (2004). While Jimena feels support from her parents to attend college, it seems that her parents have little understanding of what college life is like for her. Jimena is a first-generation college student, and her parents' images of success are narrowly defined by what they know. The dynamic between Jimena and her parent must be understood through a cultural lens. Jimena wants to please her parents while the parents want Jimena to have a financially secure life, which to them is narrowly defined by the professional careers they are familiar with. While these desires may seem contradictory in the case study, they illustrate the cultural conflicts that must be negotiated by Latino college students.

Both Jose and Jimena previously employed coping mechanisms that no longer work for them and have reached a crisis point. Jose can no longer be "color blind" and deny his status as a Mexican American and a Latino. Jimena cannot continue to choose her (narrowly defined) ethnicity over her education, because in doing so she will lose both. Consequently a culturally sensitive counselor guided by ethnic identity developmental theory can have an enormous impact on the lives of these students.

## Summary

The increase in Latinos in the United States makes understanding the ethnic identity development of these college students a critical aspect of the professional preparation of counselors. The diversity of those included within the Latino label makes it imperative that counselors understand the choices individuals make and the impact those choices have on their identity development. These choices must be understood within the context of a majority White environment that has a history of oppression of different groups and encourages the abandonment of ethnic minority culture, while idealizing majority White culture.

The case studies included in this chapter illustrate internal and external cultural conflicts that can emerge during ethnic identity formation. The theories presented can help counselors understand the dynamics as well as provide a framework for healthy resolution of these conflicts. In addition, knowledge of ethnic identity formation theories is essential for counselors so as to ensure they do not unknowing reinforce or perpetuate oppressive cultural dynamics in therapy. The chapter also provides a glimpse into the complex, multifaceted nature of Latino ethnic identity formation. It is up to the counselor to understand the depth of the choices and the importance individuals place on those cultural choices. Using ethnic identity formation theories, counselors can become advocates and agents for empowerment as Latino students develop authentic and healthy identities that encompass both their culture of origin and the culture they live in.

As we stated earlier, a counselor does not need to be Latino to understand or effectively help a Latino client. Latino culture in the United States is constantly evolving in dynamic and surprising ways. Consequently, Latino clients may need an informed and empowering guide as they try to mediate majority culture, traditional Latino culture, and the evolving U.S. Latino culture. We can think of no better guide than a counselor who is informed by ethnic identity development theory and is willing to go along on this journey.

# Annotated Bibliography

Although we have covered the major articles regarding Latino identity development within the chapter (see citations), we suggest the following readings for those interested in advancing their understanding of Latino people.

Arredondo, P. (2002). Mujeres Latinas-Santas y Marquesas. *Cultural Diversity and Ethnic Minority Psychology, 8*(4), 308–319.
Gender issues are also crucial in the Latino population, and gender roles affect development and identity. Arredondo approaches this issue from a personal perspective.

Comas-Díaz, L. (1994). LatiNegra: Mental health issues of African Latinas. *Journal of Feminist Family Therapy, 5*, 35–74.
One consequence of entering U.S. society is that Latinos are forced into the U.S. categorical system of race (Black versus White). The issue of race is one that is critical to understanding how Latinos reject or embrace U.S. categorical systems.

Delgado-Romero, E. A., & Rojas, A. (2004). Other Latinos: Counseling Cuban, Central and South American clients. In C. Negy (Ed.), *Cross cultural psychotherapy: Toward a critical understanding of diverse client populations* (pp. 139–162). Reno, NV: Bent Tree Press.
Much of the available literature is focused on the lives of Mexicans and Puerto Ricans, and because they are the two largest groups of Latinos, we feel this is rightfully so. However the issues of Latinos from other countries are often lost. In this chapter there is some context for understanding the lives of these other Latinos.

Santiago-Rivera, A. L., Arredondo, P. A., & Gallardo-Cooper, M. (2002). *Counseling Latinos and la familia: A practical guide*. Thousand Oaks: Sage.
This text is a concise and practical guide to working with Latinos in their contexts and proposes some models of identity that are highly useful, but not developmental in nature.

Torres, V. (2004). The diversity among us: Puerto Ricans, Cubans, Caribbean, Central and South Americans. In A.M. Ortiz (Ed.), *Addressing the unique needs of Latino American students. New directions for student services* (pp. 5–16). San Francisco: Jossey-Bass.
This chapter focuses on the educational and immigration differences among Latinos in the United States. It focuses on all Latino countries other than Mexico.

# References

Aboud, F. E., & Doyle, A. (1993). The early development of ethnic identity and attitudes. In M. E. Bernal & G. P. Knight (Eds.), *Ethnic identity: Formation and transmission among Hispanics and other minorities* (pp. 47–59). Albany: State University of New York Press.

Adams, M. (2001). Core processes of racial identity development. In C. L. Wijeyesinghe & B. W. Jackson III (Eds.), *New perspectives on racial identity development: a theoretical and practical anthology* (pp. 209–242). New York: New York University Press.

American Psychological Association. (2003). Guidelines on multicultural education, training, research, practice and organizational change for psychologists. *American Psychologist, 58*, 377–402.

Arredondo, P., Toporek, R., Brown, S., Jones, J., Locke, D., Sánchez, J., et al. (1996). Operationalization of multicultural counseling competencies. *Journal of Multicultural Counseling and Development, 24*, 42–78.

Atkinson, D. R., Morten, G., & Sue, D. W. (1989). A minority identity development model. In D. R. Atkinson, G. Morten, & D. W. Sue (Eds.), *Counseling American minorities* (pp. 35–52). Dubuque, IA: Brown.

Bernal, M. E., Knight, G. P., Ocampo, K. A., Garza, C. A., & Cota, M. K. (1993). Development of Mexican American identity. In M. E. Bernal & G. P. Knight (Eds.), *Ethnic identity: Formation and transmission among Hispanics and other minorities* (pp. 31–46). Albany: State University of New York Press.

Berry, J. W. (1980). Acculturation as varieties of adaptation. In A. M. Padilla (Ed.), *Acculturation theories, models, and some new findings* (pp. 9–26). Boulder, CO: Westview Press.

Berry, J. W., Kim, U., Minde, T., & Mok, D. (1987). Comparative studies of acculturative stress. *International Migration Review, 21*, 491–511.

Chickering, A. W., & Reisser, L. (1993) *Education and identity* (2nd ed.). San Francisco: Jossey-Bass.

Cross, W. E., Jr. (1971, July). The Negro-to-Black conversion experience. *Black World*, 13–27.

Cross, W. E., Jr. (1995). The psychology of nigrescence: Revising the Cross model. In J. G. Ponterotto, J. M. Casas, L. A. Suzuki, & C. M. Alexander (Eds.), *Handbook of multicultural counseling* (pp. 93–122). Thousand Oaks, CA: Sage.

Delgado-Romero, E. A. (2001). Counseling a Hispanic/Latino client—Mr. X. Counseling Racially Diverse Clients [Special issue]. *The Journal of Mental Health Counseling, 23*, 207–221.

Erikson, E. H. (1968). *Identity: Youth and crisis.* New York: Norton.

Felix-Ortiz de la Garza, M., Newcomb, M. D., & Myers, H. F. (1995). A multidimensional measure of cultural identity for Latino and Latina Adolescents. In A. M. Padilla (Ed.), *Hispanic psychology: Critical issues in theory and research* (pp. 30–42). Thousand Oaks, CA: Sage.

Ferdman, B. M., & Gallegos, P. I. (2001). Racial identity development and Latinos in the United States. In C. L. Wijeyesinghe & B. W. Jackson III (Eds.), *New perspectives on racial identity development: A theoretical and practical anthology* (pp. 32–66). New York: New York University Press.

Griswold Del Castillo, R., & De Leon, A. (1996). *North to Aztlan: A history of Mexican Americans in the United States.* New York: Twayne.

Hardiman, R. (1982). *White identity development: A process oriented model for describing the racial consciousness of White Americans.* Unpublished doctoral dissertation, University of Massachusetts, Amherst.

Hardiman, R., & Jackson, B. W. (1997). Conceptual foundation for social justice courses. In M. Adams, L. A. Bell, and P. Griffin (Eds.), *Teaching for diversity and social justice: A sourcebook* (pp. 16–29). New York: Routledge.

Helms, J. E. (1990). *Black and White racial identity: Theory, research and practice.* New York, Greenwood Press.

Helms, J. E. (1995). An update of Helm's white and people of color racial identity models. In J. G. Ponterotto, J. M. Casas, L. A. Suzuki, & C. M. Alexander (Eds.), *Handbook of multicultural counseling* (pp. 181–198). Thousand Oaks, CA: Sage.

Keefe, S. E., & Padilla, A. M. (1987). *Chicano ethnicity.* Albuquerque: University of New Mexico Press.

Marin, G., Sabogal, F., Marin, B. V., Otero-Sabogal, R., & Perez-Stable, E. J. (1987). Development of a short acculturation scale for Hispanics. *Hispanic Journal of Behavioral Sciences, 9*(2), 183–205.

McConnell, E. D., & Delgado-Romero, E. A. (2004). Latino panethnicity: Reality or methodological construction? *Sociological Focus, 37*(4), 297–312.

Phinney, J. S. (1992). The multigroup ethnic identity measure: A new scale for use with diverse groups. *Journal of Adolescent Research, 7*, 156–176.

Phinney, J. S. (1993). A three-stage model of ethnic identity development in adolescence. In M. E. Bernal & G. P. Knight (Eds.), *Ethnic identity: Formation and transmission among Hispanics and other minorities.* (pp. 61–79). Albany: State University of New York Press.

Phinney, J. S. (1995). Ethnic identity and self-esteem a review and integration. In A. M. Padilla (Ed.) *Hispanic psychology critical issues in the theory and research* (pp. 57–70). Thousand Oaks, CA: Sage.

Pizzaro, M., & Vera, E. M. (2001). Chicana/o ethnic identity research: Lessons for researchers and counselors. *The Counseling Psychologist, 29,* 91–117.

Ramirez, M., III (1983). *Psychology of the Americas mestizo perspective on personality and mental health.* New York: Pergamon Press.

Ruiz, A. S. (1990). Ethnic identity: Crisis and resolution. *Journal of Multicultural Counseling and Development, 18,* 29–40.

Shorris, E. (1992). *Latinos: A biography of the People.* New York: Norton.

Spring, J. (2001). *Deculturalization and the struggle for equality: A brief history of the education of dominated cultures in the United States.* Boston: McGraw-Hill.

Sue, D. W., & Sue, D. (1999). *Counseling the culturally different: Theory and practice* (3rd ed.). New York: Wiley.

Tatum, B. D. (1997). *Why are all the black kids sitting together in the cafeteria? And other conversations about race.* New York: Basic Books.

Torres, V. (1999). Validation of a bicultural orientation model for Hispanic college students. *Journal of College Student Development, 40*(3), 285–299.

Torres, V. (2003) Influences on ethnic identity development of Latino college students in the first two years of college. *Journal of College Student Development, 44*(4), 532–547.

Torres, V. (2004) Familial influences on the identity development of Latino first year students. *Journal of College Student Development, 45*(4), 457–469.

Torres, V., & Baxter Magolda, M. (2004). Reconstructing Latino identity: The influence of cognitive development on the ethnic identity process of Latino students. *Journal of College Student Development, 45*(3), 333–347.

Torres, V., & DeSawal, D. M. (2004, March). *The role environment plays in retaining Latino students in urban universities.* Paper presented the meeting of the National Association of Student Personnel Administrators (NASPA), Denver, CO.

Torres, V., Howard-Hamilton, M., & Cooper, D. L. (2003). *Identity development of diverse populations: Implications for teaching and practice.* Monograph for ASHE/ERIC. San Francisco: Jossey-Bass.

Torres, V., Winston, R. B., Jr., & Cooper, D. L. (2003). The effect of geographic location, institutional type, and stress on Hispanic students' cultural orientation. *NASPA Journal, 40*(2), Article 10. http://publications.naspa.org/naspajournal/vol40/iss2/art10

U.S. Census Bureau. 2001. *Census 2000 summary file 1 (SF1).* Washington, DC: U.S. Census Bureau.

Wrenn, C. G. (1962). The culturally encapsulated counselor. *Harvard Educational Review, 32,* 444–449.

# CHAPTER THIRTEEN

# White Racial Identity Development

## Jan Arminio

A number of social justice advocates have noted that U.S. society has not achieved the expected progress in civil rights though the movement occurred forty years ago (Cose, 1998; Johnson, 2001; Kivel, 2002; West, 2001). In 1941 during a speech to Congress, Franklin Roosevelt listed four "basic things expected by our people." These have come to be known as the "Four Freedoms": freedom of speech, freedom of worship, freedom from want, and freedom from fear. How can U. S. society more completely offer these four freedoms? Have all four been given equal and adequate attention? What role do helping professionals play in promoting and ensuring these freedoms?

In considering ways that our country can better ensure that all people enjoy freedom from want, freedom from fear, and freedom of expression and worship, racial identity has become a central theme. Because White racial identity provides a means by which White people can have a positive sense of self not at the expense of others' freedoms, studying and applying this theory is important to society at large but especially to those in the helping professions. Realizing that White people are the numerical majority (approximately 75% according to 2000 census data) and fill most of the influential positions in U.S. society, Helms noted that, "For racism to disappear in the United States, White people must take the responsibility for ending it" (1992, p. i). White people can "partake of White culture without insisting upon maintaining the benefits of racism for oneself and for other Whites" (Helms, 1992, p. 14).

## ABOUT THE CHAPTER AUTHOR

### Jan Arminio

Though I am currently department chair and professor of counseling and college student personnel at Shippensburg University, it was my introduction to racial identity development in my doctoral program at the University of Maryland, College Park, that began my liberation from unjust ways of being. I will be forever grateful to my teachers there and to Shippensburg students (past and present) for their trust and care.

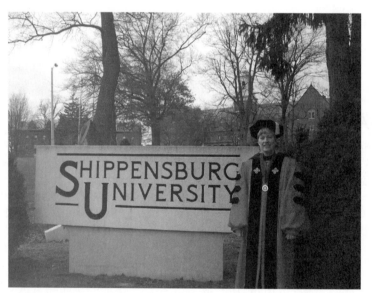

**Jan Arminio**

Particularly for helping professionals, racial identity development should be used in educational and therapeutic settings to better facilitate effective practice. Regarding counseling for clients of color, Carter (1990c) found that "racial identity attitudes led to more significant relationships than race alone" (p. 163). In other words, a White counselor is not always the best therapist for a White client, especially if the presenting issue involves race. The same is true for people of color. A counselor of color with attitudes and behaviors from a complex racial identity status could be a better counselor for a White client than a White counselor with a simple view of race. Helms (1990a) created an interaction application model to demonstrate how the racial identity development of counselor and client dyads influences the counseling process. The same could be said of teacher/student, advisor/advisee, supervisor/supervisee, and other dyads. This model is based on the framework of parallel, regressive, and progressive relationships. Racial identity theorists believe that progressive relationships lead to a stronger counselor/client relationship, are more likely to not end prematurely, and offer the most potential for client growth.

Racial identity can also be utilized to assess whether multicultural educational or training programs are comprehensive. Are programs merely to introduce students to the realization that other racial and cultural groups exist? Do the programs primarily offer food and provide demonstrations of dance and fashion? Is entertainment the sole purpose of these programs? Are there opportunities available for in-depth learning through the expression of racial experiences? Do educational opportunities push students to examine race in critical and complex ways? Are there opportunities for support and guidance of anti-racist work? How do we begin to collaborate between and within groups to promote justice for all people?

Though there are a number of racial identity theories and theorists, this chapter will focus on White racial identity development. The reader is encouraged to learn, understand, and utilize racial identity theories of other racial groups in conjunction with this one.

## The Conundrum of "Race"

Discussing race is a conundrum, a complicated phenomenon that raises more questions than answers. Race has social implications but cannot be verified biologically. Hence, in discussing race, are its oppressive tenets being perpetuated?

Many biologists, anthropologists, psychologists, educators, counselors, and others have noted that the biological concept of race is a fraud. The concept of "race" was constructed by European scientists and philosophers in the 1700s in an attempt to classify humans in biological terms as was being done with plants and animals (Hannaford, 1996). Unfortunately, such classifications were created with naive and prejudicial assumptions about what biologically differentiates humans from each other. For example, is it science that led European scientists to describe their own race as intellectual and handsome and other races less so? Today it is clear that grouping human beings by physical characteristics such as skin color, hair texture, and facial features are only superficial means of differentiation. These characteristics "were caused by recent evolution in response to climate and perhaps to sexual selection. Tests of older, more reliable genetic traits, such as certain antibodies, do not divide humans into groups that correspond to racial stereotypes" (Wheeler, 1995, ¶ 20). This fraudulent classification led to such practices as hospitals segregating patients and blood supplies by race so that patients "wouldn't be racially transformed by a transfusion" (Wheeler, ¶ 17). The study of antibodies has proven that human beings have migrated and intermixed to the point that no clear "racial" distinctions can be made (Goodman, 1994; Wheeler, 1995). In fact, there is no race gene. Consequently, there is no biological justification for racial phenotypes. Instead, biology has been used as an excuse to justify extreme forms of racism such as slavery and genocide (Riggons, 1987). Because of supposed race (and social class), some people were deemed savage and stupid needing to be controlled, while others were deemed worthy to control them, regardless of the cost to human life.

Hence, the conundrum: though the biological divisions of humans created centuries ago have proven to be unsubstantiated, the social implications of these false divisions have had and continue to have enormous social consequences. These social consequences include the ability of White families to accumulate wealth and property that is passed on from generation to generation, while families of other races have had to fight to earn the privilege to own property, obtain loans to purchase property, and to obtain life sustaining employment (Conley, 1999, 2002).

For example, my mother's ancestors arrived from Germany in the late 1880s. They came quite poor, and I have been told that the children arrived shoeless. But the family was able to purchase a small farm through government help and a bank loan. By the time I was born the family's holdings included over 1,100 acres of land, farm animals, farming equipment, a home, several barns, and a car. Though working class and without the money for my mother or her siblings to attend college or have other luxuries, when my grandfather died my mother's inheritance was significant enough to be added to my father's hard earned savings to send me to college without the need for college loans. At the same time, a Mexican American family in my community would not have been allowed to have a loan for property (the rural area banks refused to loan money to immigrants outside of Western Europe) and due to racism would not have been able to find employment other than picking tomatoes as migrant workers. If I were to be laid off from my job today, I would have my family's accumulated middle-class wealth to rely upon for assistance; a son or daughter of migrant farm workers would be less likely to have such accumulated family wealth for support.

It is these social consequences that are the basis of this chapter and the conundrum: How can I persuade people to dismantle social consequences of an erroneous biological construction without perpetuating the biological construction?

Racial identity development is a means by which U.S. society can discuss race and eventually move beyond its powerful historical influences. For counseling and people in the helping and education professions, it provides a model by which we can better understand each other's perspective and life experiences, moving from considering race as a simple concept to one that is intrinsically multidimensional. It is experienced personally, yet usually differently from person to person and group to group. How does the ways one views race influence interactions with others? How might one's view of race influence a helping relationship? How might one's view of race create a barrier to being with others?

# Overview, Background, Context

## What Is Racial Identity Development?

"I get frustrated with this [graduate] program because I feel like there is a point B that I have to be at. I really struggle with that because who is God to say that there is a point B? I am still trying to sort it out and I get angry at that. There are places I am not sure that I will ever be in. I don't think that is a terrible thing."

"What do you say about White? Is it White? I feel funny saying White! You know Caucasian seems really stupid to me."

The above quotes were from Joan, a participant in my dissertation study (Arminio, 1994) who was voicing her struggle to define herself racially. She struggled to find the words to use to describe her race and what it was for her to authentically be a White racial person. Racial identity development is the growth that occurs in negotiating such struggles.

According to Wijeyesinghe and Jackson (2001), "racial identity development has become a central theme in the study of race and race relations" in the United States (p. 1). Several theorists, including

Jackson, Hardiman, and Helms, have been instrumental in making racial identity development a central theme. Racial identity development refers "to a group or collective identity based on one's perception that he or she shares a common racial heritage with a particular racial group" (Helms, 1990a, p. 3).

According to Helms (1990a), in response to the Civil Rights Movement theorists presented frameworks that would help people be "more sensitive to racial issues" (p. 7). These frameworks could be divided into two perspectives: "client as problem" models and racial identity development models. Client as problem models exposed the faulty logic of the alleged deficiencies of the "Black personality." If the client is the problem, then what explains the healthy development of Black people in spite of living in a racist environment? Black racial identity models explained Black assertion against oppression and how Blacks could lead healthy lives despite living in a racist environment.

Unlike the experiences of Black people and other people of color, race was something that White people did not have to think about (Terry, 1975). In the 1960s and 1970s Black writers and scholars (e.g., Angelou, 1971; Baldwin, 1963; Fannon, 1967) and a few White scholars (e.g., Katz, 1978; Terry, 1975) began to call for White people to see themselves as racial beings. They felt that in acknowledging being a part of a racial collective, White people could play a pivotal role in moving society toward racial equality. Later, scholars began to explore the negative effects of racism on White people as well as people of color (Dennis, 1981).

White racial identity models (WRID) were created as a way to understand how White people "could escape from the effects of their racist programming" (Hardiman, 2001, p. 110). One of the foundations of White racial identity development is that due to socialization in a racist environment, it is difficult for White people to be immune to racist tendencies. In this regard, Tatum (2003) compared racism to air pollution; in the United States it is virtually impossible for anyone to avoid breathing in the racist notions upon which society has operated.

Initially, models of White racial identity development were based upon the biographies and interviews of White activists (Hardiman, 2001). Later Helms employed empirical means in an effort to verify her work (1990a, 1990b, 1990c; 1995), justifying racial identity development to a skeptical audience. White racial identity development models explain how White people abandon racism and come to feel positive about who they are as White people. This process occurs across the lifespan, often beginning before they reach school age.

## ABOUT RITA HARDIMAN

One of the first creators of racial identity development, Dr. Hardiman currently serves as a diversity trainer and consultant on issues of social diversity and social justice. She also is an adjunct faculty member in the department of organization and management at the Antioch/New England School of Education at the University of Massachusetts in Amherst. She has published articles on managing diversity in the workplace, racial identity development, and multicultural organizational development.

The concept of racial identity development is founded upon Erikson's concept of identity versus role confusion, his fifth psychological task necessary for healthy growth (Chickering & Havighurst, 1990). More current theorists believe that establishing identity is an ongoing process and is a primary focus of both cognitive and psychosocial development (Chickering & Reisser, 1993; Helms, 1995) occurring in adolescence on into adulthood (Baxter Magolda, 1999). According to Josselson (1987),

> establishing identity is an unconscious process that unites personality and links the individual to the social world. . . . [O]ur identity is fundamentally interwoven with others to gain meaning, contrasting ourselves with others and heightens our sense of what is uniquely individual. (p. 10–11)

Chickering and Reisser (1993) added that coming to define one's identity allows for a solid sense of self. It encourages a positive self-esteem and an overall satisfaction based on how the real compares against the ideal. One's identity is a realistic self-appraisal of oneself, allowing for greater awareness of complex reasoning and comfort with body appearance, culture, life style, and sense of self in response to feedback.

Consistent with these definitions of identity, White racial identity development models seek to explain how White people can grow to have an authentic positive sense of self by abandoning racism. This positive sense of self requires the acknowledgement of shared racial group membership. For White people this necessitates a White consciousness that is "not predicated by racial distortions" (Helms, 1990b, p. 53).

Such acknowledgment does not come easily. As with other aspects of identity development, Marcia (1966) wrote that both exploration and commitment are necessary in establishing a sense of self. A commitment can only be made when there is first a period of questioning, crisis, or challenge. Here the individual considers others' ideas about the world while determining her place in that world. This period of exploration can begin gradually or seemingly instantaneous. Such exploration could include trying on various alternative identities before committing to a sense of self. In making a commitment, an individual makes choices for herself when important goals are acted upon. Eventually there is congruence between values and behavior. White racial identity development requires exploring the concept of race and acknowledging that one is a member of the White race; negotiating with others' ideas about being White; putting oneself in circumstances where one can be challenged about the views of White people and other racial groups; and committing to act on the values of equity that lead to a positive sense of self as a White person.

In my own life this period of questioning, crisis, and challenge began in eighth grade when we were discussing whether Martin Luther King was a communist. Several students in the class said that he was not and the teacher agreed he was not. In my own extended family, I had often heard that he was a communist, rabble rouser, and troublemaker. It was my first realization that some of my family authority figures could be wrong, unkind, and unjust. I was devastated. The questioning and challenging continued throughout my schooling. After completing my master's degree I moved to the south and then to California where I could live with a variety of people. Finally, as an adult, I began to make a commitment to social justice and racial equality.

One's positive sense of self as a racial being is a combination of personal identity, reference group orientation, and ascribed identity (Helms, 1990b). Personal identity concerns one's feelings and attitudes about oneself; reference group orientation refers to the extent to which one uses a racial group to guide one's feelings, thoughts, and behaviors; and ascribed identity pertains to one's deliberate affiliation or commitment to a racial group. These components vary independently yet interact with each other. For example,

> [A] melting pot White (i.e., the person who believes everyone should be defined by the tenants of White socialization experiences) might feel good about himself or herself (i.e., positive personal identity), use Whites as a reference group for defining group behavior (i.e., reference group orientation), and feel a commitment only to other Whites (i.e., White ascribed identity).    (Helms, 1990a, p. 6)

TABLE 13.1   Helms's White Racial Identity Development (1995)

| Status | Brief Description |
| --- | --- |
| Contact | The White person becomes aware of and acknowledges that different racial groups exist. |
| Disintegration | The White person becomes aware that there is racial injustice in U.S. society. |
| Reintegration | To protect themselves from the guilt that is felt in realizing that injustice exists, White people look for means to justify their privilege and the ill treatment of others. |
| Pseudo-Independence | By connecting their own oppression to that of racial oppression or by witnessing extreme forms of racism, White people begin to acknowledge and understand the reality of racial oppression. |
| Immersion/Emersion | White people begin to understand the benefits they receive from racism and also begin to understand that they play a role in eliminating racism. Moreover, they begin to act upon that role. |
| Autonomy | White people confront racism as they encounter it by individuals and systems and come to have a strong positive sense of self as a White person. |

In my own case, my personal identity is one in which I continue to fight against the racist notions that people I grew up with own and perpetuated. I do believe that I am a White woman (reference group orientation); however, I have come to believe and have worked to ensure that all people are empowered to have equal access to high-quality housing, employment, education, health care, and other necessities (my ascribed identity). By being exposed to and trying on alternative identities I was able to find a way of being that was more authentic than the racist behaviors I had been exposed to (Marcia, 1966).

As noted earlier, Helms wrote that cognitive development influences one's racial identity development. In order to think complexly about race and oneself as a racial being, one has to be able to think complexly (Helms, 1995). To come to know through Perry's (1981) dualism or Belenky, Clinchy, Goldberger, and Tarule's (1986) received knowing is to see race as defined by others and to see race in simplistic polarized opposites: White/Black, good/bad, right/wrong.

As was made clear in Chickering and Reisser's definition of identity, realistic self-appraisal is necessary to enhance identity development.

"[I]identifications become problematic to the extent that they require denial or distortions of oneself and/or the racial groups from which one descends" (Helms, 1990a, p. 6). Denial and distortions hamper identity development. Hence, feelings of White racial supremacy hamper identity development. The website www.blackpeopleloveus.com (2006) is a satirical site that exposes the distortion some White people have regarding how they believe they are loved and appreciated by people of color. Though we may believe that others find us sincere, are we distorting how others different from us experience us?

Before I begin to describe more specific aspects of White racial identity development, Table 13.1 offers a brief glimpse of Helms's (1995) model. Please note that the creation of WRID models came in response to the racial identity development of other racial groups. This work is described in Chapters 11 and 12 in this text.

## White Racial Identity Model

The two theorists most connected with White racial identity development are Janet Helms and Rita Hardiman. Both began their work within the same five-year period (1979–1984) but did so independently. Both models propose a progression toward a personal responsibility and abandonment of racism. The discussion here focuses mostly on the work of Helms because she has attempted to verify the model through empirical research.

For White people, racial identity development involves a two-stage process. It is first necessary that a White person abandon racism (stage one) before coming to a positive sense of self as a White person (stage two). Though initially considered a stage theory whereby a person moves through a "linear process of increased acknowledgement of racism and consciousness of Whiteness" (Helms, 1990b, p. 53), Helms replaced the word *stage* with *statuses* to better communicate that people could act and have attitudes at all levels simultaneously, but have one status from which a person behaves most comfortably. The word *stage* often depicts a too linear progression or a static condition, whereas racial identity is a "dynamic interplay between cognitive and emotional processes" (1995, p. 183), as depicted in Figure 13.1. Think a measuring container of liquid, such as water. The small circles are drops of oil in the liquid, representing behaviors within the White racial identity statuses. In this example the bulk of the behaviors hover in the emersion area; however,

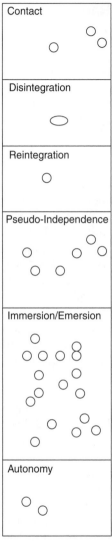

Contact

Disintegration

Reintegration

Pseudo-Independence

Immersion/Emersion

Autonomy

FIGURE 13.1    Bubbles of
Oil in a Beaker of Water

behaviors can come from a perspective of any status at the same period in one's life. I also refer to
these droplets as "moments."

For example, though the bulk of my behaviors at this point in my life are consistent with
the emersion status, when I am well prepared,
feeling confident, and in a surrounding with
which I am comfortable I have the competence
to behave consistent with the autonomy status.
This is an "autonomy moment." Contrarily, the
next day I may be in unfamiliar surroundings,
may be pressured by an authority figure, or may
be feeling ill and behave in a way less competently than I know how. For example, though I
teach courses in multicultural issues, have conducted research on multicultural topics, have
mentors of diverse backgrounds (emersion and
autonomy behaviors), when walking down the
sidewalk of an unfamiliar street and an expensive
car goes by with a Black male driver wearing
a gold necklace, immediately I think "drug
dealer." This stereotyping is a reintegration
behavior and moment. The following instant I
am aware of the stereotyping and feel remorse (a
pseudo-independence behavior or moment). I
next begin to contemplate from where such a
thought came and how to overcome such stereo-
typical thinking in the future (an emersion
behavior). Because of this dynamic nature of
WRID, many White multicultural educators
refer to themselves as "recovering racists."

One's racial identity is influenced by a complex mixture of environmental forces (e.g., familial attitudes, geography), individual attributes
(e.g., cognitive development) and personal life
experiences. However, the most influential aspect
of racial identity for White people is being a
member of the numerical majority and the socioeconomic and political
dominant group (Helms, 1990b). Consider the specific statuses of
Helms's model.

## Progression Through White Racial Identity Development

There are two phases of racial identity development: overcoming racism and developing a positive sense of self as a White person. The statuses in the abandoning racism phase are contact, disintegration, and reintegration. The statuses of pseudo-independence, emersion, and autonomy lead one to a positive sense of self as a White person.

### Contact

According to Helms, contact describes White people who are becoming aware that different racial groups exist. Depending on where the White person lives, this could occur at a very young age or not until early adolescence. Certainly television has allowed White people in secluded areas to become more aware of people of other racial groups earlier than in the past. Racial naiveté could be a simple description of contact. Even if people do realize that people of other races exist, people in contact do not believe that there are consequences of one's particular racial group. Common contact statements include: "I'm color blind," "I don't see race," or "I belong to the human race." All the while this person is benefiting from racism. Consequently, he remains satisfied with the racial status quo and judges people of color according to White cultural criteria. The longer the White person remains segregated from people of color, the longer a person will be most comfortable in acting from a contact perspective. A contact moment in my own life occurred during a diversity training session when the facilitator asked who in the group had friends who were people of color. I did not raise my hand. A Japanese American colleague said, "Am I not your friend?" I replied, "I don't see you as a person of color, I just see you as Nancy." She responded, "But I want you to see me as Japanese American. I am proud of it. My parents survived internment camps."

Counselors should encourage their clients, whose attitudes and behaviors come from the status of contact, to increase their knowledge of and exposure to various cultural groups. This will highlight how culture and history influence current perceptions and behaviors, and though there are common qualities to all humans, there are also important distinctions.

### Disintegration

Eventually, because of socialization with people of color, White people usually discover that in the United States not all people are treated equally and that differences in treatment are often determined by racial

## ABOUT JANET E. HELMS

Often considered the foremost researcher on cultural identity development, Janet Helms grew up in Missouri and struggled to overcome racism and oppression. She currently serves as professor in the department of counseling, developmental, and educational psychology and the endowed Augustus Long Chair in the Lynch School at Boston College, where she founded the Institute for the Study and Promotion of Race and Culture. Her area of expertise is the measurement of racial and cultural constructs. She has been a prolific writer and researcher on that topic and most recently on unfairness and discrimination in the testing industry. She has served as a mentor and teacher to a number of scholars who are also now are engaged in the exploration of racial identity development.

group. For example, when accompanying a friend of color into a store, a White person may notice how quickly the person of color is followed. Or the White person may notice how often colleagues of color are stopped for speeding, asked to speak on behalf of their race, or singled out because of their race. The White person may begin to feel guilty and anxious about such realizations. As these negative feelings increase, some White people may attempt to alleviate the guilt and anxiety by avoiding any occasion to witness these inequities or by beginning to blame people of color for the inequities. More over, the desire to be accepted by one's own White racial group influences the "content of the person's [racial] belief system" (Helms, 1990b, p. 60).

As a college student I lived across the hall from two African American students. Though not friends with them, I was friendly. One day someone wrote racial epithets on their door. I was shocked, but felt incredibly anxious about the incident. I did not discuss my feelings with the two women or other residents in the hall, nor did I attempt to find who committed the act. Instead I avoided the two women. It seemed the best way to avoid future anxious feelings about racial incidents.

Encouraging clients to discuss and make meaning of their feelings seeks to prevent these feelings from becoming overwhelming. Counselors should continue to support increased learning, especially related to the contradictions of myths and historical inaccuracies.

## Reintegration

Sometimes people enter the "racist" status. To avoid guilt and anxiety, White people consciously acknowledge a White identity where they idealize people of their own race and grow intolerant of people in other racial groups. From the status of reintegration, White people not only believe that bad things happen to bad people but also that perhaps bad things should happen to people of color. Perhaps that person of color deserved to be followed in the store or profiled? White people in this status believe that White culture is superior and that White people are superior. Helms (1990b) noted both a passive and active aspect of reintegration. Reintegration behavior not only entails outrageous and criminal behaviors such as joining hate groups and attending cross burnings (active reintegration) but also reintegration behaviors that can be more subtle, such as telling racist jokes, not welcoming people of color into one's community, only reading literature of one's cultural group, and only advocating for one's own needs (passive reintegration).

Unfortunately, I grew up with several authority figures who not only told racist jokes but also refused to hire any people of color. A year before I moved to my current neighborhood, there was a cross burning on the lawn of an Army officer and his wife, a school teacher. Several years later they divorced and moved away. These are behaviors that come from a reintegration perspective.

I was oblivious to my own reintegration until fairly recently when a group of colleagues and I were discussing whether we had been taught by any teachers of color. I stated that not until my doctoral program had I been taught by a person of color. Yet as soon as I said it, I knew it wasn't true. I spent the next couple of days searching my memory and finally recalled a psychology professor I had in college who was African American. Why had I not remembered him? In continuing my behavior of avoiding people of color due to the potential for "racial anxiety," I unexpectedly had been placed in this man's class. My movement from disintegration into reintegration progressed as I came to believe that this man was not worthy of my consideration. Though never disrespectful to him, I never interacted with him before or after class. I certainly never sought his advice or assistance. Yet, even worse, I never thought him worthy of any of my attention or remembrance.

Counselors should allow clients an opportunity to reflect on the foundation of their feelings and opinions. Rephrasing statements may help expose their racist qualities. Counselors should encourage valuing the self but not at the expense of others. Counselors could also explore the relationship between self-esteem and attitudes toward others. Be prepared to contradict inaccurate information.

## Pseudo-Independence

Luckily, many White people can come to see, act, and behave beyond reintegration, often through witnessing racist events or connecting racism to their own experiences of oppression (i.e., sexism, homophobia, classism, ableism). Through these connections, White people begin to understand the reality of oppression. This reality first occurs as an intellectual exercise. White people often begin to read about race and racism. They attend lectures and contemplate racial issues as they pertain to society at large. However, because at this point the White person has no "visible standards against which to compare and/or modify his or her behavior" (Helms, 1990b, p. 61); rather than reforming society, White people from a pseudo-independence status often want to help people of color become more like White people. For example, a college student stated, "I want to reach out and help people of color, but they just brush my hand away." Her hand was pointing down indicating a desire to "lift up" people of color onto her level. In this status, White people are more concerned with changing people of color to act more White, than changing racist beliefs of White people.

My own rescue from identity behaviors that were primarily in the reintegration perspective came as a result of my experience of being a victim of sexism. After having interviewed for a job, I was told that I would not be hired because I had a boyfriend and "would just run off and get married." I was devastated. Soon afterward I was walking down a sidewalk and passed four African American college students and realized what I had experienced was oppression. For me my own oppression legitimized other forms of oppression, including racial oppression. I no longer needed to avoid cross racial interactions or the powerful emotions these interactions could initiate. I began reading books by authors of color to learn about others. However, I was not yet ready to learn about my racial self.

It will be beneficial for clients to reflect on their personal commitment and individual responsibility to social justice. Gradually turning dialogue from academic aspects of racial identity to more personal responsibility will enhance growth. Participating in psychoeducational or growth groups such as "Whites only" groups will assist clients in exploring their individual responsibility to eliminating oppression.

## Immersion/Emersion

It is in immersion/emersion status when White people begin to understand their own individual responsibility for creating a more just society, the ways they personally benefit from racism, and their own redefinition of Whiteness. They begin to reflect upon their own racist behaviors and those of people around them, as well as the systematic nature of racism in U.S. society (the immersion aspect). From this perspective, White people read biographies of White people who are antiracist activists, find mentors who are antiracist activists, and join groups that promote antiracist work. In addition, they assess their individual actions and contemplate how they must change their behaviors to create a more just society. White people learn skills to confront others' racism and in doing so begin to take on a positive racial identity. In fact, some White people feel liberated from previously held distortions of themselves and other racial groups (emersion). I think of this status as immersing or diving into one's racial group and then learning from that to work with other racial groups (diving from one's own group).

Luckily for me I found several mentors, both White and people of color, who were patient role models in teaching and challenging me about my own role in working to make social justice a reality. My White mentors challenged me to acknowledge my privilege. My mentors of color challenged me to become aware of their life experiences. I read books, joined a social justice support group for White people, and participated in interracial dialogues.

Clients should continually be exposed to White role models as well as people of color who are committed to acting to achieve social justice. Encourage clients to enhance their growth by participating in multicultural groups where White people participate but do not dominate.

## Autonomy

Though a very difficult status from which to behave consistently in this society, people in the autonomy status work in collaboration with others to eliminate racism, not only individual racism but also racist systems (e.g., predominately Western European school curricula, unequal funding of neighborhood schools, unsafe neighborhoods, racial profiling, sentencing differences dependent upon racial group). People who behave from an autonomy perspective become aware of White privilege and work to give up their unearned assets (McIntosh, 1997). To act in autonomy means to go against the status quo of White superiority. It means to confront racist practices, including those of supervisors, family members, friends, teachers, and the like. One's commitment to confront racism can be measured by what one is willing to risk on behalf of it; in autonomy, White people take risks. In doing so, they can feel positive about being White.

In the status of autonomy, people use internal standards for defining themselves and they have the "capacity to relinquish the privileges of racism" (Helms, 1995, p. 185). They take advantage of opportunities to learn from other racial groups and become increasingly aware of the oppression of other stigmatized groups. As is implied here, autonomy requires ongoing learning and action.

Though I am still growing in my racial identity development, I have been able to confront racist practices and encourage others to do so as well. For example, I was purchasing a snow scraper for my car when the sales clerk asked if I was traveling far. As I indicated my destination was Providence, Rhode Island, she rolled her eyes and began telling to my watch out for "those people." I calmly told her that I did not share those beliefs and in fact my experiences were quite the contrary. She seemed to listen and internalize what I said. I didn't want to demean her, but instead wanted to communicate to her in a way she would embrace to change her own attitudes and behaviors. White people acting from the perspective of autonomy break what Sleeter (1996) called White silence. They speak and act against racist practices.

Addressing the racist notions of a sales clerk is not as risky as addressing the racist notions of an employer or supervisor. Remember, one's commitment to social justice is measured by what risks one is willing to take to achieve it. During my tenure year I confronted a colleague who had a direct bearing in the decision as to whether or not I would receive tenure. He had used a derogatory term to refer to a Black colleague. This was an autonomy moment for me. People behaving from the perspective of autonomy take on such risks.

Because social justice advocacy necessitates an incredible amount of courage, energy, and time, counselors should support clients who take on such risks and be knowledgeable about groups that support people engaged in these efforts. Counselors should encourage clients to take on leadership roles in such efforts and should model behaviors that eliminate oppression. Efforts of clients and counselors should be integrated across a variety of groups.

Now that the reader is more familiar with the model, it is prudent to contemplate on how White racial identity development can assist helping professionals in serving others.

## White Racial Identity Theory as Embedded in Our Profession

White racial identity development not only describes a model by which a White person can overcome racist attitudes and behaviors and come to have a positive White identity, it also provides a means to better serve clients and students in a variety of settings, including schools, colleges and universities, community mental health agencies, and even businesses and nonprofit organizations. Because we live in an increasingly diverse society and because making social justice a reality requires it, there is a need for the general population to become multiculturally competent. White racial identity development offers a model upon which multicultural education can occur intentionally.

### Interactive Dyads

In exploring ways to better facilitate effective counseling for clients of color, Carter (1990) found that "racial identity attitudes led to more significant relationships than race alone" (p. 163). In other words, depending on the racial identities of those involved, it is not always more effective to have a same race client/counselor dyad. One's racial identity is more indicative of one's crosscultural effectiveness than solely race. Helms (1990c) created an interaction application model to demonstrate how the racial identity development of counselor and client dyads influences the counseling process. This model is based on the framework of parallel, regressive, and progressive relationships because "participants' role expectations are not violated" (p. 178). A progressive relationship, the interaction dyad with the largest potential for growth, is where the person with the most influence (i.e., the counselor, supervisor, or teacher) has developed a more complex racial identity than the person with less power (the client, student, or employee). For example, this would occur when a counselor is most often behaving from the status of autonomy and the client is most often behaving from the status of contact, disintegration, or reintegration in White racial identity or in the encounter stage for people of color in racial identity development (see Chapters 11 and 12). Racial identity theorists believe that progressive relationships lead to a stronger counselor/client relationship, are more likely to not end prematurely, and offer the most potential for client growth. This underscores how critical it is for counselors to grow personally so that their work with clients can produce growth.

A regressive relationship occurs when the person with the most influence or power in the relationship has a less complex racial identity. In this relationship the client's growth is stifled. You have probably heard of a number of instances where teachers, professors, or counselors made racist comments to students of color. An African American student shared with me that she had asked a professor if she could borrow a book. The professor answered, "Yes, but don't take it back to African with you." Though perhaps intended as a joke, the comment serves to racialize and demean the request. Would he have ever said to a White student, "Yes, but don't take it back to England"? At best, the comment demonstrates a naiveté to racial issues (contact) or at worst an inferior attitude toward the student (reintegration). Because people of color typically learn about race and racial consequences earlier than White people, because 75% of the population is White, and because most people in the helping professionals are White, many helping dyads are unfortunately regressive with the White "helper" having a less sophisticated racial identity than the student or client of color. These relationships can be stifling if not harmful to clients of color. Helping professionals should work diligently to avoid regressive dyads.

Lastly, a parallel relationship is when the client and counselor share a racial identity worldview. It is the least contentious of the three types of interactions; however, there is little potential for growth. The counselor, teacher, or supervisor is unable to challenge the client, student, or employee to think more complexly about race.

## Other Applications

This interaction model could also be helpful in other interactive dyads, such as on college campuses in trying to understand conflicts that arise between residence hall roommates, students, and staff in judicial hearings, faculty and students in academic advising relationships, and in the mediation of grievances (Wing & Rifkin, 2001). How might differing perspectives on race be influencing these conflicts? It also has been advocated as a model on which to create leadership education programs (Arminio, 1993).

Racial identity can also be utilized as a means to conduct an environmental assessment to determine whether multicultural programs or trainings are comprehensive. For example, by assessing the publicity of campus multicultural events along the racial identity model, an institution can assess the comprehensiveness of its multicultural programs.

Hyman and Arminio (2000) found that a preponderance of programs advertised as "multicultural" were designed to merely introduce students to the realization that other racial and cultural groups exist. These programs were primarily festivals offering food, dancing, and fashion shows. They could be considered programs that advocate a "contact" perspective. Though nothing is wrong with these programs, at many schools and institutions there is a preponderance of contact multicultural programs and a dearth of other types of programs offering more complex representations of race. Lectures can sometimes offer a more sophisticated view of race than the programs described above, but if the audience is solely encouraged to intellectualize about race, the perspective is from the pseudo-independence status. At some institutions there are few opportunities available for in-depth learning through emersion experiences with others. These emersion programs could encourage students to examine race in critical and complex ways, allow students to view the world through others' perspectives, and provide opportunities for support and guidance of antiracist work where people already engaged in such work serve as role models. Chavez, Guido-Brito, and Mallory (2003) called these more complex learning opportunities risk taking and exploration of otherness. Such programs allow students to temporarily leave behind their own culture and race and experience aspects of another group. Interestingly, most emersion type programs are sponsored by organizations made up of primarily people of color (Hyman & Arminio, 2000).

The most complex programs would be those that encourage collaboration between and within groups to promote justice for all people. These come from the perspective of Helms's autonomy status in White racial identity development. Chavez et al. (2003) called these integration and validation activities. These occur often through service learning programs, community rallies, and other means of advocacy. Programs from this status perspective encourage and demonstrate how one can choose to connect with communities of identity as a way of life. Participants learn how to validate the differences and similarities of others into numerous, if not all, aspects of one's life.

In essence, a campus, community, or organization could use racial identity development as a model to assess from what perspectives their trainings and programs are grounded. Are educational offerings grounded in complex racial identity statuses or primarily simplistic ones? What types of offerings should be increased? As the reader might expect, the response to the creation of racial identity models has been significant but not without controversy.

## Theory Validity

When Helms first proposed her White racial identity development model, it was not surprising that White people in particular found fault with the reintegration aspect of her model. Not many White people were willing to admit that they do or did act from the status of reintegration. Some White people rejected the idea of reintegration because they did not join hate groups, burn crosses in lawns, or use racist language. They failed to consider the more subtle and common forms of racial bias as behaviors and attitudes encompassed in reintegration. Subsequently, more current authors and researchers have acknowledged the validity of both active and passive reintegration.

Though her model is readily accepted as a theoretical model (Mercer & Cunningham, 2003), the instrument most associated with measuring White racial identity, the White Racial Identity Attitudes Scale (WRIAS) (Helms & Carter, 1990), has come under scrutiny for psychometric reasons (Mercer & Cunningham, 2003; Miville, Darlington, Whitlock, & Mulligan, 2005). When tested using factor and component analyses, the WRIAS scales do not consistently hold up independently, and it has been reported that the factors do not correspond to the theory (Mercer & Cunningham). In response to these criticisms, Helms transitioned the theory from one of a stage model to the concept of statuses (that White people can behave from several statuses but from one primarily). Yet, some researchers still find that the scales correlate too closely. Hardiman (2001) believed that though the terms have changed, the essence of Helms's descriptions of the phenomenon is unchanged from her original work.

However the WRIAS has yielded adequate reliability estimates to measure White superiority/segregationist ideology, perceived cross-racial competence and comfort, interest in racial diversity, reactive racial dissonance, and positive dimensions of White identity (Mercer & Cunningham, 2003). In essence, although the WRIAS has psychometric problems in measuring White racial identity development, it does measure important constructs of the theory.

Questions also surround whether White identity development is a theory of what White people should do and feel, or rather what White people are meant to do. As Hardiman noted, "the WID [White Identity Development] stages were and still are more of a prescription for what I felt Whites needed to do than a description of experiences of what Whites shared" (2001, p. 113).

Furthermore, some question the conceptualization of Helms's White racial identity theory in that it was formulated on grounding similar to Cross's Black racial identity development. Because the Black model was created as a reaction to racism, is it appropriate to suggest that it can inform a White model that described the attitudes and behaviors of a dominant group?

Recent research in identity development has recognized that identity is lived in multiple dimensions simultaneously, though often studied and theorized separately (Jones, 1997). The salience of different dimensions of identity intersects and diverges depending on various factors, including environment and circumstances (Jones & McEwen, 2000; Miville et al., 2005). For example, the case below reveals the influence of social class on racial identity.

Regardless of the above psychometric concerns, recent research, and ongoing disagreements about the theoretical model, there is no doubt that the theory "has had a major impact on the field of counseling psychology . . . by challenging the unmarked, dominant, and normative character of the White group against which all other races are measured" (Hardiman, 2001, p. 117). I firmly believe that the WRID model offers a useful theoretical approach on which to ground practice. How is it that White racial identity is lived and how can helping professionals use the model in specific instances to assist student and client growth?

## White Racial Identity Case

"I understand why there are scholarships for minorities, to compensate for past discrimination, but I wish there were scholarships for White people. There weren't scholarships for me when I was looking for them. This is reverse discrimination you know," Rita stated boldly in a graduate master's counseling class.

I first met Rita when she sought to change her graduate work emphasis from community mental health counseling to college student personnel work at the institution where I teach. This institution is a regional, public, comprehensive institution located in a rural area. She appeared to be confident, bright, and enthusiastic. When I asked her to tell me about herself and her motivation for changing her graduate programs, she relayed the following.

> After graduating from college with a foreign language degree, but not in education, I searched for teaching positions and was able to find several long-term substitute positions in this geographic area. After the substitute positions ended, I was able to find a

teaching position at an alternative school for adjudicated youth. I work there now. But the management frustrates me, so I wanted to look for something else, but I have few options. I decided to look into graduate programs. This is the best graduate department at this institution, so I decided to begin taking classes here. However, I was speaking with someone in athletics about his job as an academic advisor. As we talked, he said that he thought my interests were more in line with college student personnel. So, I decided to come and see you.

When I asked Rita what she saw herself doing in college student personnel she replied, "I am not exactly sure. There are many areas, but my interest seems to be in academic advising or learning assistance." After reviewing her application materials to graduate school and her academic record, I saw that Rita was thirty-one years old, had earned acceptable grades as an undergraduate, had transferred from a liberal arts college to our regional public institution, and had worked in a variety of long-term substitute teaching positions, mostly in poor rural areas. Rita was allowed to enter the college student personnel program the following semester and enrolled in one of my classes. In the beginning of the semester we met to formulate her academic coursework for the next two years. She told me,

> I am eager to finish my graduate work. I have not been able to save much money for graduate school, so I have a graduate assistantship to pay for my tuition. Plus, I am engaged to a soldier who may be transferred soon and I want to follow him when he does.

I asked her to clarify that indeed she had a full-time job, graduate assistantship (that requires her to take three graduate classes), and a serious relationship. She responded, "Yes, but it is not a problem. I have always had a lot of energy and during undergrad I had several jobs at one time." I expressed my concern about taking on a number of commitments simultaneously. She rebuffed my concerns by stating, "I can handle it, believe me. I am old enough to know what I can handle. I am older than you think."

Consequently, Rita maintained her full-time job teaching adjudicated youth, her graduate assistantship, her full-time course load, and her relationship. By taking classes in the evening and working her graduate assistantship hours at night and on the weekends, she was able to complete required tasks, but I suspected with great stress.

Rita's academic work, though not stellar, was adequate until toward
the end of the semester when several times she stated that she forgot
her assignment and would send it via e-mail after class. When I read
her written assignments, it was obvious that they were completed hur-
riedly. I asked Rita to come see me. I asked her about the declining
quality of her work. She explained,

> I am not sure if you are aware of this, but my finance was trans-
> ferred a couple of months ago. Soon afterward he wrote me a let-
> ter breaking off our relationship. I have been in a whirlwind about
> it. I am sorry but it has been difficult to concentrate. I need a
> couple of weeks to recover and then I will be okay.

Rita did complete the course satisfactorily, but I asked to see her again,
soon after the course ended to discuss her goals for her first internship.
She said,

> In searching for an internship site I found that a nearby small,
> private liberal arts college has an opening for a summer job work-
> ing with a conference program of graduate students from all over
> the world. I have decided to apply for it and if I get it, I will quit
> my job at the alternative school. It sounds very interesting and
> would provide housing for the summer.

I asked if this was to be her proposed internship site. She stated, "No,
I have decided to intern here at this institution in the Admissions
office." I then asked if the summer job with international students
would replace her assistantship. "Oh, no, I still need that to pay for
tuition." Again, I expressed my concern about the number of large
responsibilities she carried. Again, she brushed off any concerns.

It was in weekly individual supervision with Rita and in the weekly
class meetings with other student interns that I became increasingly
concerned about Rita. Her strong opinions did not allow her to establish relationships with student peers easily. I noticed that at times the
body language of her peers indicated discomfort when she spoke. In
supervision with other students, some would comment on Rita's abra-
siveness. We would discuss strategies of how to share with Rita our
experiences of her. Also, Rita became noticeably abrasive to Laquita, an
African American woman in the class who is a single mother and works
full time in a social service agency.

When discussing the topic of creating inclusive communities in class,
Rita remarked frequently about incidents from her undergraduate

experiences that she believed were "reverse racism." For example, while Rita was an undergraduate student, a Black woman was elected homecoming queen (the third in the institution's history). However, during the homecoming parade several people along the parade route in town yelled racist epithets at her. In addition, there were no pictures in the student newspaper showing the homecoming queen, as was customary. Black students protested these events by burning student newspapers on the campus grounds. These students were punished through the campus judicial system, but many Black students felt their punishments were far more severe than White gay students who had burned the student newspaper for the printing of homophobic editorials. Later that same year, the Black Student Union decided to hold a Miss Black pageant as a Black woman had never been selected as the winner of this institution's beauty pageant.

Though these incidents had happened several years ago, Rita excitedly discussed them as if they occurred recently. She described the newspaper protests as "foolish" and stated that it should be obvious that there was no racism on campus because there had been three Black homecoming queens elected. Interestingly, Laquita remembered these incidents as she, too, was an undergraduate student at this institution when they occurred. She briefly offered her point of view but bridged those experiences with current ones as well as the topic of inclusive communities. She mentioned support efforts to recruit and retain a diverse student body. Rita responded stating,

> I understand why there are scholarships for minorities, to compensate for past discrimination, but I wish there were scholarships for White people or other forms of assistance. There weren't scholarships for me when I was looking for them. This is reverse discrimination, you know.

Several of her classmates challenged Rita on her belief in reverse racism, pointing out the total number of scholarships and the wide range of criteria for scholarship selection. Students also commented on how unwelcoming the rural campus and community have been for students of color. They also asked why these incidents of several years ago still mattered so much to her.

During our next individual supervision meeting I asked Rita to tell me from where her feelings and opinions on race have been generated.

> I grew up a town of about 30,000 people. My father was a banker and we did okay. I applied and was admitted to a reputable small

private institution. I loved it there. However, during my sophomore year in college my father left us. My mother found a job as
a secretary, and I had to find a part-time job as my dad stopped
paying my tuition. I applied for financial aid and scholarships but
I didn't get any. I'm White, and there are none for Whites. I had
to leave that school and come to this one. I worked as an RA and
several other jobs to make ends meet.

"That must have been difficult for you" I responded. Rita replied,

Not really. I got over it. It just makes me mad that minorities
have it so easy. They don't have to work like I do. Plus, it's like
some of these graduate students I work with in the summer
conference program. Several of them, the Black ones, don't try to
get along with anyone else. They stand out like sore thumbs. One
wears African garb that you can't miss and the other expects me
to serve him. Plus, one's skin is so black that you can't help but
notice him. They should try better to fit in.

I tried to contradict Rita's broad generalizations about people of
color. "Do you really believe that all people of color have it easy and
don't have to work hard?" Rita countered with, "Yes, like my new boss
at my assistantship. He is Latino and has threatened to fire me because
I have had to miss some of my shifts due to my summer campus conference job." I decided that I needed to think more of how best to
address Rita's distortions using White racial identity as a guide.

## Analyzing Rita's Case

It is unfortunate that Rita conducted her graduate work at a rural institution. Because there were few students, faculty, and staff of color, she
saw Laquita, her adjudicated students, and her Latino boss who threatened to fire her as "representing their race." She saw all people of color
similarly, mostly according to stereotypes. In essence, she saw what she
believed. She discounted other more recent events and interactions that
might have offered a broader perspective about race and instead connected race with past events. She faulted the international graduate students at the summer grant-funded program for their inability to "fit in"
while missing the stares the Black graduate students received from
White people in the community. She did not consider that the stares

communicated to these students that they did not fit in and that subsequently they responded accordingly. Additionally, Rita expected these students to act, dress, and talk like her.

Rita assumed that because she did not receive scholarships, that they are only offered to "minorities." She failed to realize that her father's high salary and her average grades prevented her from receiving both merit and need-based aid. She felt a need to blame others for her predicament rather than her father. Her unresolved issues of abandonment by her father and her boyfriend made learning new insight difficult.

According to Helms, Rita could potentially behave from all of the statuses simultaneously, but behaved from one primarily. Rita had attitudes and behaved from disintegration, reintegration, and pseudo-independence perspectives. However, she was most comfortable in behaving through reintegration. She blamed people of color, particularly Black people, for taking scholarships that she felt would have made her life easier. As a White person (and upper middle class), she expected and felt that she deserved an education, and ultimately success, without the burden of struggling to pay for it herself. She resented having this financial burden. Consequently, Rita saw people of color as the culprit in any incident involving race, and in particular for preventing her from receiving her "American dream."

Rita recognized that some scholarships were established because of the inequities of the past. The recognition of an inequitable society is an attribute of disintegration. However, her own demotion from upper middle class to working class and her inability to pay for higher education made people of color—in Rita's eyes less deserving but nonetheless achieving an education—a threat. To eliminate the anxiety created by her recognition of racism, she blamed people of color, particularly Black people. It also became easy for her to blame them for her financial problems. Material in Rita's classes forced her to think about herself as a racial being. Course discussions provided the opportunity for her to articulate her feelings and for classmates and faculty to offer alternative points of view.

## Implications of Racial Identity Development

In order for Rita to work with people of color justly, it was imperative that she move from the reintegration status. Her insight was not only in response to my questions but also by her continued study of race, racism, and racial identity, and in particular interactions with White peers who were committed to antiracist work. Developmental goals were established that were aligned with the racial identity model. Specific goals and objectives along racial identity lines supported and challenged

Rita to understand her connection to race and her racial group in more complex ways. This led to more just ways of being in the world.

## Using the Model to Increase Racial Understanding Among White People

Below are some suggestions for ways that educators and helping professionals can use the White racial identity development model as a guide to increase the racial understanding of White people. Means of supporting and challenging clients and students are noted for each racial identity status.

### Contact

These programs introduce students/clients to a variety of cultures. Begin with fun activities like food and dancing then move on to discussions regarding the history behind cultural holidays (e.g., not only eat tacos on Cinco de Mayo but also discuss the historical significance of the day and what is being celebrated). Expose contradictions and myths regarding justice in the United States. Show movies that expose students/clients to other cultures and the issues of oppression these groups face.

### Disintegration

Provide opportunities for students/clients to discuss and process their feelings (especially, guilt and anxiety). Encourage students to manage and learn from these emotions so they will not become overwhelmed. When are these feelings occurring? What prompts them? What might that be about? Encourage clients/students to journal about these feelings and encourage continued learning about how racial groups were and are being treated in the United States. Encourage continued interaction with people of color.

### Reintegration

Allow students/clients an opportunity to reflect on the foundation of their opinions and feelings. Rephrase statements of students exposing their racist qualities. For example, when a students says, "All Hispanics are illegal immigrants," respond by noting, "Really, all of them, even Alberto Gonzalez, Rebecca Lobo, Ellen Ochoa, and Antonia Novella?" Expose students' and clients' inaccurate assumptions and contradictions. Explore the relationship between self-esteem and attitudes toward people of color. Provide accurate and current statistical information regarding poverty, class, and affirmative action (i.e., White women have been the largest beneficiaries of affirmative action or the dramatic increase in salaries of White male corporate executives). Provide life stories of real people's victimization (i.e., Malcolm X, James Byrd, and interned Japanese Americans). Use White allies who are committed to eliminating oppression as co-facilitators.

## Pseudo-Independence

Ask students and clients to reflect upon their own personal commitment to racial justice. Expose students to the concept of White privilege by having them take White privilege self-assessments and encourage participation in White privilege exercises. Move discussions away from academics, history, or arts/literature to personal responsibility. Introduce students and clients to famous White role models who have served as allies for oppressed people (e.g., Sophie Scholl, Morris Dees, Eleanor Roosevelt, Henry O. O. Howard) as well as local allies. Encourage participation in "White" groups that are committed to eliminating oppression.

## Immersion/Emersion

Continue to encourage participation in "White groups" or at least use White role models to increase the opportunities to identify racism, one's own and that of others. Provide resources that inform students and clients about White people and people of color who are working together to eliminate oppression. Encourage participation in difficult dialogue groups or organizations in which Whites participate but do not dominate (Sleeter, 1996).

## Autonomy

Provide information on opportunities to work in collaborative groups to eliminate oppression. These groups should be opportunities for White people to participate but not dominate (Sleeter, 1996). Encourage students/clients to become advocates on behalf of all the oppressed. Advocate for change in institutional oppression. Encourage students and clients to serve as leaders of efforts to eliminate oppression and be role models for those in preliminary development statuses.

# My Specific Work with Rita

In individual supervision meetings with Rita, I offered her opportunities to discuss her feelings of resentment and encouraged her to consider the source of these feelings. I also assigned her readings on sexism, classism, and the intersections of class and race. I said to her,

You use "every" and "all" when speaking about people of color. Is that what you mean? Let's name together people who do not fit these generalizations. How might your family experiences be influencing your generalizations? In your situation I would feel anger and resentment toward my father. Do you? I have looked at the large list of scholarships for this institution, I see that some are geared specifically for musicians, students from particular communities, students interested in particular majors, and other areas. They are not limited to people of color. Why might it appear otherwise to you? In reading the assignments of working-class White people in graduate programs, are there any connections for you? If so, in what ways? Who are your role models?

I told her that I believed that she had not "gotten over" the financial difficulties that plagued her while earning her degrees. I also asked if her resentment was misplaced. She did admit that indeed she struggled to finance her education. Plus, she admitted her father's role in her misfortunes.

In additional to these discussions and readings, I encouraged Rita to seek counseling regarding abandonment issues related to her father and ex-boyfriend. I also personally invited Rita to campus antiracist events.

Rita transitioned her personal, reference, and ascribed identities from the privileges of being upper middle class to acknowledging her struggles of being working class and trying to afford a college education. She realized that blaming people of color was not going to help her solve her money woes and in fact was separating her from her potentially supportive classmates. She was able to lessen the distorted implications of her father leaving the family and his refusal to help her financially. She also came to see how she could recognize her racial group affinity through a positive sense of self, rather than through racist attitudes.

## Summary

White people typically have not considered themselves as having a race, though their ancestors constructed the concept of race. White racial identity development offers a way for White people "to understand the psychological meaning of race" (Carter, 1997, p. 199). It has become the central theme in current discussions on race in the United States and is pivotal in promoting antiracist work. The notion of identity development comes from lifespan development work of Erikson. Racial identity was born from the work of Cross (1971) and Jackson (2001) in the 1970s, both of whom sought to describe the "conversion experience for Black people in the 1960's" (Jackson, p. 8). White racial identity is a reflection of their work, though it describes the developmental experiences of the dominant group. Racial identity is also related to cognitive development in that one cannot consider race complexly without cognitive complexly.

Racial identity describes the connection one feels to one's racial group. For White people racial identity requires that they abandon notions of superiority, subsequently having a positive sense of themselves as racial beings. Within that process there are identity statuses that describe increasingly complex attitudes, feelings, and behaviors. These statuses are contact, disintegration, reintegration, pseudo-independence, immersion/emersion, and autonomy. The process begins at naiveté and progresses to a sophisticated understanding of the self as a racial being skilled in working competently with diverse others for social justice.

This model initially was used to provide a means for more effective and ethical counseling between White counselors and clients of color. Since its inception, it has also been used to increase understanding of and competence in a variety of interracial dyads in education, business, and social service agencies. Specifically, in the case provided here, White racial identity was used to provide guidance in encouraging a thirty-one-year-old counseling graduate student to recognize her misplaced resentment of her father toward people of color.

Many White people are defensive when reading about White racial identity. Many become angry at the notion that they are not colorblind and in fact have racist tendencies. However, it is my hope that the reader will first walk around in the model as one would a fine pair of new shoes. There is some discomfort at first, but after walking around and reflecting upon the possibilities of taking us new places, White racial identity can offer important insights and skills imperative for ethical practice.

## Annotated Bibliography

Fine, M., Powell, L., Weis, L., & Wong, L. M. (Eds.). (1996). *Off White: Readings on race, power, and society.* New York: Routledge.
This book offers intriguing chapters on how White people from a variety of groups (e.g., White working class men, White people outside of the United States, White lesbians, White allies of people of color) construct their

identities. It includes a chapter by Robert Carter in which he discusses expressions about race along the White racial identity model.

Helms, J. (1990). *Black and White racial identity: Theory, research, and practice.* Westport, CT: Greenwood Press.
This text brought White racial identity to prominence. It includes definitions of racial identity and other related terms and offers the instruments Helms used to conduct research on both Black and White racial identity theory. This text still offers necessary information on how racial identity influences the counseling process.

Helms, J. (1992). *A race is a nice thing to have: A guide to being a White person or understanding the White persons on your life.* Topeka, KS: Content Communications.
Written with the general public in mind, this small workbook is filled with exercises demonstrating the founding principles of White racial identity development. It also provides a brief first glimpse at White racial identity. For those new to racial identity development, it is a wonderful starting place. Now available at www.emicrotraining.com/books.html.

Helms, J. (1995). An update of Helms' White and people of color models. In J. G. Ponterotto, J. M. Casas, L. A. Suzuki, & C. M. Alexander (Eds.), *Handbook of multicultural counseling* (pp. 181–199). Thousand Oaks, CA. Sage.
Written for an informed audience, in this update Helms discusses her use of the term "socio-race" and also why she replaces the word *stage,* used in her earlier work, with *status.*

Tatum, B. D. (2003). *Why do all the Black kids sit together in the cafeteria?: And other questions about race.* New York: Basic Books.
Written for a general audience, this book presents a childhood-to-adulthood perspective on racial identity development. It includes the poignant personal experiences of Dr. Tatum and her children growing up. More specific to teaching than counseling, it presents insight into the engagement or lack of engagement of students of color and how the racial identity of White teachers, classmates, and administrators influences that engagement. Also, offers advice for White parents adopting children of color.

Wijeyesinghe, C. L., & Jackson, B. (2001). *New perspectives on racial identity development: A theoretical and practical anthology.* New York: New York University Press.
Rita Hardiman authors a chapter here on her groundbreaking work. She also clarifies the similarities and differences between her work and that of Janet Helms. This text also offers a noteworthy chapter by Leah Wing and Janet Rifkin in which they present a case study of how racial identity development was used to increase the understanding of a faculty member and a student involved in a mediation process.

# References

Angelou, M. (1971). *Just give me a drink before I die*. New York: Random House.

Arminio, J. W. (1993, March). Racial identity as development theory: Considerations for designing leadership programs, *Programming Magazine*, 40–46.

Arminio, J. W. (1994). *Waking up White; A phenomenological journey into racial being*. Unpublished doctoral dissertation, University of Maryland, College Park.

Baldwin, J. (1963). *The fire next time*. New York: Vintage.

Baxter Magolda, M. (1999). Constructing adult identities. *Journal of College Student Development, 40*, 629–642.

Belenky, M. F., Clinchy, B. M., Goldberger, N. R., & Tarule, J. M. (1986). *Women's ways of knowing: The development of self, voice, and mind*. New York: Basic Books.

blackpeopleloveus.com/about.html (2006). Available GOOGLE: http://www.blackpeopleloveus.com/about.html.

Carter, R. T. (1990). Does race or racial identity attitudes influence the counseling process in Black and White dyads? In J. Helms (Ed.), *Black and White racial identity: Theory, research, and practice* (pp. 145–164). Westport, CT: Greenwood Press.

Carter, R. T. (1997). Is White a race? Expressions of White racial identity. In M. Fine, L. Weis, L. C. Powell, & L. Mun Wong (Eds.), *Off White: Readings on race, power, and society* (pp. 198–211). New York: Routledge.

Chavez, A. F., Guido-Brito, F., & Mallory, S. L. (2003). Learning to value the "other": A framework of individual diversity development. *Journal of College Student Development, 44*, 453–469.

Chickering, A. W., & Havighurst, R. J. (1990). The life cycle. In A. W. Chickering (Ed.), *The modern American college* (pp. 16–50). San Francisco: Jossey-Bass.

Chickering, A. [W.] & Reisser, L. (1993). *Education and identity* (2nd ed.). San Francisco: Jossey-Bass.

Conley, D. (1999). *Being Black, living in the red: Race, wealth, and social policy in America*. Berkeley: University of California Press.

Conley, D. (2002). *Wealth and poverty in America: A reader*. Walden, MA: Blackwell.

Cose, E. (1998). *Color-blind: Seeing beyond race in a race-obsessed world*. New York: Perennial.

Cross, W. E., Jr. (1971). The Negro-to-Black conversion experience: Toward a psychology of Black liberation. *Black World, 20*, 13–27.

Dennis, R. (1981). Socialization and racism: The White experience. In B. Bowser & R. Hunt (Eds.), *Impacts of racism on White Americans* (pp. 71–80). Beverly Hills, CA: Sage.

Fanon, J. R. (1967). *Black skin, White masks*. New York: Monthly Review.

Goodman, A. H. (1994, September, 7). The study of racial differences [Letter to the editor] [Electronic version]. *The Chronicle of Higher Education*. Retrieved May 6, 2006, from http://chronicle.com/che-data/articles.dir/articles-41.dir/issue-02.dir/02b00301.htm.

Hannaford, I. (1996). *Race: The history of an idea in the west.* Baltimore: Johns Hopkins University Press.

Hardiman, R. (2001). Reflections on White identity development theory. In C. L. Wijeyesinghe & B. W. Jackson III (Eds.), *New perspectives on racial identity development: A theoretical and practical anthology* (pp. 108–128). New York: New York University Press.

Helms, J. (1990a). Introduction: Review of racial identity terminology. In J. Helms (Ed.), *Black and White racial identity: Theory, research, and practice* (pp. 3–8). Westport, CT: Praeger.

Helms, J. (1990b). Toward a model of White racial identity. In J. Helms (Ed.), *Black and White racial identity: Theory, research, and practice* (pp. 49–66). Westport, CT: Praeger.

Helms, J. (1990c). Applying the interaction model to social dyads. In J. Helms (Ed.), *Black and White racial identity: Theory, research, and* practice (pp. 177–187). Westport, CT: Greenwood Press.

Helms, J. E. (1992). *A race is a nice thing to have: A guide to being a White person or understanding the White persons on your life.* Topeka, KS: Content Communications.

Helms, J. (1995). An update of Helms' White and people of color models. In J. G. Ponterotto, J. M. Casas, L. A. Suzuki, & C. M. Alexander, (Eds.), *Handbook of multicultural counseling* (pp. 181–199). Thousand Oaks, CA. Sage.

Helms, J., & Carter, R. T. (1990). Development of the White racial identity inventory. In J. Helms (Ed.), *Black and White racial identity: Theory, research, and practice* (pp. 67–80). Westport, CT: Greenwood Press.

Hyman, K., & Arminio, J. (2000, September). The influence of students' racial identity on campus programming. *Programming Magazine,* 58–60.

Jackson, B. W. (2001). Black identity development: Further analysis and elaboration. In C. L. Wijeyesinghe and B. Jackson III (Eds.), *New perspectives on racial identity development: A theoretical and practical anthology* (pp. 8–31). New York: New York University Press.

Johnson, A. (2001). *Privilege, power, and difference.* Boston: McGraw-Hill.

Jones, S. R. (1997). Voices of identity and difference: A qualitative exploration of the multiple dimensions of identity development in women college students. *Journal of College Student Development, 38,* 376–386.

Jones, S. R., & McEwen, M. K. (2000). A conceptual model of identity development in women college students. *Journal of College Student Development, 41,* 405–414.

Josselson, R. (1987). *Finding herself.* San Francisco: Jossey-Bass.

Katz, J. (1978). *White awareness.* Norman: University of Oklahoma Press.

Kivel, P. (2002). *Uprooting racism: How White people can work for racial justice* (rev. ed). Gabriola Island, BC: New Society.

Marcia, J. (1966). Development and validation of ego-identity status. *Journal of Personality and Social Psychology, 3,* 551–559.

McIntosh, P. (1997). White privilege and male privilege; A personal account of coming to see correspondences through work in women's studies. In

R. Delgado & J. Stefancic (Eds.), *Critical White studies: Looking behind the mirror* (pp. 291–299). Philadelphia: Temple University Press.

Mercer, S. H., & Cunningham, M. (2003). Racial identity in White American college students: Issues of conceptualization and measurement. *Journal of College Student Development, 44,* 217–230.

Miville, M. L., Darlington, P., Whitlock, B., & Mulligan, T. (2005). Integrating identities: The relationship of racial, gender, and ego identities among White college students. *Journal of College Student Development, 46,* 157–175.

Riggons, M. (Producer/Writer/Director). (1987). *Ethnic notions* [Documentary]. (Available at California Newsreel, U.S.)

Perry, W. G. (1981). Cognitive and ethical growth: The making of meaning. In A. W. Chickering (Ed.), *The modern American college* (pp. 76–116). San Francisco: Jossey-Bass.

Sleeter, C. E. (1996). White silence, White solidarity. In N. Ignatiev & J. Garvey (Eds.), *Race traitor* (pp. 257–265). New York: Routledge.

Tatum, B. D. (2003). *Why do all the Black kids sit together in the cafeteria?: And other questions about race.* New York: Basic Books.

Terry, R. (1975). *For Whites only.* Grand Rapids, MI: Erdmans.

West, C. (2001) *Race matters* (rep. ed.). New York: Vintage. (Original work published in 1993 by Beacon Press)

Wheeler, D. L. (February, 7, 1995). A growing number of scientists reject the concept of race. *Chronicle of Higher Education.* Retrieved May 30, 2006, http://chronicle.com/che-data/articles.dir/articles-41.dir/issue-23.dir/23a 00801.htm.

Wijeyesinghe, C. L., & Jackson, B., III (2000). Introduction. In C. L. Wijeyesinghe and B. Jackson III (Eds.), *New perspectives on racial identity development: A theoretical and practical anthology* (pp. 1–7). New York University Press: New York.

Wing, L., & Rifkin, J. (2001). Racial identity development and the mediation of conflicts. In C. L. Wijeyesinghe and B. Jackson III (Eds.), *New perspectives on racial identity development: A theoretical and practical anthology* (pp. 182–208). New York: New York University Press.

# CHAPTER FOURTEEN

# Spiritual Development: Focusing as a Gateway in Counseling

## Kathryn K. Brooks

In this chapter, readers will notice a very broad and inclusive approach to the notion of spiritual development. Throughout I invite and encourage you to hold on to any spiritual concepts, any faith traditions, and any personal experiences that are meaningful to your lives and/or your work as counselors. Carry them with you as you read on. Allow them and the following material to engage and enliven one another. More importantly, I urge you to continually ponder how to do the same for your clients, that is, to create the widest possible opening in your minds and hearts for the diversity of their spiritual lives. With that in mind, allow me to suggest some simple working definitions of spirituality, spiritual development, and religion. *Spirituality* is a connection to something greater than oneself. *Spiritual development* is a process of growth occurring in connection to something greater than oneself. *Religion* is an organized set of beliefs and practices pointing the way to such a connection and/or such development.

My choice to leave the definition of spiritual development as broad as possible is a purposeful one. It is my sincerest hope that this chapter will contribute to a process of ongoing expansion within each of you: an expansion of your ability to respect and support the diverse ways spiritual development may be manifest within the counseling process. I ask you to use such a wide-angle lens that you make room as well for growth that clients may not name as spiritual per se; and in these cases name it whatever feels right to the client.

424

## ABOUT THE CHAPTER AUTHOR

### Kathryn K. Brooks

I have enjoyed the opportunity share with you about focusing as a process of spiritual development. From my first exposure to focusing, it seemed somehow familiar—as if it was something I already recognized on some level and innately trusted. At the same time, it seemed to hold the promise of meeting a need for something I was missing, something that was very important both personally and professionally. I hope that it resonates with you in similar ways, helping you to feel more grounded in where you 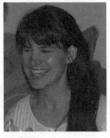 are, while also providing something you need to continue on your own journey. Equally important, I hope it helps you to do that for your clients as well. I believe you will find focusing well-suited to facilitating both aspects of spiritual development.

*Kathryn K. Brooks*, Ph.D., LPC, NCC, ACS, Certified Focusing Trainer, Certified Imago Therapist, is a counselor and assistant professor at the Shippensburg University Counseling Center. In addition to focusing and spirituality, her professional interests include couples therapy, women's issues, and the counseling process. In addition to her counseling center work, she has practiced in outpatient, inpatient, day treatment, and private practice settings. She lives in Shippensburg, Pennsylvania, with her husband, daughter and two cats.

**Kathryn K. Brooks**

Psychiatrist M. Scott Peck (1978) makes no distinction between mental and spiritual growth in his best-selling work *The Road Less Traveled*, beginning instead with the assumption that the two are one and the same. Could the same thing not be said for emotional growth, psychological growth, or interpersonal growth as well? Perhaps any genuine growth, any form of human development, *is* spiritual. Perhaps not. In either case, I invite you to consider the key qualities that constitute *spiritual* growth. On a personal note, at the time of this writing, I am reflecting on how much my daughter has grown in the first year of her life, and her development seems more than purely physical, mental, or social to me. So does my own development as her mother, for that matter. I could sit with that felt sense of "more," and describe qualities that I consider to be spiritual. I will, however, leave each of you to draw upon your own life experiences to ponder for yourselves what qualities constitute spiritual growth and how much of human development might also be spiritual.

This chapter rests on a more limited assumption, which is simply that all of human experience has a spiritual *dimension* that is accessible within the context of the counseling relationship. Toward that aim, I will introduce you to Eugene Gendlin's model of accessing the experiential realm through a process he termed *focusing* (1981). It is a body-centered approach to counseling, so this chapter will be examining the body as a gateway to a spiritual dimension and therefore spiritual development. Clearly, from this perspective, the body is not only a physical machine or a collection of flesh and bone. It is in continual interaction with the environment, affecting it and being affected by it. As such, a great deal of information registers on a bodily level, much more than we are consciously aware of.

We can enter into that "more" by directly connecting with an internal sense of an issue as it is felt on a visceral or bodily level in the here-and-now. The ability, "the internal equipment needed to perform the act" (Gendlin, 1981, p. 9) is within everyone, though few know that it can be deliberately used. Fewer still know that the step of connecting with a felt sense can begin a process of unfolding meaning. I believe you will find this process particularly well suited for accessing a spiritual dimension and for doing so in a way that is uniquely inclusive and respectful of diversity and individual differences. A focusing-oriented approach to counseling, particularly for spiritual issues, recognizes that counselors can facilitate the process, but the content must originate within each client. To the degree that the process is recognizable or familiar to you, perhaps by another name or from another field of study, feel free to incorporate other terms or language throughout the discussion that follows.

## First, an Experience

Let's pause for a moment, before going any further. I would not be doing justice to the topic to write *about* it without offering you an opportunity to *experience* it. With that in mind, I invite you, the reader, to try a couple brief exercises. Take a moment to let go of mental activity, and let your awareness drop down inside your body, resting in the area between your throat and your lower belly. Some attention to your breathing may help.

Closing your eyes (after reading each bit of instruction) may help as well. Now take a moment to reflect upon how your life is going. You might begin with a question like "How am I, right now?" or "What am I holding on to here inside?" or perhaps "What is the main thing for me right now?" Allow a response to come from inside, without exerting any particular effort, and just notice whatever comes into your awareness. Try to suspend mental analysis and refrain from going into all the details. Instead, simply notice the felt sense of the whole thing. Take your time with this. Next, check if there's a word, phrase, or image that captures that felt sense. This may take a moment as well. Don't rush. Next, check inwardly if that word, phrase, or image fits just right. Perhaps you get a sense of "yes, that's exactly it" or "no, it's more like such-and-such." Give yourself a minute or so for this inner checking. Next, try asking inwardly "What is it about [the issue] that gives it that [word, phrase, or image] quality?" Allow some time for a response to come. Finally, I ask you to suspend any tendencies to criticize or dismiss or minimize what came, and instead simply appreciate it.

For the next exercise, I invite you to take a moment to reflect specifically upon your spiritual development, in whatever way you might define it. This process will be similar to the first one, but the content may be different. Bring your awareness into your body in the same way. This time begin with a different question. Try asking inside "How am I, right now, spiritually?" or "What is the main thing for me right now in terms of my spiritual development?" or perhaps "Where am I right now on my spiritual path?" If you can't connect with any of these questions, create one of your own that you can connect with. Move through each of the same steps outlined above, assuming a patient and receptive stance, allowing whatever comes to come without forcing it. Notice what comes. Notice the felt sense of it. See if there is a word, phrase, or image that captures the whole thing. Check that word, phrase, or image against the felt sense to see if it fits. Ask what it is about the issue that gives it that quality. End by appreciating what came.

If anything at all happened for you in the first exercise, you've had a taste of focusing. If something happened for you in the second one, you've had a taste of focusing specifically with spiritual issues. If you had trouble with either one, don't worry, many people do at first. I assure you that you can focus, and certainly would with a bit of assistance and support from someone familiar with this process. In any case, I propose that both exercises tap into a spiritual realm. In other words, with or without religious or spiritual content, the process is one that reaches into a spiritual dimension.

## Focusing as a Key Ingredient in Successful Counseling

We can thank Gendlin and his colleagues at the University of Chicago for "discovering" the process as they attempted to explain why it is that not all clients benefit from counseling. The crucial difference concerns what clients do within themselves (or not) from the beginning. Consequently, we now know that some clients can tap into that bodily level, directly accessing their inner experience of an issue or concern, and reap the benefits in terms of better counseling outcomes. Other clients don't seem to know how, and don't spontaneously learn to do so; they tend not to benefit from counseling. In other words, some clients need to be taught how to be clients, how to access their inner lives, so they can make better use of the counseling process.

Focusing has expanded to a wide range of specific applications in within counseling. In light of this, Gendlin was asked what was "absolutely essential" to focusing, what he wouldn't want to be lost or altered. He said,

> I always say that focusing is just paying attention to something unclear that you directly feel in your body, which has something to do with some situation, some thing in your life. Every wonderful thing that comes on the other side of that is what you get when you go through the door. (E. T. Gendlin, personal communication, 2004)

He said further, "It seems that that can be combined with anything, and can deepen anything, and can profit from anything else that ever helped anybody" He wants to be clear that he is not saying anyone has "a hotline to God" or access to universal truth through focusing, but he is saying "that what we sense the situation to be has a certain validity." In fact, new steps can emerge from tapping into this bodily realm, the "murky zone," with any topic or context one has lived with or been immersed in. The applications of his philosophy have extended to many fields other than counseling and psychology. For instance, recent research findings from neurology, genetics, paleontology, and other fields are supporting the concepts in his process model.[1]

---

[1]Quotes by E. T. Gendlin are from a series of phone conference conversations between the author, other Focusing Institute trainees, and Dr. Gendlin during the 2004 Spring Valley, New York, Institute.

## ABOUT EUGENE T. GENDLIN

Eugene T. Gendlin earned his Ph.D. from the University of Chicago and was a professor of psychology there. In collaboration with Carl Rogers, he was able to articulate what the *client* was doing when empathic conditions were present (reference) and therapeutic change was happening. Gendlin founded *Psychotherapy: Theory, Research and Practice* and served as its editor for many years. He also received the first Distinguished Professional Psychologist award from the Psychotherapy Division of the American Psychological Association. He is a prolific writer, having authored many books and articles, and he continues to be active in sharing focusing with an expanding international focusing community. The Focusing Institute has two locations: Chicago and Spring Valley, New York.

Gendlin's original way of describing and teaching focusing was through the following "six steps." As a kind of preliminary first step, it can help to "clear a space," which is like taking an internal inventory of present difficulties, but simply noticing and acknowledging each of them without making any contact yet. (We skipped this step in the above exercises). Choosing one issue, connecting with it, and sensing the quality of it, is the second step, "getting the felt sense." A felt sense is an awareness of something unclear just beneath what one is aware of. It is also underneath the usual mental static and inclinations to analyze. It is more vague and subtle, more holistic. Finding a word, phrase, or image that fits it, is the third step, "getting a handle." The fourth step is a matter of checking inwardly if the handle fits the felt sense. This is called "resonating." It's like holding up the handle and asking the felt sense "Is that right?" In doing so, the handle can change, so there is a fluid process of finding language to fit the felt sense. It is like a "zigzag" between the "something" that is directly sensed and our capacity for language/thought (Gendlin, 2004). The fifth step is asking the felt sense a question, and then waiting, which often opens a kind of inner dialogue. For instance, one could ask what it is about the issue that gives it that quality (the handle). Patient waiting is key. Answers that come quickly are usually from our heads rather than from the felt sense. The sixth step of receiving and appreciating what came from the focusing process may occur spontaneously, but it can be helpful to do consciously. It is sometimes also necessary to protect what came from critical thoughts and questions that intrude. "Don't let them dump a truckload of cement on this new green shoot that just came up" (Gendlin, 1981, p. 61). In light of the fact that focusing could often continue indefinitely, it also sometimes helps to "mark your place" in a sense, knowing that you can return to that place inside later. Marking your place might mean getting a new "handle" (word, phrase, or image) that captures your current sense of the issue. You might also envision giving the felt sense whatever protection, care, or containment it needs.

## Focusing as a Process of Spiritual Development

I often notice the intersection of focusing with spirituality. Many times, a distinctly spiritual quality to my own focusing process arises as a pleasant surprise. Just as often, I enjoy sharing in another's recognition of something inherently spiritual about focusing for them. Both have frequently happened within my focusing partnerships, which are simply relationships in which each person takes turns focusing with the benefit of the other's listening. One such moment came when a focusing partner of mine had "cleared a space" and spontaneously noticed how her experience in that moment resonated with something she read in Christian theology. She said, "Ah, this is what they call 'practicing being in the presence of God.'" I now realize that my focusing partners and I aren't the only ones to notice that focusing can be more than a tool for emotional or psychological growth and problem solving.

Some focusing practitioners consider focusing itself to be a spiritual practice. Several examples of this include the following: One group in Boston explores ways that focusing and meditation complement one another (Lennox, 2001). *Changes* meetings in New York City have an interest group that practices focusing in conjunction with meditation. A member of the Religious Society of Friends articulates a number of ways that focusing converges with Quakerism (Saunders, 2003). For instance, from both perspectives, truth is within each person and can be experienced directly there. Also, the individual looks within rather than to external authorities for truth and guidance. She notes that "focusing seems to bring one closer to a point of spiritual alchemy, whereby body transmutes into soul and soul into body" (p. 2). Rabbi Goldie Milgram (2005) describes how focusing "synergizes beautifully" with Judaism as well. For instance, traditional Jewish texts and teachers describe the process of learning to listen for the deeper, more subtle voice within and illuminate how it gives rise to passion and clarity when one listens to it, but depression and confusion when one does not. She utilizes focusing in bar/bat mitzvah preparation to find "the prayer of one's heart" and highlights how focusing can help synagogue services to be more meaningful and beneficial. I shall elaborate on the intersection of focusing and specific faith traditions later.

I think it is important to note that Gendlin does not directly refer to focusing as a process of spiritual development per se, although many others have made this connection. Expanding on the way that a felt sense grows out of an individual's relationship with his environment, Gendlin (personal communication, 2004) reminds us that we (i.e., human beings) are all "already part of the universe, already part of a huge context, already immersed in living from . . . like a plant living from wherever plants live from . . . wherever life originates." He also describes how, even when focusing begins with personal content, it characteristically moves to a wider perspective of more freedom and less fear, and "you discover yourself part of this much bigger thing, and some of these things are stated of course in various traditions" (E. T. Gendlin, personal communication, 2004). Although he acknowledges that he is describing territory some would call spiritual, he seems to prefer pointing to the huge context *there* and inviting others to *go* there, with whatever language helps them to do so.

## The Scope of Focusing Across the Lifespan

It is worth noting that Gendlin's book *Focusing* is written for the general public, and the process has wide applicability that includes but is not limited to counseling and spiritual development. It can help with "stuckness" of any kind in life and can even assist in cultural change. In the broadest sense, it can bring fresh life and direction into any area in which old forms and patterns don't fit. It seems to be a universal human capacity, albeit one that may lie dormant or untapped. Thus its applicability is as broad as human experience across the lifespan, including clients of all ages, from children (Blanco & Pascual, 2004; Bowers, 2002; Klein, 1998; Olafsdottir, 2002) to older adults (Sherman, 1990).

## Underlying Theoretical Assumptions of Focusing

The early theoretical work on focusing, particularly how it operates within the context of counseling, is articulated in Gendlin's (1964) theory of personality change. Notice how the very notion of "personality change" suggests changes that are deep and substantive. I propose that the depth of self-examination and personal work involved in substantially altering one's character or personality structure must certainly tap into the spiritual realm. This particular theory is unique in the way it works to incorporate two common clinical observations about how change occurs, namely that it involves an intense feeling process and that it happens within a relationship. The feeling process is an inwardly felt reworking that counselors notice in a client who is "really" working on or facing something, as opposed to "merely" talking about it. The personal relationship is also frequently cited as the context within which personality change occurs, without describing *how* it makes such a critical difference. Gendlin's theory is unique in its attention to the change *process*, and the constructs of *experiencing* and *focusing* are central in this formulation.

*Experiencing* is an ongoing process of inner experience that can be sensed or felt in the body. I liken this process to an underground stream of life energy, always present and continually flowing inside each of us, whether we are tuned in to it or not. Interestingly, the metaphor of an "underground river" is one that was used by Meister Eckhart to capture how, in silence, the Spirit of God could "bubble up" into our psyches (Punshon, 1987). When and if one pays particular attention to something within this flow of experiencing, that becomes what Gendlin calls a *direct referent*, which holds complex felt meanings. That "something" that we are aware of in the form of a felt sense is often likened to the tip of an iceberg, because it is connected to much more just beneath our conscious awareness. In the process of finding words to symbolize it, we make some of the meaning explicit. We might say that we become acquainted with more of the iceberg by sensing further into it and describing what we sense.

It is important not to take this iceberg analogy too literally, however. In Gendlin's theory, the implicit meanings are preverbal, preconceptual, not-yet-formed meanings, as opposed to preexisting but somehow hidden units of meaning. We're not taking the lid off a box to see what is inside. It would be more accurate to say the implicit meaning is *carried forward* in the interactive process of finding words or symbols for a felt sense. There seems to be a creative quality to this process, because the way it is carried forward cannot be known in advance. Focusing, then, is the process of paying attention to something specific within one's bodily felt flow of experiencing and interacting with it through words or symbols, thereby carrying it forward.

The movement that occurs during the process of focusing is a self-propelled feeling process, in contrast to the distinct lack of movement when talking "at" oneself. The latter is like trying to force change from the outside, which paradoxically reinforces the status quo, and usually bad feelings about it. On the other hand, the stance of "being with" and "interacting with" a felt sense engages the self-propelled feeling process that Gendlin describes as the "essential motor of personality change." It is more like being a willing participant in a natural change process, and is at the heart of *how* change comes about.

Take the common clinical observation that change occurs within the context of a personal relationship. Gendlin articulates *how* by contrasting the kind of listener with whom one's experiencing is more constricted from the kind with whom it becomes more vividly alive. Note that he is not simply describing differences in how much someone is willing to share with another, but is actually saying that the experience itself is quite different with a better listener. It is fuller, more intense, expansive, and alive. The person thinks of more to say, has more patience with herself, has more access to emotions, and is less hindered by secondary emotions (such as guilt, shame, anxiety, disgust, annoyance). Thus, a better listener helps someone reach further into the experiential realm where change can occur. This gives fresh meaning to the notion that a good counselor can help clients to "open up."

## How Focusing Embraces Diversity

We truly honor our clients' inner wisdom when we look to their felt sense for the answers to their questions, for the right direction in their lives, or for deeper understanding of their spiritual concerns. In doing so, we embrace the cultural context without losing sight of clients' individuality. Discussing the philosophical underpinnings of focusing, Gendlin describes how the postmodern perspective, which recognizes that there is no absolute truth or knowledge, results in a kind of dead end for some as far as what they can think or say with confidence. He credits Wittgenstein for articulating a contextual philosophy of language that shows how "any set of words depends for its meaning on the context." The focusing process picks up from there by adding a way of "referring directly to a person's sense of the context" (E. T. Gendlin, personal communication, 2004), a context that includes cultural differences such as those stemming from language, social class, and personal history. In other words, focusing is reaching into one's felt sense of all-of-that, a sense that includes the cultural context. Keep in mind that the particulars of that context may or may not be well-articulated on a conscious level for any given client. Thus, working at a felt sense level provides a way for clients to clarify key cultural influences as well as how those influences intersect with current concerns.

Moreover, going into the wider context of a felt sense, one often gets an intricacy beyond the differences due to culture or personal history. For example, the experience of living in another culture typically brings an understanding that "has something further in it" than a linear combination of the two cultures. The "more," the "something further," in Gendlin's philosophy, is a natural part of being alive, in contrast to scientific concepts that separate living things as if they were static and isolated entities. Because we are living things, "everything we say and think is really a product of a relationship, of a connection, of an –ing, of some sort of activity" (E. T. Gendlin, personal communication, 2004). From this perspective, culture is a part of the context of someone's life without defining it, in the sense of binding or limiting it, because living things still generate their own next steps. When someone is focusing, reaching into their present felt sense of any particular thing, not only can we trust that the whole cultural context is "in there" in the process, we can also trust that the process will result in some forward step that is not a simple combination of the person and their culture. Rather it is a dynamic interaction of that individual's immediate experience and the whole cultural context of his life.

## The Experiencing Scale

At this point, it is probably apparent to the reader that focusing is not a process that easily lends itself to description in terms of distinct stages. The development that occurs during the process is more fluid and organic than stage-like. Much of what we know about its relevance to counseling outcome, however, comes from research with The Experiencing Scale (Klein, Mathieu, Gendlin, & Kiesler, 1969), which operationalizes the experiencing construct in terms of seven stages. These are distinct levels of access to the experiential realm as verbalized by clients. Excerpts from the manual appear in Table 14.1.

Keep in mind that you do not have to be a researcher for knowledge of these stages to be useful. They also serve as a valuable heuristic for counselors interested in helping their clients to access deeper levels of their inner resources. Note that while clients begin to refer to feelings

TABLE 14.1 Seven Stages of Experiencing

| Stage | Description |
| --- | --- |
| 1 | The content is not about the speaker. The speaker tells a story, describes other people or events in which he is not involved, or presents a generalized or detached account of ideas. Nothing makes the content personal. |
| 2 | The association between the speaker and the content is explicit. Either the speaker is the central character in the narrative or his interest is clear. The speaker's involvement, however, does not go beyond the specific situation or content. All comments, associations, reactions, and remarks serve to get the story or idea across but do not refer to or define the speaker's feelings. |
| 3 | The content is a narrative or a description of the speaker in external or behavioral terms with added comments on his feelings or private experiences. These remarks are limited to the events or situation described, giving the narrative a personal touch without describing the speaker more generally. |
| 4 | The content is a clear presentation of the speaker's feelings, giving his personal, internal perspective of feelings about himself. Feelings or the experience of events, rather than the events themselves, are the subject of the discourse. |
| 5 | The content is a purposeful exploration of the speaker's feelings and experiencing. There are two necessary components. First, the speaker must pose or define a problem or proposition about himself explicitly in terms of feelings . . . Second, he must explore or work with the problem in a personal way. |
| 6 | The content is a synthesis of readily accessible, newly recognized, or more fully realized feelings and experiences . . . The speaker's immediate feelings are integral to his conclusions about his inner workings. . . . His manner may reflect changes or insights at the moment of their occurrence. |
| 7 | The content reveals the speaker's expanding awareness of his immediately present feelings and internal processes. . . . Manner at this stage is often euphoric, buoyant, or confident; the speaker conveys a sense of things falling quickly and meaningfully into place. |

in the third stage, the direct reference to a felt sense that would be considered *focusing* does not begin until stage four (Hendricks, 2001).

I propose that spiritual development begins at the same point, stage
four, when a personal inner perspective emerges, and not before. Keep
in mind that the content is not the determining factor, but the manner in which it is being discussed. For instance, if a client tells a story
about something she observed in church or relates a Biblical story in
an impersonal way, it remains at a level one. The same kind of content
reaches a level two if the client demonstrates more personal involvement, perhaps by describing a conversation she had with her minister
or by sharing an opinion about a Biblical passage. Level three is reached
with the introduction of feelings, such as "I felt validated by my minister;" or private experiences such as "It occurred to me that we were
becoming friends, and that made me feel important."

As feelings and personal experiences move more to the foreground,
the client is communicating at stage four, where focusing—and spiritual development—can begin. The content might be a discussion of
experiences in prayer, meditation, or worship. It might be a discussion of feelings of connection or disconnection from something sacred
or divine. It might be about the client's experience of an interpersonal conflict. Whether the content is religious, spiritual, both, or
neither, I am suggesting that a process of spiritual development is
occurring if the focus of the client's attention is on her inner life. The
same is true for stage five, which is characterized by a more deliberate exploration of a particular inner issue. Perhaps the client wonders
aloud why she has such personal difficulty with a tenet of her church,
and actively explores that with sustained inner attention. Alterna-
tively, perhaps the client is in a job or relationship that is depleting
or feels damaging on a spiritual level, and is exploring that in a similar manner. Stage six is reached when the client's inner attention cul-
minates in answers or insights. The tone and process at stage seven
is even more expansive.

## The Critical Relevance of Focusing
## Within Counseling

If success in counseling can be predicted from clients' initial experiencing levels (Focusing Institute, 2002; Hendricks, 2001), then it matters a great deal whether or not our clients are able to access their
bodily felt sense. If they can not do so on their own, it is up to us to

help guide them. Certainly, then, one way of doing that is to teach focusing directly to your clients, perhaps using the traditional "six steps." You might offer the rationale that this process will likely help them to make better use of their experience in counseling. This would be particularly appropriate with clients who come in speaking at lower experiencing levels, "story-telling" if you will, i.e., not knowing how to speak from their own experience. The whole notion of teaching focusing presents a challenging kind of dilemma, however, that of how to offer without imposing something "from outside" in the hope that the client may better connect with that which comes "from inside." One way to handle that is with tentative bits of instruction, and with ample room for the client to see what comes inwardly in response (Gendlin, 1996).

Another way to bring focusing into your work is to recognize an opening for focusing as it naturally occurs in the flow of the counseling process, know that this is a delicate opening, and take care to nurture it without getting in the way. You can often tell that you're at that kind of a juncture by a shift in the way the client is talking. Having told their story, clients often reach a point where the words aren't coming as quickly or clearly, because they've come to the edge of what they already know about the issue. There may be silence or incomplete sentences, as if they're groping for words. As a counselor, you can help them across the bridge to "the more" within the felt sense that is not yet known. How? First, you must recognize that the gap is not an empty one, but "the language is implicit in there," implicit in the felt sense. Gendlin said, "The trick is to stay with, close, next to, return to, come back to, that sense, until the language rearranges itself to form fresh sentences" (personal communication, 2004). Help the client to slow down and spend time with the felt sense. Reflect back key words, which can help the client resonate them against the felt sense. Attend to the something *there*, which helps the client to attend there as well. Notice aloud the distinct *something* that is without words as of yet, and patiently encourage the client to find words. It is critical to recognize that other ways of "trying" to be helpful can actually be counterproductive. In our anxiety to do a good job, we may impose *our* concepts or techniques, which break the client's connection with the felt sense, thereby inadvertently squelching their process. In fact, another significant finding from research with the Experiencing Scale concerns those clients who come into counseling knowing how to process in a focusing manner. For them, the process is deepened when working with a counselor who also knows how to process in that manner, but flattened over 80% of the time when working with a counselor who doesn't (Focusing Institute, 2002; Hendricks, 2001). Thus, the most important "tool" we can carry into our day-to-day work as counselors is an awareness of this level of process that can be experienced directly in the body, some familiarity with it from our own experience, and a readiness to attend to it within our clients. If you can do that for your clients, you are in a very good position to facilitate a process of spiritual development for them. Yes, spiritual development. I suggest that the felt sense dimension is a spiritual one. Therefore, I am also suggesting that when change in that dimension is happening, spiritual development *is* happening. I realize this notion may seem radical to some, because I am essentially saying that counseling involves the spiritual dimension whether we are conscious of it or not. There are also many ways that focusing can be used consciously for spiritual development. I shall share just a few.

## Focusing and Native American Spirituality

The first connection I became aware of was the remarkable similarity between how Gendlin describes a felt sense and how "Grandfather," an Apache elder describes "inner vision" to Tom Brown Jr. in his book *The Journey* (Brown, 1992). Recall Gendlin's point that making direct contact with a felt sense is very different from thinking about it on an intellectual level. Similarly, Grandfather points out the difference between rational language and the language of "Inner Vision [which] does not communicate to us in the words and concepts of man but through the language of the heart. Inner Vision speaks to us only through feelings and emotions, symbols, signs, dreams, and waking visions" (Brown, p. 37). Inner vision and focusing both must be experienced. They cannot be understood mentally alone.

Grandfather tries to teach Tom Inner Vision by asking him for something at a time when he was preoccupied (so he would be likely to forget it) and then later asking, "Haven't you forgotten something?" The question evokes a gnawing sensation in Tom's gut until he remembers. Grandfather uses this to explain,

> The tightness in your gut when you tried to remember but could not was your Inner Vision trying desperately to talk to you. . . . That tension, that deep gut feeling, is exactly how our inner vision tries to talk to us. Thus when the answer is finally found on a logical level, the gut reacts with the release of tension. Your greater

self is so relieved that you have found an answer, an answer that it knew all the time." (Brown, p. 42)

Gendlin provides a strikingly similar illustration of the characteristics of a felt sense using a familiar human experience:

the odd feeling of knowing you have forgotten something. . . . You are troubled by the *felt sense*. . . . Notice that you don't have factual data. You have an inner aura, an internal taste. *Your body knows but you don't.* . . . Then suddenly, from this felt sense, it bursts to the surface [remembering what you forgot]. Somewhere in your body, something releases, some tight thing lets go." (Gendlin, 1996, pp. 37–38)

Whatever language we use to describe it, there seems to be a universal human process at work here. Receptive attention to a bodily felt tension invites the underlying meaning to rise to the surface of one's awareness.

## Focusing and Early Quakers

Another example of remarkable similarity between focusing and spiritual process can be found in Rex Ambler's (2002) experience. He seeks, for personal and intellectual reasons, to better understand some of the concepts early Quakers wrote about, particularly "the light" and "the truth," so that he too can access "that of God" within. He is struck by how the Quaker practice of "dwelling in the light" is essentially describing the passive attention cultivated in meditation, and proceeds to break that practice down into four steps. He makes the first step, that of paying attention to the light in one's own conscience, very concrete and accessible this way: "We have only to stop and consider if there is anything in our lives we feel uncomfortable about and we can feel a twinge or niggle about something or other" (p. 17). This is very similar to how many begin focusing, by asking if there is anything standing in the way of feeling completely okay (Hinterkopf, 1998b). It is the same kind of receptive attention to inner tension described earlier.

The second step Ambler describes is opening one's heart to the truth, with a receptive attitude and a willingness to see beyond fear, pride, and preexisting ideas about oneself. The third step is waiting, or standing still in the light, in a detached manner, with "a kind of distance between us and the problem" (p. 19), allowing one to see it whole. This is very similar to others' attention to getting the "right distance" from a felt sense (Gendlin, 1981; Hinterkopf, 1998a; Weiser Cornell, 1996). The fourth step is submitting to the truth, which Ambler says is not a matter of giving up responsibility or accepting dictates of anyone, but is more a matter of accepting what one comes to see through the previous steps, relinquishing resistance and any conflicting or self-deceptive ideas or stories. When he remarks to a friend "that the first Quakers found a therapeutic process which didn't need a therapist" (p. 25), that friend recognizes the process to be very similar to what Eugene Gendlin describes as focusing.

Upon reading about focusing and trying it himself, Ambler has to agree that it resonates very much with his own journey of rediscovering what the early Quakers had found and written about. That in itself seems remarkable to him since focusing isn't a spiritual practice per se. Thus, Ambler comes to view focusing as a tool or skill that can be utilized with a wide range of issues and situations, some spiritual, some not. (This diverges slightly from the premise of this chapter, that focusing is a process of spiritual development.) To use it for spiritual development, Ambler finds that "there had to be a desire for wholeness and healing, a readiness to face truth that might be painful, and a willingness to let go my ego which so likes to think it has the answers already" (p. 29). Clearly, those conditions will greatly enhance the process and the degree of development it brings. Further, he finds focusing extremely helpful for accessing "the light" or the "voice of truth" within, through stillness, quiet, being receptive, and listening to the body. He sees this as particularly helpful and necessary in modern times, which emphasize mental activity, rationality, conscious thought, and control.

## Focusing and Buddhist Practice

David Rome shares about the integration of focusing into Buddhist practice in the *Shambhala Sun* (Rome, 2004). He notices that the emphasis in focusing upon "repeatedly letting go of conceptual activity and returning to the body sense" (2004, p. 61) is similar to the Buddhist practice of attending to the present moment and suspending mental activity. He cites the key importance in focusing of cultivating an attitude of "self-empathy" or "caring feeling presence," and notes how these ways of befriending oneself are very similar to what Buddhists refer to as *maitri* or loving kindness. He sees this kind of attitude as particularly helpful, even necessary, in accessing "more embryonic or emergent or delicate kinds of going-on in the body," which can be inhibited "in the Western psyche [by] a very strong critical voice or superego," or in some Buddhist traditions by "a very strong emphasis on discipline [which] can be characterized by a certain harshness of attitude" (2004, p. 63).

In addition to these ways the two practices overlap, Rome shares several ways that focusing can enrich Buddhist meditation practice and serve as a "wonderful companion" to it. He notes that Robert Aitken Roshi, dean of American Zen masters, regularly recommends focusing to students as well. The step of clearing a space can be a helpful precursor to meditation. Focusing also can substantially enhance the experience of meditation, better incorporating the "much more" that lies beneath the surface of conscious awareness, which may be missed in the meditative practice of "bare attention" to whatever appears in one's awareness. Focusing offers a "middle path" of noticing and sensing life issues more wholly, without discursively going too far into them. It also narrows the gap that often exists between contemplative practice and the challenges associated with "living in the world." Whereas meditation doesn't aim to solve personal problems per se, focusing offers a way of connecting quite directly with life issues, bringing about more understanding and insight, as well as specific action steps. Thus, focusing can be an "antidote" of sorts to the way that spiritual practice may sometimes, and perhaps inadvertently, "bypass" personal and emotional issues that need to be addressed (D. Rome, personal communication, 2004).

In addition to the intrapersonal ways focusing can enhance Buddhist practice, Rome sees an important interpersonal piece inherent in the value and depth of the kind of empathic listening cultivated in focusing partnerships, which are based upon reciprocal exchanges of focusing and listening to one another. While Buddhist meditation cultivates attunement and sensitivity to one's own inner processes, it doesn't necessarily cultivate the same attunement to others', or at least not as directly. Focusing partnerships not only develop the capacity to be highly present for another (fitting well with Buddhist compassion practice) but also the capacity to do so "without losing track of ourselves" (2004, p. 62). Rome appreciates that focusing does not pretend or even try to be a "complete path," but rather interacts and joins beautifully with many other practices and fields, including "of course, spirituality." Some learn meditation first and then discover how to incorporate focusing and/or other forms of psychological work. Others learn focusing first, and from there, "I think, in a sense, it's almost inevitable that they start to enter into territory that we might describe as more spiritual" (D. Rome, personal communication, 2004).

## Focusing and Christianity

Peter Campbell and Edwin McMahon emphasize the spiritual relevance of focusing crossculturally as well as for Christians in particular in their book *Bio-Spirituality* (1997). They not only emphasize the human capacity for bodily experience of spirit, but also see it as "ultimate common ground" that holds great potential as a force for peace and connection underneath the multitude of religious and other differences in the world. They also provide a vision of what a healthy spiritual practice in any faith should look like. It should assist you in entering into and processing your feelings rather than suggesting you substitute more "acceptable" ones. It should not only affect you on a level of ideas and thinking but also on a level of bodily experience. The means of growth should be characterized by openness and surrender to change, as opposed to will or self-control.

In the way Campbell and McMahon teach focusing, direct assistance to clients in silently entering their bodies and owning their feelings is even more important than active listening. They also emphasize surrendering and letting go, so that one may experience *grace*, which feels like easing, life energy, relief, change, and movement toward wholeness. Another emphasis in their bio-spiritual approach is that of creating a *caring-feeling presence* inside (similar to the more secular terminology of "friendly focusing attitudes") to assist someone in being with a difficult issue by giving it more gentleness and caring. For instance, approaching it as a "teacher" (as opposed to an "enemy") might help. Approaching it with the tenderness you would feel toward a child who is hurt or scared would be another way. A particular strength of the bio-spiritual approach is the respectful stance toward defenses and resistance, seeing them as "doorways not walls, if you know how to be drawn through them" (p. 154). For instance, after noticing an issue that is present and before getting a felt sense of it, Campbell and McMahon recommend asking, "Is it OK to be with it right now?" If something inside says *no*, you can ask if it's OK to be with *that*, the sense of not-right or not-OK to be with the original issue. If the inner response is still *no*, you can ask what it *is* OK to be with right now. This respectful stance without external pressure extends throughout the process to the end. In the event that it hasn't yet moved toward something that feels better, you can let it know you will come back to it and remain open to it, or ask how it needs you to be with it in the meantime. Finally, Christianity can fit nicely in a round of focusing at the end, during the "nurturing period," a time of quiet reverence that is akin to Gendlin's sixth step of receiving. One might notice and appreciate "God's grace" or "God's life-giving presence," or take a few minutes to be "in Christ" or say "thank you" in whatever way feels right.

## Differentiating Spiritual Development from Arrested Development and Pathology

As we have discussed, one way of responding to an uncomfortable or even painful feeling is to acknowledge it, sit with it, approach it with friendly curiosity, take time to sense what it is all about, and allow its implicit meaning to unfold from inside without external pressure. From this perspective, any feeling—or more accurately, the holistic felt sense of any feeling—is an opportunity for spiritual growth. Campbell and McMahon would say it's an opportunity for grace. Moving away from it, avoiding it, or trying to control it instead misses the opportunity for that process of growth to occur. Gendlin uses the term *process-skipping* to describe this, and Campbell and McMahon see it as an underlying mechanism of unhealthy spiritual practices. They illustrate with an example in which someone draws from the image of Jesus on the cross to help them forgive someone for hurting them. The likely result of praying for forgiveness in this way is further rejection of one's feeling of anger (which remains unprocessed and further denied) and an effort to substitute love and compassion in its place. "If Jesus could be an encouraging presence, accompanying the person as he or she enters into and owns real inner feelings, then this could be a prayer that leads toward healing and wholeness" (p. 192). Otherwise, there is a missed opportunity for spiritual development.

Let's go a step further and consider process-skipping *structures*, which are habitual ways of avoiding uncomfortable feelings. This essentially describes an addiction in Campbell and McMahon's view, which may take the form of an addiction to drugs or alcohol or sex, but may also be to socially acceptable activities like work, pleasing others, or even prayer. "Most people, in my experience, at one time or another use religion and their relationship to God as just one more way of numbing and escape" (p. 180). Now we are talking about more of a pattern that amounts to arrested spiritual development. It is true that attending to a bodily felt sense can be extremely difficult when one's ego structure or belief system is designed for protection from the very pain or weakness the felt sense is tapping into (Sears, 1997). If a religious practice is driven by the need to protect oneself from pain, it most likely will reinforce it instead. Religious fundamentalism, for instance, could be considered a form of arrested spiritual development in which one holds tightly onto a belief system as a way to avoid "going inside."

The violence that can stem from a fundamentalist belief system could then be considered an extreme expression of the inability to own one's own pain and an extreme form of spiritual pathology. Campbell and McMahon (1997) point out the relevance of focusing to the worldwide problem of "violent religious fundamentalism" and "simplistic religious solutions to complex social problems as well as the growing use of political power to impose those interpretations and solutions" (1997, p. xix). The presence or absence of an inner process (i.e., focusing or process-skipping) offers a compelling way of distinguishing religious practices that are a force for peace and unity from those that create divisions and fuel conflicts. Responding to spiritual pathology in the social and political spheres is an immensely complex issue, but not entirely beyond the scope of this chapter. "Social and political action from an inwardly connected place creates new possibilities" (Hendricks, 2005). Let us consider the wider applications of the principles we've been discussing.

## Spiritual Development in Social and Political Spheres

It is a misnomer to view focusing as a purely introverted activity. "Our felt sense is OF our lived situations" (Hendricks, 2005). "Interactive focusing" (Klein, 2001) is one application that brings the depth of focusing into interpersonal situations. One person focuses on an issue between them while the other listens. This is followed by a step in which the listener first sits with "all of that" and then puts words or an image to the essence of it. This is called the "double empathic moment" because the focuser also sits with "all of that," practicing self-empathy. The final step is a relationship check in which each person shares how he is now with himself and with the relationship. The process is very similar to the couple's dialogue process utilized in imago relationship therapy (Hendrix, 1998) in which one partner assumes the role of "sender" while the other is the "receiver" who simply mirrors (i.e., reflects) the communication back throughout, completing the process with validation and empathy. While these processes appear simple, they share common elements which may account for why they are often experienced as quite powerful.

The "something" one is aware of when beginning a round of focusing is connected to much more on the edge of one's awareness, just as the discomfort or pain one is aware of in an interpersonal conflict is often connected to much more, usually from unprocessed past experiences. The safety of being heard and validated helps the speaker/focuser access more of "the more," and each step of putting language to preverbal visceral experience is an instance of the very spiritual growth we've been talking about. Such processes offer an alternative to conflicts characterized by reactive postures, power struggles, and good/bad right/wrong dichotomies. Hearing and honoring an individual's inner experience as it is without having to agree makes understanding and connection possible between two (or more) people with very different experiences. There is even some growing recognition in the field of interpersonal neurobiology (Mulhern, 2006; Siegel, 1999) that such processes are reflected in our physiology, for example, in the form of integration of various parts of the brain and the rewiring of neural pathways. Furthermore, this openness to seeing beyond one's own perspective, and to sitting with whatever inner resonance or dissonance that brings, is likely to stimulate spiritual growth for the listener as well.

Let me share an example that goes a step beyond a dialogue between two people. In response to an incident of tragic violence in an abortion clinic, one organization invited five pro-choice and five pro-life women into dialogue with each other over a period of years (Hunt, 2006). The process created strong relationships across the significant divide of political and ideological differences, although none of the women changed their beliefs in the end. This illustrates how the notion of "going inside" and communicating from there can facilitate spiritual development for groups as well as individuals. It also illustrates how "going inside" requires courage and a willingness to face a great deal of fear and pain at times. The notion of utilizing focusing beyond an individual counseling relationship might translate to facilitating interactive focusing between individuals or adapting it to groups. It could also translate to acting from an inwardly connected place in your own social and/or political life. At one time or another, I imagine you have felt some dissonance between your relationships with clients that are a source of healing and even spiritual development for them (perhaps even for you) on the one hand and some of the other professional and personal relationships in your life on the other. There may be many reasons for the difference, but I propose that much of it can be explained by the willingness and ability to "go inside" versus the unwillingness or inability to do so. I have observed the mechanism of "process-skipping" (talking or moving right past a bodily felt sense) to be quite common, even normative, in most groups and institutions. Just imagine the degree of change possible if we made more room for the felt sense dimension within the structures of our daily lives.

## Focusing in Practice with Diverse Religious and Spiritual Issues

The above are just a few examples of how focusing resonates with particular spiritual and religious practices and processes. One explanation for this complementarity is the uniquely holistic nature of focusing, which also makes it useful in counseling.

> The goal of counseling is the development of the whole person: mind, body and spirit integrated together. Focusing is the sine qua non of holistic therapy. It is not just body plus mind plus spirit together. The Focusing Method helps us access that which is whole in us *before* it is split apart." (Hinterkopf, 1998b, p. xxii)

Earlier, we discussed how focusing embraces diversity more generally. Here we turn to Hinterkopf's very helpful guidance in utilizing focusing specifically in relation to the diverse manifestations of spirituality within counseling (1998b). Focusing is broad and inclusive enough to be useful with clients who present with a wide range of religious or spiritual issues. It even offers spiritual benefits whether clients are defining their issues in those terms or not. For instance, the exercise of clearing a space can be a spiritual experience of entering a more centered, expansive, and peaceful dimension. Using the word *whole* also tends to access a transcendent dimension, e.g., setting the *whole* thing aside, noticing the felt sense of the *whole* thing, et cetera. Following the direction inherent in a felt sense without controlling the process or forcing steps or solutions is also inherently valuable and resonates with spiritual principles from a variety of disciplines.

Spiritual growth can come from focusing on the positive aspects of religious or spiritual experiences, and by attending to the felt sense and asking what is best or most meaningful or most important about the whole thing. Often, however, focusing begins with uncomfortable feelings that shift or ease as the felt sense unfolds. Indeed, some religious experiences have been painful or abusive, and focusing provides a means of examining whether a religious experience of a particular client's was abusive or not, quite separately from whatever the counselor's opinion or value system might be. The client can take any experience, "check inside" in a bodily way, and notice if the inner response is one of easing and more life energy. Hinterkopf also describes how focusing can help integrate conflicting aspects of religious experiences, e.g., painful and positive aspects.

Hinterkopf (1998b) wants counselors to know that they can respond to spiritual process and thereby facilitate growth for clients even if they are ignorant of the particular spiritual content the client refers to. Not realizing this, counselors unfortunately may instead ignore or judge that with which they are unfamiliar. If the client fills in the content with a particular religious term that has meaning for him or her (e.g., the word *God*), it can be quite helpful for the counselor to use it as well, whatever meaning the words have (if any) to the counselor. Focusing is delicate. Focusing on religious or spiritual content can be particularly so. When particular words resonate with a felt sense, even slightly different words may not resonate at all.

## Focusing in Various Practice Settings

Most of what we've discussed about focusing applies to counseling adult clients, whether in a college counseling center or in a community mental health agency. School counselors can also employ some of the creative applications of focusing for working with children. For instance, "clearing a space" can be made more concrete via words or pictures on pieces of paper. Getting a felt sense can be made more tangible by sitting in "the seat of looking at yourself inside." Drawing pictures can be incorporated as part of the process of resonating (Blanco & Pascual, 2004). Teachers of grades one through five can use a focusing-based Social and Emotional Learning (SEL) program entitled "Inside-Me Stories: Something Is Happening Inside-Me!" (Klein, 1998). Children can play a game of pretend "elevator rides" inside, pushing buttons to see how different parts of their bodies are feeling. They can also press a special Story button for "stories that live inside our bodies." They can be encouraged to be gentle, like they would be with a puppy or a kitten, for any hard parts (Bowers, 2002). A nursery school in Iceland has integrated focusing into its daily routine through activities such as noticing the body in both stillness and motion, drawing, talking about feelings, "focusing play," and checking with "the place that knows what is best for us" (Olafsdottir, 2002). Applications of focusing with children are expanding, as evidenced by the emergence of International Focusing with Children Conferences.

Focusing is very well-suited to working with adolescents as well, particularly those who are acting out in any number of ways. "Violent teenagers are full of feelings . . . If anybody says, 'What are you feeling here in the middle of your stomach?' they're surprised that anybody wants to know, but they can talk from there" (E. T. Gendlin, personal communication, 2004). One focusing trainer (Rosenblum, 2004) shared how readily focusing fit into a spontaneous group activity she tried with adolescents in a day treatment program. One day when a patient happened to have a keyboard, some brief attention to her own felt sense led her to drop her plan for the day and invite the group to write a song together. Their curiosity about what she'd just done when she closed her eyes evolved into each of them using a similar process to contribute to the song: "take a breath, drop down inside, ask the question 'what wants to be written about?' and listen for the response" (p. 4).

## Listening Attitudes

Bringing focusing into your work with clients is more a matter of attitude than techniques. I love Ann Weiser Cornell's (1996) metaphor of approaching a felt sense as one might approach a shy animal at the edge of a forest, because it captures many of the essential listening attitudes. These include curiosity, wonder, gentleness, patience, respect, and a presence that is receptive but not imposed or forced. She is actually describing how to focus alone (later extending this to focusing with another person or within a counseling relationship), but those inner attitudes are ones we can strive to help clients cultivate within themselves and useful attitudes to have ourselves in our relationships with our clients. These attitudes are valuable for their own sake, particularly to the extent that they differ from clients' typical ways of responding to themselves (Hinterkopf, 1998a). Distinguishing these attitudes from those of an "inner critic" can be illuminating as well. The latter can be recognized by the response it elicits: a sense of constriction, hiding, and defending inside (Leijssen, 1998). In counseling, the client can be invited to set it aside, attending instead to the felt sense. In my experience, this often leads to a discussion of how ever present the critic is in a client's life. More importantly, it points to an alternative, an innate capacity that is already there, perhaps dormant and ready to respond to gentle attention.

## Finding the Right Distance

The clients who feel "easy" to us as counselors are probably the ones with the ability to connect with a felt sense, while those who feel "tough" instead repeatedly cycle through the same emotions or stay in their heads (Weiser Cornell, 1996). Some of the challenges you encounter as a counselor working with these tougher clients fall into two broad categories. Either they are too far from a felt sense or too close to it. There is a certain optimal distance for holding a felt sense—close enough to be in contact with it but far enough to keep it in focus. The same is true with respect to spiritual experience. A client may be overwhelmed and preoccupied with spiritual material that is not yet integrated or digested on the one hand or may be disconnected from a spiritual dimension on the other. (Hinterkopf, 1998b).

A client who is too far from the experiential realm may come to a session not knowing what to talk about, with nothing in particular wanting their attention. With this person, you might pose a statement such as "I feel totally well" or "all my problems are solved," which often evokes an inner protest (Gendlin, 1981). As the client is sharing about an issue, seeming too distant from it, you can attend to slight bodily movements you notice but the client isn't aware of. You could also invite the client to put a hand on the spot where the issue is felt to literally "hold onto it" or breathe into that place (Leijssen, 1998). With clients who have difficulty accessing feelings at all, Weiser Cornell (1996) suggests an "attunement" exercise, gently guiding their attention into the body and asking what's presently there. Another possibility is to ask if the client can sense any difference between the feeling in one part of the body and another. Also, the notion of an "inner child" having feelings may help some clients to access them (Hinterkopf, 1998b).

On the other end of the continuum clients may be too close to the issue, stuck or mired in the feelings. Emotions are narrower. Focusing is more holistic. When a client is too close, Hinterkopf (1998b) suggests he imagine observing the inner experience from a distance, for instance, from the perspective of a "neutral reporter" or a fly on the wall. A client may have a surprisingly specific sense of how far away the issue needs to be in order to interact with it without extreme discomfort. Imagining it in a picture frame, behind thick glass, under lock and key, and the like may also help. You might encourage or "give permission" to put the whole thing outside his body, separating "I" from "it." The client may find it helpful to distinguish parts of himself, relating to those parts in whatever way is needed, whether it's having more control or giving more care (Leijssen, 1998; Weiser Cornell, 1996). A subtle way of getting a bit of distance is a more linguistic approach, noticing aloud that the client is "sensing something in you which feels . . ." (Weiser Cornell, personal communication, 2004).

# Sharon

In sharing the following example of my work with a client, I hope to bring this discussion of focusing to life for you as well as bring the theory down to earth and into the trenches of day-to-day clinical work. In my college counseling center work, some clients have certainly been more receptive to "focusing invitations" than others, but each has presented unique challenges for me to learn from. Sometimes I wonder if the academic setting makes it more difficult for my clients to let go of mental activity and listen to their bodily felt sense. Then again, many of us (I include myself) can have difficulty accessing this inner resource, even when we know it is there.

Although some background information is provided, keep in mind that the most relevant context is always the immediate one, whatever arises in the process of the interaction in counseling and most importantly, from within the client. In the transcript that follows, brackets [] will be used to provide any additional information needed to understand the dialogue, or to abbreviate portions of the session. I will also omit some content that is not critical to understanding the dialogue, using ". . ." Interspersed throughout, I will offer commentary on what's happening from a focusing perspective.

## Sharon, Part I: Seeking the Right Distance from Worry

The following is one of my earliest efforts to introduce focusing to a client, who I'll call Sharon. A nineteen-year-old single White female in her junior year of college, she was originally "strongly encouraged" to come in for counseling following an episode of self-injury. She subsequently gained some insight into how and why emotional disconnection was a trigger. For instance, conflicts in her family frequently resulted in emotional cut-offs, her parents divorced when she was young, and she had no contact with her biological father until she was eighteen, apparently because of sexual abuse which she cannot recall. She continued counseling by choice after the initial referral, and begins this session describing how "stressed out" and worried she feels about academics and her other responsibilities.

*Sharon:* I just wish it would be over . . . But it's still there. Like I guess I don't really have to worry about it. I just feel like I have to worry about it.

*Kathryn:* Ooh, that's interesting. You feel like you have to worry . . . but you don't.

*I also could have said "something in you feels like it has to worry."*

*S:* Like, I don't think that I should be worrying about it . . . [provides rationale for not worrying] . . . but I just feel like I have to worry about it. 'Cause it's not here yet, and it's not all over with . . .

*K:* So that's part of this "I want things to be over with fast" 'cause you worry until . . .

*I'm trying to understand her inner process, incorporating information from previous sessions.*

*S:* I worry until things come and then they're over. Then I'm done worrying. I worry a lot. I worry about everything.

*K:* Hm

*S:* [She gives another example.] I look at my planner like ten times a day, and I make sure I know everything that's coming, so then I know what's going on. And then I'll worry about every single thing 'til they're over.

*K:* Until it's over, ahh

*S:* So it's kinda like I'm constantly worrying about things.

*K:* Hmm

*S:* I don't like that.

*K:* Wow, that helps me understand a whole lot better what goes on inside you. I'm not sure I quite got that before.

*I want her to know that I'm interested in her internal process, and that it makes sense.*

*S:* Yeah, I guess. I never really thought about it. But I guess I worry 'til things are over. So I constantly am worrying about something. I don't like that though. (laugh). I don't wanna have to. I think that I should just be more relaxed. 'Cause my friends are always like, they're like, "Sometimes I just wish you would relax for once."

'Cause I think that I'm so, like, uptight about things. And I'm always worried about something.

*K:* Mhm

*S:* And I never relax. And I think I would just like to relax for once.

*K:* Well, maybe we can try.

*I could address the energy of the inner critic which seems to be present. Instead, I decide to take this as an opportunity to teach the skill of "clearing a space," which also works nicely as a stress-management technique, as well as accessing a transcendent dimension (Hinterkopf, 1998).*

*S:* Like how?

*K:* . . . See if you can find, inside, something that you're worried about right now.

*S:* What am I worrying about right now?

*K:* Yeah, what worry are you carrying around right now?

*S:* I have to pick a little {a little sister in her sorority}. And I have first choice. Which is a good thing. But I'm worried about it because . . . I want a little sister that is nice and sweet and (pause) like me (pause) and we get along and talk. [She elaborates a bit.]

*K:* Mm. So you're worried about making the right choice, of someone you click with.

*S:* Right. But do I have any worries right now, at the moment, today? No, no, not today. Tomorrow. . . .

*K:* Well, let's just stick with right now.

*S:* Yeah, that's what I'm worried about.

*K:* Okay, now take that one thing, and then kinda like, see if you can get a little distance from it. Even use your imagination to come up with [images] . . . putting it in a drawer or something, or putting it on a shelf.

*S:* I don't know if I can put it away though. I don't know how to. Do you know what I mean? 'Cause it's like constantly there, and I'm like "oh geez."

*The whole process of clearing a space is new to her, but she seems willing to try.*

*K:* Okay, maybe not away, maybe just a little bit outside of you . . . We're trying to get to a place inside where there's a nice clear space for you to be in, with this stuff in your life just a little bit outside.

*S:* Okay, so I have to put myself, and put my stuff like a little bit outside of me.

*I cringe now at her words "have to." I want it to feel more like an invitation.*

*K:* Yeah. See if you can take that worried feeling, and just get a little bit of space between you and it. So it's still there, but you're not, like, *in* it. You're just kind of a little bit outside of it.

*S:* Like looking at it?

*K:* Yeah.

*S:* Well, I think I can do that . . . I can look at it, but . . . it's out there . . . I'm not really worried about it. I feel more relaxed.

*K:* Hm. Do you feel that now? You're getting a feel for that now?

*S:* Yeah, yeah. But it's the kind of thing that . . . You remember how I told you how I used to see this counselor that I hated?

*K:* Uh huh

*S:* . . . That's how I felt when I was in her office. And I don't think I like that feeling.

*Her present feeling is reminding her of a past experience that was uncomfortable in a way that's hard to put in words.*

*K:* You felt . . . like what?

*S:* Okay, when I sit here and I think about everything being outside, and I know where it is, and I feel relaxed, I feel kinda like dazed.

*K:* Oh, like it's not a good feeling?

*I'm wondering if she's talking about a dissociative experience, given the possible history of childhood sexual abuse. Focusing is a way of being grounded in the body, not dissociating. At the same time, I want her to decide if "dazed" is good or not.*

*S:* Well, I don't know . . . It's kinda like not me . . . I'm relaxed. But I just feel like I'm dazed, and a weird feeling. And that's how I felt when I would go see this lady. But I didn't like this lady. (laugh). . . . She was nice. I just didn't like going to her. I just always felt like . . . I was in this trance or daze, like I had to say all these things that . . . felt right, that was right. You know what I mean?

*K:* Like there's something you were supposed to do in there.

*S:* Right, like I tried to make her happy.

*K:* Oh. Mhm.

*S:* That's kind of how I felt then.

*The vague-but-distinctly-felt quality seems to be a felt sense, so I decide to teach her a bit about focusing. My hope is to help her to develop some trust in her own body and to experience some safety there.*

*K:* Well, see this thing . . . that's what focusing is. Focusing is tuning into something that you know is there but it's sort of like unclear at first . . . And it seems kinda like you're on the edge of something like that right now. It's this feeling, something like kinda dazed, something like . . .

*S:* I feel like too relaxed.

*K:* Mm

*S:* Like I could, well I could just fall asleep, but kinda like that. Like my whole body just feels like relaxed. But it's too relaxed. I don't know.

*Now I wonder if it feels "too" relaxed because it's so unfamiliar to experience relaxation in her body, or to be in her body at all. I trust her body to know what's good for it, so I continue offering some key words to resonate against her felt sense.*

*K:* Kinda dazed, kinda relaxed, but too relaxed. . . .

*S:* Like, it's kinda like, well, when I think about when I let everything outside, I feel like . . . I can feel everything, like, relaxing, like my whole body.

*K:* Hmm

*S:* You know what I mean?

*K:* Yeah. I mean, I'm glad you can do that. I think that might be a good thing.

*S:* But I don't know if I like it.

*K:* Hmm

*S:* I just don't feel like myself. I feel like I have too many things to worry about, that I shouldn't do that. Because . . . then what if I forget about something? And then, you know, it'll just hit me . . . and then I'll be confused . . . It comes back to planning. I like to be planned.

*K:* Hmm

*I'm silently empathizing with how worrying and planning have probably been important coping skills for her and noticing how they've been incorporated into her sense of who she is. It is not uncommon for clients to be identified with processes that are actually obstacles to focusing, e.g., the inner critic.*

*S:* But I would like to feel relaxed, but not so relaxed. Like my stomach always has like this knot, 'cause I'm always worried about something. [She gives an example.]

*Already her body is pointing her in the direction of what's needed: something in between the ever-present knot and "too relaxed." She seems ready to move on from clearing a space.*

**K:** Hm. Wow. There's a whole lot . . . Just to tell you how focusing works. First you try to clear a space, and get everything out there. Then you kinda like ask inside, 'cause only you can really know, which thing is the most important thing right now. And then you sort of bring it back into . . . bring it back in, I guess . . . and feel what it feels like. It's not like you're trying to stay distant from everything.

**S:** Oh, okay

**K:** It's kinda like getting some clear space until you can choose which is the most important, or what wants my attention most right now.

**S:** Right, I can do that. I can take it and see everything, and I know what's pointing at me right now. [She elaborates on how the most important thing would've been different yesterday, and will be something different tomorrow.] But right now, it's this little [sister] thing. I have to pick a little . . . When I put it back in, you want me to, like, feel like I have it again?

**K:** Well, it seems like you had a nice clear space, and you're saying, yeah, the thing that wants my attention most is this little . . .

*Although I'm helping to guide, I want her to know we're following her inner direction.*

**S:** Yeah, it's kinda like I can see a light bulb on it, kinda. Like I can sit here and see all my things. And then I can see that that is brighter than the rest of them.

**K:** Wow, this is really cool.

*Even though I know the capacity for focusing is universal, I often feel like I'm rediscovering it freshly each time.*

**S:** You know what I mean? 'Cause like, that's what I'm worried about now.

**K:** Mhm. Well, let's sit with that whole thing a little bit . . . and try to get what they call a "felt sense" of the whole thing. It's like sometimes you get caught up in all the details of something, and sometimes it helps to kind of sit with the whole thing, and how that whole thing about choosing a little feels inside.

[S proceeds to elaborate some of the issues within her worry about choosing a little sister. She sees that, from a wider view, it doesn't matter as much to her life. Yet she would still like a close relationship with her little sister. She notices how some of this is connected to having a "horrible," uninvolved big sister, and wanting to do a better job.]

## Sharon, Part II: Feelings Without Memories

*I had the opportunity to see this particular client several years later when she entered graduate school. This time, she wanted to focus more specifically on her patterns in relationships and her childhood abuse. She begins by lamenting that she remembers none of the abuse and none of the court proceedings that prohibited her father from contacting her until she was an adult.*

**Kathryn:** I think . . . you can get where you need to get by starting with what you do remember and what you do feel . . .

*I could have reflected her distress about what she can't remember. I opted instead to point in the direction of what* is *there inside for her, rather than what's missing.*

**Sharon:** Even if I don't remember.

**K:** Yeah.

**S:** I know, but I wish I remembered it. Cause that would make it easier . . . I wish I had a movie of my life . . . because I would know exactly what happened . . . but I don't think I am going to remember.

**K:** Well, say this scene that your mom and sister described [of her being very upset at the courthouse] to you is a scene in that movie. What do you feel now, looking back at this image of you at six years old?

**S:** Yeah, that's the thing . . . I feel this stuff. That's why I'm so confused, because I do see what they tell me and I do remember certain things and they run through my head, and I think about them . . . I think that's why I'm so confused as to what I want to do and how I want to feel about all this.

*Her mental confusion seems to be an obstacle to accessing whatever feelings or body sense is there.*

**K:** It's sorta like you don't know what to feel if you don't know what happened.

**S:** Right. Sort of . . . I like concrete answers . . . They [her mom and sister] weren't there. They don't know everything . . . Somehow if I could figure all this out, and I could make sense of it for myself, then maybe . . . Maybe it would affect other parts of my life, where I have issues with being assertive, and feeling bad about telling people no, and the fear of loss of relationship . . . I guess I kinda know how it all interconnects, but maybe if I figured out one part, I would figure out the rest of the parts, and I could maybe fix them?

*She seems to be "talking at" herself. Her analysis of issues that stem from her abuse may be accurate, but has a tone of inner criticism. Rather than joining in this process of psychological fault-finding, I try to reflect the "life forward" part of all this . . .*

*K:* So there's a real . . . wanting things to be right again.

*S:* Right. And I just want to figure it out for myself . . .

*I missed, however, the impulse to "make sense of it herself" as part of the life-forward direction, so she repeats it.*

*S:* And I don't know what to do about my father. 'Cause I don't know how I feel. I feel one way but then I feel another way. And I don't want to totally lose him, but I don't want him to think it's okay. 'Cause it's not okay.

*K:* Those are alive right now, those feelings. I don't want him to think everything's okay, 'cause it's not. But I don't want to lose him.

*S:* They're recent feelings. Cause I didn't really ever have them. I just wanted . . . I think I just wanted my father in my life so much that I just wanted it to be normal . . . But now . . . I'm starting to think a little differently about it . . .

*There is subtle but significant movement inward as Sharon acknowledges some of the reasons that it has been difficult to 'go inside' up to this point.*

## Summary

I hope the above example has demystified what focusing might sound like in an actual counseling setting. It is admittedly mysterious in some ways, but it is also perfectly natural and accessible to all of us and to all of our clients. We've probably all experienced it to some extent, without calling it "focusing," and without knowing we could pay attention "there" on purpose. Every time we have a sense of something we want to say (or write) and let the words come as we open our mouths (or sit with pen in hand), we're speaking (or writing) from a felt sense. Whenever we experience a sense of recognition that we've met someone before but can't place where or when, there's a felt sense of how-we-know-that-person. Most of us have also felt the difference between a silence with unspoken words and feelings in it versus a silence that's more neutral. In fact, with any person we know, we could bring to mind many details about them, but there is also a wider felt sense of the whole person that contains all those details. Even with someone we've just met, we might get a felt sense about them, which obviously is not coming from anything we already know. Any time we pay attention to a felt sense like that, we're focusing. The "body" we're referring to is more than something "inside the skin envelope" (E. T. Gendlin, personal communication, 2004), more like another dimension of the physical body we know, a dimension that is always in process, containing neither subjective perceptions nor objective reality but a more inclusive whole. This chapter proposes that dimension is a spiritual one.

Integrating focusing into your work as a counselor need not be complicated. It can be as simple as inviting a client to slow down and share what they're noticing on a bodily or visceral level as they speak. It can be a matter of recognizing when a client has shared all of what they already know, yet has an unclear sense of something more there, then helping him or her to pay attention there, saying back key words to resonate with the felt sense, or perhaps directing a question there if that feels right. By integrating focusing into your work as a counselor, you are helping your clients to cooperate with their innate capacity for growth and development, which includes spiritual development. Focusing is also an ideal way of helping clients with specific religious and spiritual concerns, by pointing to the process without supplying the content. Focusing rests on a foundation of skillful listening, and upon attitudes of open curiosity and patient receptivity toward your clients' experiences, as well as encouraging them to adopt those attitudes toward their own experience. As in the case of Sharon, it might involve a bit of teaching about focusing.

## Annotated Bibliography

Campbell, P. A., & McMahon, E. M. (1997). *Bio-Spirituality: Focusing as a way to grow* (2nd ed.). Chicago: Loyola Press.
Peter Campbell and Edwin McMahon, both priests, teachers, and researchers, first offered this book integrating focusing with Christianity in 1985. It has since become a spiritual classic, apparently meeting a strong need among both Christians and non-Christians alike for a more embodied spiritual discipline that is a force for unity and peace.

The Focusing Institute website. http://www.focusing.org
The Focusing Institute website is rich with focusing-related resources, including information about focusing partnerships, focusing training, Gendlin's philosophy, felt community, and various applications of focusing. These resources also include counseling and spirituality, trauma, body work, research, children, medicine, creative process, and science. The section on

focusing and spirituality has links to an online discussion group, to find a focusing partner who shares a background in meditation, to get a focusing coaching session by phone with an experienced focuser and Buddhist practitioner, or to read a variety of articles.

Gendlin, E. (1981). *Focusing.* New York: Bantam Books.
Gene Gendlin makes focusing accessible to the general public in this popular book that has been published in twelve languages and has sold over 400,000 copies. He describes the "inner act" he discovered to be at the heart of successful counseling, points out that anyone can do it, and illustrates with numerous examples how to find, recognize, approach, and listen to a bodily felt sense, tapping into this source of direction and healing in life. He highlights focusing as a way of moving beyond the limits of traditional ways of viewing oneself and others to discover a depth and richness that is too often obscured by standard roles and routines.

Gendlin, E. (1986). *Let your body interpret your dreams.* Wilmette, IL: Chiron.
Gendlin outlines a method of dream interpretation that is essentially "focusing plus questions," keeping in mind, of course, that a felt sense stirs or responds to certain questions more than others. Some of the questions specifically concern spiritual development, while other questions (about the place, plot, characters, or symbols) can certainly access spiritual issues as well. He illustrates how dreams are not only a rich source of the gifts focusing has to offer but may also be pointing toward a growth direction in the last place we're inclined to look for it in the dream, if we can open ourselves to see beyond our usual biases and judgments of good or bad.

Hinterkopf, E. (1998). *Integrating spirituality in counseling: A manual for using the experiential focusing method.* Alexandria, VA: American Counseling Association.
Elfie Hinterkopf describes the many benefits that come from integrating focusing into the counseling process and illustrates how well-suited focusing is for addressing the whole spectrum of ways that individuals may experience spirituality. The clarity with which she distinguishes the "still small voice" of a focusing process from the "inner critic" is particularly helpful, as are her discussions of friendly focusing attitudes, ways of keeping the right distance, and asking the most effective questions. She describes how to work with spiritual process as well as content, tying this endeavor to counselor competencies endorsed by the Association for Spiritual, Ethical and Religious Values in Counseling (ASERVIC).

The Reclaiming Judaism website. http://www.ReclaimingJudaism.org
The Reclaiming Judaism website offers retreats, programs, and resources to help those seeking more fulfilling Jewish spiritual practice. Programs are available for prayer and meditation, Jewish health care professionals, and Torah Commentary for Jewish women and girls, and for bar/bah mitzvah preparation. Resources are provided for daily rituals, holy days, study of

sacred text, and more. Several books by Rabbi Goldie Milgram are also available, including *Reclaiming Judaism as a Spiritual Practice—Holy Days and Shabbat, Meaning and Mitzvah*, and *Make Your Own Bar/Bah Mitzvah*.

Weiser Cornell, A. (1996). *The power of focusing*. New York: MJF Books. Ann Weiser Cornell, one of Gendlin's students, offers a practical, readable, down-to-earth way of walking the reader through the steps of finding a felt sense, "having a conversation" with it, and receiving the gifts. She illustrates some specific uses of focusing, such as working with addictions, decision making, physical symptoms, writer's block, and interpersonal situations. She also addresses some common difficulties and questions one might have: getting nothing or a blank, how to distinguish what comes from the body versus the head, wondering whether you're "making it up," or fear of what may emerge.

# References

Ambler, R. (2002). *Light to live by: An exploration in Quaker spirituality*. London, U.K.: Quaker Books.

Blanco, P. C., & Pascual, A. G. (2004, January). How does the process of body-focusing happen in children? *Staying in Focus: The Focusing Institute Newsletter, 4*(1), 1–2 & 4.

Bowers, L. (2002). Elevator rides help children learn focusing. *Staying in Focus: The Focusing Institute Newsletter, 2*(1), 1 & 6.

Brown, T., Jr. (1992). *The journey*. New York: Berkley Books.

Campbell, P., & McMahon, E. (1997). *Bio-Spirituality: Focusing as a way to grow* (2nd ed.). Chicago: Loyola Press.

Focusing Institute. (2002). *Focusing* [video]. (Available from the Focusing Institute, Spring Valley, NY)

Gendlin, E. (1964). A theory of personality change. In P. Worchel & D. Byrne (Eds.), *Personality change* (pp. 100–148). New York: Wiley.

Gendlin, E. (1981). *Focusing*. New York: Bantam Books.

Gendlin, E. (1986). *Let your body interpret your dreams*. Wilmette, IL: Chiron.

Gendlin, E. (1996). Focusing-oriented psychotherapy. New York: Guilford Press.

Gendlin, E. (2004). Five philosophical talking points to communicate with colleagues who don't yet know focusing. *Staying in Focus: The Focusing Institute Newsletter, 4*(1), 5–8.

Hendricks, M. N. (2001). Focusing-oriented/experiential psychology. In D. Cain & J. Seeman (Eds.), *Humanistic psychotherapy: Handbook of research and practice*. American Psychological Association. Retrieved from http://www.focusing.org/research-basis.html.

Hendricks, M. [N.] (2005, March). *Grass roots globalization: Creating free, self-organizing spaces in the social body*. Keynote address given at the 17th Annual Focusing Conference, Toronto, Canada.

Hendrix, H. (1988). *Getting the love you want.* New York: Holt.

Hinterkopf, E. (1998a, March). *Experiential dream interpretation.* Presented as a Learning Institute at the American Counseling Association Conference, Indianapolis, IN.

Hinterkopf, E. (1998b). *Integrating spirituality in counseling: A manual for using the Experiential Focusing Method.* Alexandria, VA: American Counseling Association.

Hunt, H. L. (2006). Faith and feminism. Presented on "Think Tank" telephone bridge. New York: Imago Relationships International.

Klein, J. (1998). *Inside-me stories: Something is happening inside-me!* Hypoluxo, FL: The Inside-People Press.

Klein, J. (2001). *Interactive focusing therapy: Healing relationships.* Evanston, IL: Center for Interactive Focusing.

Klein, M. H., Mathieu, P. L., Gendlin, E. T., & Kiesler, D. J. (1969). *The Experiencing Scale: A research and training manual.* Madison, WI: Wisconsin Psychiatric Institute.

Leijssen, M. (1998). Focusing microprocesses. In L. Greenberg, J. Watson, & G. Lietaer (Eds.), *Handbook of experiential psychotherapy.* New York: Guilford Press. Retrieved from http://www.focusing.org/micro.html.

Lennox, S. (2001). Focusing and spirituality. *Staying in Focus: The Focusing Institute Newsletter, 1*(1), p. 5.

Milgram, G. (2005). Judaism and the focusing process. *Staying in Focus: The Focusing Institute Newsletter, 5*(2), 1–6.

Mulhern, D. (2006, March). *Transformation, evolution and healing. What might be happening in the brain?* Presented on "Think Tank" Telephone Bridge. New York: Imago Relationships International.

Olafsdottir, V. (2002, September). Focusing project in a nursery school in Iceland. *Staying in Focus: The Focusing Institute Newsletter, 2*(3), 1–2.

Peck, M. S. (1978). *The road less traveled.* New York: Simon & Schuster.

Punshon, J. (1987). *Encounter with silence: Reflections from the Quaker tradition.* London, U.K.: Friends United Press.

Rome, D. I. (2004). Searching for truth that is far below the search. *Shambhala Sun,* September, pp. 60–63, 91, & 93.

Rosenblum, R. (2004). Unexpected focusing moments in a psychiatric hospital. *Staying in Focus: The Focusing Institute Newsletter, 4*(3), 4–5.

Saunders, N. (2003). Focusing on the light: A modest proposal. *Staying in Focus: The Focusing Institute Newsletter, 3*(2), 1–2.

Sears, R. T. (1997). Forward. In P. Campbell & E. McMahon, *Bio-Spirituality: Focusing as a way to grow* (2nd ed.). Chicago: Loyola Press.

Sherman, E. (1990). Experiential reminiscence and life-review therapy with the elderly. In G. Lietaer, J. Rombauts, & R. Van Balen (Eds.), *Client and experiential psychotherapy in the nineties* (pp. 709–732). Leuven, Belgium: Leuven University Press.

Siegel, D. J. (1999). *The developing mind: Toward a neurobiology of interpersonal experience.* New York: Guilford Press.

Weiser Cornell, A. (1996). *The power of focusing.* New York: MJF Books.

# Name Index

## A

Aboud, F. E., 366
Ackerman, D, 295
Adams, E. M., 332, 341–342, 356, 368
Adler, A., 164, 170, 174
Ainsworth, M. D., 168
Alexander, F., 174, 189
Allison, S., 130
Alvarez, M., 130
Ambler, R., 439
American Academy of Pediatrics, 295
American Counseling Association, 267–268
American Psychiatric Association, 241
American Psychological Association, 268, 376
Anastasi, A., 239
Anderson, W. T., 138
Angelou, M., 394
Apfelbaum, E., 25
Arimino, J. W., 393, 407–408
Arredondo, P., 376
Artistotle, 236
Athanasiadou, C., 235
Atkinson, D. R., 368, 377

## B

Baker, M. J., 180–181
Baldwin, J., 338, 394
Baltes, P. B., 53, 55
Bandura, A., 98
Bannock, J. C., 284
Bar-Yam, M., 130
Barret, B., 298
Basseches, M., 134
Baucom, D. H., 180–181
Baxter-Magolda, M., 137, 378, 383, 395
Beard, J., 295, 308
Beaudoin, M., 33
Bebeau, M. J., 137, 143
Becker-Schutte, A., 262
Belenky, M. F., 137, 218, 353, 397
Beneson, J. F., 239
Benshoff, J. M., 143
Berenbaum, S. A., 237

Bernal, M. E., 366
Berry, J. W., 366–367
Besley, T., 33
Beukema, S., 130
Beutler, L. E., 180–181
Bieschke, K. J., 262, 273
Binder, J. L., 168
Binner, V. F., 130
Bird, L., 10, 12–14, 16, 18, 23
Blanck, G., 96
Blanco, P. C., 431, 447
Blehar, M. C., 168
Blunt, J., 236
Borders, L. D., 143
Bowers, L., 431, 447
Bowlby, J., 168
Boyd, C. J., 288
Bracho, A., 33
Bradford, J., 261
Braeck, M. M., 143
Brannock, J. C., 265–266
Breuer, J., 169
Briggs, M. K., 49
Bringaze, T. B., 272
Bronfenbrenner, U., 54, 56, 60–61, 62, 64–66, 81
Brown, J., Jr., 330, 438–439
Brown, L. M., 208, 240–241
Brown, L. S., 271
Brown, S., 376
Brown-Collins, A. R., 353
Browning, C., 308
Bruner, E., 31
Bruner, J., 21, 23–24, 30, 92–93
Buhrke, R. A., 262
Burman, E., 10, 14, 16–18, 22, 37, 242
Burr, V., 11, 28–29
Burt, J. M., 338–339

## C

Caird, E., 89
Cairney, J., 235
Calhoun, K. S., 180–181

# Subject Index